BLOOMING BIRTH

blooming
birth
how to get the
pregnancy and birth
you want

LUCY ATKINS & JULIA GUDERIAN

Collins

First published in 2005 by
Collins, an imprint of
HarperCollinsPublishers
77–85 Fulham Palace Road
Hammersmith
London w6 8jb

The Collins website address is www.collins.co.uk

11   10   09   08   07   06   05
7   6   5   4   3   2   1

Editor: Joanna Carreras
Design: Mark Thomson, Sara Soskolne
Illustrations: Amanda Williams

A catalogue record for this book is available from
the British Library.

ISBN 0-00-718401-8

Printed and bound in Great Britain by Clays Ltd,
St Ives plc

Contents

Introduction

When I was pregnant for the first time, I was your typical swotty mother-to-be. *What to Expect When You're Expecting* was my bible. I diligently attended childbirth classes, toured my local hospital and performed regular antenatal yoga exercises. I was supposed to push the baby out *with my breath* but ended up with every intervention known to modern obstetrics (at least that's how it felt). I was healthy, educated and - supposedly - informed but still the reality of childbirth floored me. And I'm not alone. One 2005 survey of 3,000 first-time mothers found that for the majority of women giving birth in the UK today, childbirth is a scary ordeal that leaves us in a state of shock. Eight out of ten of us say we were frightened at some point during labour, and that giving birth was more painful than we had ever imagined. One-third of us, meanwhile, say ante-natal classes didn't prepare us for the reality of childbirth.[1] Our preparations, it would seem, are not exactly hitting the mark.

When I got pregnant for the second time, I was really scared about the birth. I had just moved to the States where doulas - women who are trained to give you emotional and practical support during pregnancy and childbirth - are widely available and people kept telling me I should hire one. Figuring I had nothing to lose I started to interview doulas. There was something about Julia that stood out - a combination of practicality, pragmatism, realism and genuine empathy. She also has impressive credentials. Julia is a mother of two, a doula and childbirth teacher, trained and certified by the world's largest doula organisation (DONA International) to give women emotional and practical - but not medical - support before, during and after childbirth. She has 14 years' experience of helping women through pregnancy and birth and is a certified counsellor and hypnotherapist. She has also worked with all kinds of mothers: she founded and ran the The New Hope Doula Project in Seattle, connecting volunteer doulas with women giving their babies for adoption. She also founded a non-profit support group for women who have had caesareans (and are upset by them) and she designed and set up a popular network of mother's groups - helping women connect with one another for support, companionship and ideas across the States. Julia was, to put it mildly, a lucky find.

She worked closely with me for the rest of my pregnancy and showed me that truly preparing for childbirth is about admitting what scares you, making good choices, staying open minded and learning brilliant ways to cope with whatever labour throws at you on the day. It's about understanding, and accepting the areas over which you have no control - without becoming a fatalistic loon about the whole thing. When I went into labour for the second time, I was prepared to handle whatever happened (including my worst case scenario). My son's birth was an amazing, positive experience. As a journalist used to disseminating information, it amazed me that I'd come across no book or resource that could compare with the work Julia did to help me prepare for childbirth. It was clear to me that her methodology and experience could - and should - be made available to any woman who simply wanted to have a better birth. Julia's work with me -

and with countless other mothers and mothers-to-be over the years – forms the backbone of this book. It will be relevant to you whether this is your first baby, or you have a whole brood already. *Blooming Birth* is for any woman who simply wants to give birth without feeling shocked, terrified, upset or horrified by the experience.

Though doulas are becoming more and more popular in Britain, they are still a relatively new phenomenon here. Not all of us can afford, or find, one where we live. This book will give you some useful doula tricks for coping during childbirth. It will also show you what your partner – and anyone else who'll be supporting you during this birth – can learn from doulas.

The actual writing of this book was my department. As a health writer for newspapers like *The Guardian*, I'm used to grappling with ideas, interviewing experts and translating their arcane medical jargon into something that normal people can actually understand. Since I specialise in writing about pregnancy, birth and babies I'm also used to finding the best expert, support group or information source for these particular issues. This is where my professional skills come in but, above all, I'm writing this book as a mother. I have three children (my third baby, Ted, was born somewhere around Chapter 5 so I'm certainly up to date on birth in Britain). I am, then, your average 'punter'. I'm not a childbirth expert, a childbirth nut or medically trained in any way: I'm a mother like you, who simply wanted and got a better experience of childbirth. I used the ideas in this book to prepare for, and cope with, Ted's birth: they worked brilliantly (again).

This is not a medical book, but we have worked closely with doctors, midwives and other experts to give you the basic facts. You should see *Blooming Birth* as a springboard when it comes to medical matters – we show you what preparation means and the details are up to you. To help you do this, we've given you book lists and online resources so you can find the more detailed or specialist information you need.

We have unashamedly set out to give you the nitty gritty of birth here, not some neat, textbook version. We don't talk about 'discomfort', we talk about pain because if you're to cope with it you need to know about it. Between us Julia and I have certainly run the gauntlet of birthing experiences – from prolonged labour, failure to progress, epidurals, forceps delivery, a broken tail-bone, a 4th-degree tear, an infected scar and an emergency caesarean to drug-free labour, vaginal birth after caesarean, homebirth in a tub and homebirth on dry land. We've also interviewed over a hundred women from brand-new mothers to grandmothers about pregnancy and birth: you'll learn what worked, and didn't work, for them and you'll learn the tips, strategies and awakenings that come from simply getting babies out.

Or witnessing this – *Blooming Birth* is for blokes too. Virtually every man we spoke to for this book said he, too, felt utterly unprepared for the reality of his baby's entry into the world. If properly prepared, your baby's dad can have a hugely positive influence on how you experience this birth. So, even if he's not an avid reader of birth books, at the very least get your partner to read Chapter 8: Blokes, Birth and Babies.

By the time you finish reading this you may not actually be looking forward to giving birth but you'll certainly feel more confident about it. You'll know you can't control everything that happens, but you'll understand more about what might. You'll understand the maternity system and how to negotiate it so it serves you best. You'll know how to get the support you need, before, during and after the arrival of your baby. And you'll know where to go, what to read and who to talk to if you need more help or information.

Finally, we don't have any hidden agenda here. Neither Julia nor I are obsessed by natural birth and New Age philosophies have largely passed us by (we will not, for instance, be asking you to mould your vagina in clay or write poetry to your fetus). We genuinely do not care if you want an elective caesarean, an epidural at the first twinge or a troupe of nuns in your delivery room singing *Land of Hope and Glory* as you push – as long as it's a genuinely informed choice, based on what you know about yourself, and about your realistic options. We want you to cope brilliantly with this birth – whatever crops up – so that you can become a healthy mother (of one, two or more) with no regrets or lingering upset. We want you, in short, to become the kind of mother who forgets that she ever needed a book like this.

Chapter One:
Pregnancy for busy women

'Nobody can really tell you what to expect
when you're expecting because every
woman feels it differently. My sister adored
her expanding belly and said she felt like
a sexy goddess throughout her pregnancy.
I felt like an increasingly mad, swelling
gorilla.'

FAITH, 32, MOTHER OF HARVEY (2)

1 **Your love for this baby** one day will be stratospheric.
2 **People will treat you as if you are deeply special** (well sometimes, at least).
3 **You are not alone.** Around 596,000 other women in England and Wales alone are having a baby this year too.
4 **You have maternity choices and rights** like never before. You have the right to question your caregivers, change hospitals, midwives or doctors, see your records and make informed decisions.
5 **The laws on maternity leave have never been more in your favour** and there are organizations to help you sort out what you're entitled to if you're confused. (See Resources, page 50.)
6 **You are giving birth as the 'doula' movement is taking off** in Britain – you can now find one-to-one emotional and practical support throughout this pregnancy and birth, even if the NHS can't provide it.
7 **You can still be glam:** clothing companies are finally waking up to the fact that you may not want to wear leggings and bloke's t-shirts for nine months. High street shops like Hennes, Dorothy Perkins and even Mothercare are coming up trumps; designer maternity lines are springing up all over the place and online maternity shopping is a constant temptation. (See Resources, page 49.)
8 **You can look forward to nine months free** from tampons, pads, PMT and condoms.

Welcome to the Alarmist Club

Brace yourself. You are pregnant. You're probably floating in a world of stupendous self-admiration right now (you're growing an actual, real BABY in there). But you may also have noticed that people now want to start scaring you about all the things that could go wrong. This will get worse. Over the next nine months you will be fed a load of neurosis-inducing claptrap about what you must eat, drink, breathe, think and do to keep that baby 'safe'. There will be some good, solid, sensible information in there – things you really need to know – but it can be hard to isolate this from the endless conflicting advice you'll get on how to 'optimize' your chance of producing a healthy baby. Pregnancy, these days, has become pathology. Friends, relatives, colleagues, books, websites, health professionals and even complete strangers will conspire to fill you with fear, guilt and self-doubt. You'd think it was some insane, risky, reckless ordeal you're embarking on, not something basically ordinary, that women have successfully achieved since time began. In this chapter we'll give you the 'need to know' information, and hopefully lay some of the neuroses to rest.

We won't provide you with medical minutiae about obscure conditions or rare complications. Other books have done this far better than we ever could (though we'll give you resources and ideas of where to look if you need to know more). Instead, we're going to give you a solid sense of some of the oddities you might experience over the next nine months, along with practical tips from professionals and other women about how to handle them. We'll show you that you can, indeed, have a basically healthy pregnancy whilst remaining a viable member of ordinary society.

Goddess or gorilla

Pregnancy can make you feel unbelievably beautiful; replete with hope and womanliness. It can be a blissful time, not least because those of us who've spent the last ten years trying to disguise our flabby bellies get to show them off in tight tops. Pregnancy can be a time when you're treated like a goddess by your partner; a time when blokes in white vans look on protectively as you cross the road; when people give you seats on the bus (well, occasionally) and when strangers congratulate you. You may, as the months go by, look more and more fantastic, and feel amazing: have thicker hair, better skin, stronger nails and a beatific glow. It's a time, in short, when you feel that life is the oyster inside the pearly shell that's you.

But this may not be the whole story. For most of us, pregnancy doesn't feel like glorious fruition **all** the time. At times it can feel distinctly disempowering to be up the duff. You can't control what's happening to your body and you may feel as if you've been hijacked by medical professionals and, indeed, a small alien. You may be constantly vomiting. You may have mood swings. You may feel shattered. You may also swell to the size of a house, sprout varicose veins and become a borderline psychotic. Pregnancy involves huge contradictions – physical and mental. Pregnancy books often use words like 'blessing', 'joy' and 'gift'. A pregnancy may be all of these things but at times you can feel more like an overstuffed mammoth than a fecund goddess; more axe murderer than earth mother. Much of this is hormonal. Much entirely reasonable, all of it normal.

Staying sane in pregnancy

The good news is that though you can't do much about the hand your pregnancy deals you, you **can** influence how you react to this manic, blissful, awful, amazing, fundamental new condition.

YOU CAN CHOOSE TO:

- become well-informed but not obsessed.
- take what people tell you with a pinch of salt until you know it's true.
- research and understand important medical matters that affect you.
- embrace what works for you and reject what doesn't.

Most of all, you can remind yourself, when you are being prodded, poked, advised and bossed, that it is still your body and your life – even if you do look like an inflatable hippo when you're in the bath.

That blue line

Julia's heard some odd stories about how her clients know they're pregnant:

'It's not always the obvious things that make you aware you're pregnant – aching boobs, test kits, or late periods. Many of my clients tell me they knew they were pregnant when smells became stronger. Many – particularly second time mothers – tell me they had weird dreams that made them rush out and buy a test kit. And more than once I've heard of women dreaming about giving birth to a squirrel or mouse and discovering the next day that they're pregnant.'

Finding out you are pregnant, however you do it, is a moment you'll remember forever. The pictures of each of my three test sticks with the thin blue lines are stamped in my mind like little Polaroids. I remember where I was sitting, how I felt, what I did when I saw each one. (One thing that's worth knowing is that while negative pregnancy tests in the very early days can be wrong, positive ones rarely are.) It can be a moment of exquisite happiness to find out you're having a baby, but also a huge shock. Most of the literature on pregnancy assumes that you'll simply pat yourself on the back at this point and become a saintly consumer of organic-only foodstuffs. But even if you planned meticulously, took your own temperature and peed on ovulation sticks for weeks on end, actually becoming pregnant can feel quite intimidating. Suddenly, your life (and soon your body) has taken on a shape all of its own. There's a baby in there and it's only going to get bigger. And it has to come out. And then you have to look after it for 18 years or more. If you're used to at least a superficial sense of control over your own destiny, that moment of discovery can be daunting.

Going it alone

Facing motherhood alone can be a panicky, if exciting, time whether you have deliberately chosen to do this, or not. Your pregnancy may have come as a surprise, or it may have been a longed-for result: these days, more and more single women in their thirties and forties are choosing motherhood alone, sometimes using donor insemination. Telling people you're pregnant can sometimes be tricky, whether the baby is planned or not, but the good news is that there is plenty of support and advice available. While one in four families in Britain today is headed by a single parent[1] (that's 1.75 million families) most of these happen because of marriage breakdown (usually once you have kids). You may, then, find it helpful to seek out specific support if you are single and tackling pregnancy and birth on your own. Even if you're not a 'joiner', building up some kind of network once you are a parent can make a huge difference.

Where to go for help:
One Parent Families 020 7428 5400 www.oneparentfamilies.org.uk
Parent-run charity **Gingerbread** 020 7488 9300 www.gingerbread.org.uk

Further reading:
Single Mothers by Choice: A Guidebook For Single Women Who Are
Considering or have Chosen Motherhood by Jane Mattes (Three Rivers Press, US,
1997) This is an American book, but many issues are the same, wherever you are in
the world. www.mattes.home.pipeline.com

Unplanned pregnancy

About one in five pregnancies is unplanned. If this fetus is the result of some
Chianti-fuelled madness, or if you thought you practised the contraceptive
equivalent of Fort Knox, discovering you're pregnant can be distressing. Many of
us won't admit to such thoughts – it feels shameful even to consider not wanting
a baby when other women out there are devastated by infertility. But many of us –
at least initially – do feel this way. *'My first baby, Mia, was five months old,'* says
Kate. *'She hadn't slept for more than two hours at a stretch, screamed all the time,
and we were shattered. One night, we drank a bottle of wine and had reckless sex –
some kind of stress relief I think. Conrad was the result. When I discovered I was
pregnant again I sat on the bathroom floor and cried. Mia cried next to me. Jim came
in, and cried too. It was like some kind of Greek tragedy.'* They all came round to it
in the end, of course, and Conrad is the light of their lives but really, pregnancy
test kits should carry a mental health warning.

HEALTHY PREGNANCY: WHAT TO STOP DOING RIGHT NOW

STOP:

- smoking cigarettes. Cigarette smoke contains more than 4000
  chemicals that cross the placenta into your baby's blood. It can lower
  your baby's birth weight by 12 to 18 grams per cigarette consumed per
  day and doubles your chances of having a premature baby. It is
  associated with bleeding, pre-eclampsia, stillbirth and miscarriage.
- taking over the counter drugs (without a doctor's advice). Though
  paracetamol is considered safe to take in pregnancy, anti-inflammatory
  pain medication like ibuprofen can increase your risk of miscarriage.
  Best to check with your midwife before you take anything.
- taking all recreational drugs (including cannabis)
- taking all street drugs
- drinking more than a couple of glasses of wine a week
- soaking in saunas or hot tubs
- having x-rays (unless suggested by your obstetrician)

Where to go for help:
QUIT helpline 0800 002200 www.quit.org.uk
NHS Pregnancy smoking helpline 0800 169 9 169
American Lung Association (us) www.lungusa.org/tobacco/

Less positive emotions

Depression

Everyone expects you to feel elated and special but you just feel even less like getting out of bed in the morning. Depression can be particularly isolating in pregnancy, yet it's rarely talked about. One recent study found that not only is antenatal depression considerably more common than was previously thought – around 10 per cent of pregnant women, the study found, are depressed – it is mostly missed by doctors. In the study, only five of the 41 women with antenatal depression were identified by their GP as depressed.[2] Depression can have serious effects on your health and that of your baby: depressed women may be less likely to keep antenatal appointments, eat well and do what's best for their baby. There is also thought to be some link between antenatal depression and postnatal depression. You should always tell your midwife or doctor if you are feeling depressed as you may need their help.

If you are already depressed and taking antidepressants you're hardly alone: according to mental health charity MIND, between 1990 and 1995 the number of prescriptions for antidepressants such as Prozac rose by 732 per cent in England alone. Being pregnant does not necessarily mean you have to ditch your meds and feel suicidal for nine months: some depression drugs are considered safe to take in pregnancy but others are not. So talk to your doctor the minute you know you're pregnant.

Where to go for help:
Start with your GP, midwife or health visitor.
The Depression Alliance provides information for mothers and pregnant women who are isolated and lonely or experiencing depression. 35 Westminster Bridge Road London SE1 7JB. 0845 123 23 20 www.depressionalliance.org (ask for their booklet *Depression During and After Pregnancy*)
Meet-a-Mum Association Postnatal Illness Helpline can also help with pregnancy depression. 0845 120 3746
The mental health charity **MIND** has an online information service for users of mental health services, carers and other groups. For information on types of mental distress, treatments, therapies and legal information: 08457 660163 (9.15am–4.45pm everyday) www.mind.org.uk

Online:
www.depression-in-pregnancy.org.uk

Further reading:
Antenatal and Postnatal Depression by Siobhan Curham (Vermilion, UK, 2000)

Just feeling low

Milder 'feeling down' moods are also very common in pregnancy. This can be particularly overwhelming in the early stages when your hormones are flying all over the place. No matter how many times people say 'hormones' to you, you still think it's life, not chemicals, that is making you feel so low. Your partner may find this disconcerting (my husband, having been through two previous pregnancies with me, was still unnerved by my dismal mood in the early stages of my third pregnancy). He may have no idea what to do to help you, so spend some time thinking about what you need from him then try to talk to him about it – if possible at a time when you're not feeling murderous. Tell him that feeling low in pregnancy is common, chemical, but no less powerful or real for that. Suggest ways that he can help you (even if it's just to leave you alone, buy you chocolate or give you a massage). The good news is that your dismal moods should pass. Talk to your midwife about this, or your GP or the Health Visitor at your doctor's surgery. If your mood doesn't alleviate, see above for where to get help.

Specific worrying

Even if pregnancy makes you basically happy, you may find yourself plagued by worries. Anxiety, like depression, is common in pregnancy and takes many forms.

WORRY THAT A PAST PROBLEM WILL RECUR | Some serious medical issues in the past (such as infertility, miscarriage, birth defects or other complications) can make your worries pretty specific and understandable. Many women who have had a miscarriage in the past, for instance, worry furiously up to the point at which the previous miscarriage occurred (and sometimes beyond). Get the most up to date information on whatever condition or event you fear. Ask questions, get referrals and second opinions. Start with your GP or midwife and don't rest until you have answers. Information will not eradicate worry but it may help. Learning relaxation techniques may also help you to manage your more panicky moments. (See Find Out More, Chapter 4: Fear and Pain, page 108, for ideas and techniques.)

WORRYING ABOUT THE BIRTH | The vast majority of us (most studies put it at around 80 per cent) are scared of giving birth. We fret, often aimlessly, about this: will the birth be traumatic? Painful? Disastrous? Easy? Will it be like that horrendous one on ER last night? The good news is that pregnancy gives you time to prepare yourself mentally for giving birth. You can use this time to decode your fears, worries and preconceptions so that you can make intelligent choices about how, when and with whom you want to give birth. This book will show you how.

Generalised worry

There's nothing like impending motherhood for bringing out the paranoid within. The world, suddenly, is filled with peril: pollutants, aggressors, toxins, accidents waiting to happen. *'Throughout my pregnancy I worried the entire time about chemicals in body lotions harming the baby,'* says Jazz, mother of Karim (2). *'I think I read it in some newspaper somewhere. It didn't stop me putting lotion on every day, but it really bothered me.'*

The rule is: if you find yourself worrying about some half-reported issue, physical twinge or weird feeling discuss it with your GP or midwife, no matter how mad or silly you feel. If they are vague or don't have the answer, ask them where you can get it. For a good midwife, no question is too silly. If your general anxiety is stopping you sleeping, eating or otherwise preoccupying you, talk to them about the anxiety itself. Counselling, as well as treatment for more serious anxiety disorders, is available and now is a good time to get it (parenthood is unlikely to make it go away).

The root of worries

Much of this kind of paranoia boils down to the basic belief that pregnancy (and by implication birth) is both scary and dangerous. From TV, film, newspapers and magazines, you'll absorb frightening images and stories of pregnancies that go disastrously wrong. This makes great TV and copy, but serious, life-threatening pregnancy complications are rare (how do you think we all got here?). Your 'pregnancy/birth is unsafe' mindset is not going to help you when you are in labour. For the vast majority of us pregnancy and birth are healthy, normal events. They're neither threatening nor perilous.

Stress

'Stress is definitely something pregnant women need to get to grips with. But you can do it. I have seen highly anxious, stressed out women at the beginning of pregnancy become, by the end, calm, relaxed and prepared simply by refocusing and making even slight changes to their busy lives,' says midwife Jenny Smith. If your days are spent juggling million pound budgets, wiping your toddler's bottom or – God forbid – doing both, you can still have a healthy pregnancy and be in good physical and mental shape for this birth.

We're a stressed bunch these days: one survey of about 5,000 women[3] found that women who work full time say they still do most of the household chores. Only 37 per cent of working couples share jobs equally around the home, and only 3 per cent of men do more ironing and washing than their partners. If you've already got children, the chances are you're even more frazzled: the same survey found that 93 per cent of mothers feel stressed out, trying to cope with all the demands made on their lives. Add pregnancy to this and you get a heady cocktail of neurosis.

We stress about our inability to eat balanced portions of home-prepared food, our failure to attend a regular antenatal exercise class, to be productive enough at work, to get enough sleep or to relax – especially when we're supposed to be relaxing. And then we worry that we're worrying too much. The key question here is: will your stress harm the baby? The answer: it is extraordinarily unlikely to.

A handful of studies have suggested that a *very high* level of stress can increase your risk of having the baby too early, or having a low birth-weight baby by sparking off certain hormones.[4] Certainly, if you are extremely stressed you are more likely to skip meals, reach for ciggies, booze or even drugs at the end of the day, all of which have been linked to low birth-weight (alcohol and drugs are also linked to birth defects). If any of this sounds familiar to you, don't brush this under the carpet. Talk to your GP, Health Visitor or midwife.

TEN QUICK WAYS TO MINIMISE STRESS

1 **Learn 'mini' stress relieving techniques.** These can be very useful for labour, not to mention further down the line when you have an illogical toddler on your hands.

2 **Make a list** of things that, in the past, have reduced your stress levels, and do some of them if you can (leave anything chemical, nicotine-related or alcoholic off this list for obvious reasons).

3 **Become an idler:** leave the washing, let the carpet stay dirty, ask for deadline extensions and generally give yourself a break. Now is not the time to 'prove' anything to anyone.

4 **Throw money at the problem.** If you can't do the above, and can possibly afford it, get a cleaner, get a cleaner more often or even bung a teenager a few quid after school to do 'maid' type duties for an hour or so. If you've got no money, divide your tasks into small, manageable chunks and plan meticulously for them: e.g. laundry (day 1), floors (day 2), bill-paying (day 3).

5 **Negotiate divisions of labour** with your partner. If studies are right, he probably does a fraction of what you do around the house, even if you are both working outside it. Inequalities like this will only be exacerbated when you have babies to cope with. He needs to be roped on board even (or perhaps especially) at this stage. Be aware that his standards and yours may differ (this does not mean it is his fault). He may in fact be exceptionally glad to feel useful at this point in your pregnancy.

6 **Do small, beneficial things** for yourself. Eat a yogurt before bed (calcium), keep fruit on your desk for snacks (and a water bottle), book yourself a lunch-hour massage (enforced relaxation), buy posh bath oil and use it religiously, at least once a week, and – why not? – treat yourself to an hour in the Waterstones café with a chocolate muffin and a good book.

7 **Book an alternative therapist.** Even if you're a sceptic, things like massage or aromatherapy can help us all, at least temporarily. Sometimes just being listened to and pampered for an hour with smelly oils can really turn things around.

8 **Get support:** family, friends, neighbours can all be drafted in, even if just in small ways around the house, garden or with your other kids. But this involves asking for help. Which means no longer seeming perfect.

9 **Try gentle exercise** (if ok'd by your doctor or midwife). It is clinically recognized to lower stress levels. You don't have to go to the gym but when you want to bludgeon a colleague or spouse, take a walk round the block. Ideally, join a pregnancy yoga class. Or try and walk for half an hour a day. But don't beat yourself up about it if you can't. You may just want to lie in a darkened room with earplugs in. That's fine too.

10 **Get help:** counselling or even life-coaching can help you decode your stress and work out how to handle it better.

Career worries

Worrying that your career will evaporate when this baby arrives is also common.

'Most women need to remember that their careers do not necessarily go away when they have children,' says midwife Jenny Smith. 'Maternity leave actually goes very quickly: to have 6–8 months off is nothing in terms of one's whole life and what is most important right now is preparing your body and mind to nurture this baby. It's a shame so many women ruin this precious time by worrying about work.'

If your pregnant-and-working life, like your belly, is starting to strain at the seams the hardest thing can be finding time to do something about it. The first thing to do is stop meta-worrying. Stress is a known part of pregnancy and to some extent we all feel it. But going into labour in a frazzled state is not ideal: you'll have fewer physical reserves, be less able to relax during contractions, potentially have less endurance and then not be in the best position to cope with pain. **A crucial part of your childbirth preparation should be to make stress-relief a priority.** One way to start is by sorting out the practicalities of your maternity leave and eventual return to work so you can stop worrying about this for now.

Where to go for help:
Working Families is an organisation that gives practical help and information for parents about choices in childcare and employment rights; it also campaigns for changes in the law, and persuades employers to adopt practices which work for them and you alike. 020 7253 7243 www.workingfamilies.org.uk
Also try the webzine **Mother@Work**: www.motheratwork.co.uk. This is a good place to get a sense that other women are struggling with the same issues.
The Daycare Trust This national childcare charity, promoting high quality affordable childcare, can help you find out more about childcare for when you return to work. 21 St George's Rd, London SE1 6ES 020 7840 3350 info@daycaretrust.org.uk www.daycaretrust.org.uk

Further reading:

Balancing Pregnancy and Work: How to Make the Most of the Next 9 Months on the Job by Nancy Hall (Rodale Books, US, 2004) is worth a look, as is:
Working Woman's Pregnancy by Hilary Boyd (Mitchell Beazley, UK, 2004)

A WORD ABOUT TWINS AND MULTIPLE BIRTHS | In the UK about one in 35 babies is born a twin or triplet (in 1980 the figure was one in 52; the rise is mainly due to fertility treatments). There are nearly 10,000 multiple births in the UK every year. About a third of twins born in the UK are identical and two thirds are non-identical. Having twins can be a very different experience from your 'average' pregnancy but equally, you don't want to end up feeling that nothing applies to you. *'If you are carrying twins, you get a lot of fuss made of you by friends and colleagues and by the medical profession, but I also felt rather excluded from the "baby club",'* says Rachel, 36, mother of Nick and Ella (4). *'It started when we were told by the medics that "twin births are not normal" and then all the books I'd been religiously reading as a first timer stopped really applying. Even though I was getting excited about having two rather than one, I began to feel a bit of an outsider.'*

Most of the issues we cover in this book should be as relevant to you as they are to singleton mothers. It is just as important to prepare for this birth if you are carrying more than one baby; to face your fears, understand your options, inform yourself, have a meaningful plan and good support. But as a healthy mother of twins or multiples you may face certain specific challenges. One of these is that your experience of pregnancy is likely to be more 'medical' than it would if you were expecting a single baby. You may have more frequent antenatal checks and your babies will be scanned regularly – very regularly towards the end of the pregnancy – to monitor their development. This is because pregnancy complications are more common with multiple births, such as pre-eclampsia, pre-term labour, anaemia or exhaustion.

'We went for the first (of many) scans at twenty weeks and I think the nurse thought we must already know. She said, "There's the baby" and gave us our first sight of Nick and then said "and there's the other baby" meaning Ella, and Martin and I just looked at each other and laughed. I remember thinking "this is like a film" and I felt like everything had changed. I went home to bed and lay there thinking about two of every-thing, names and cots and buggies. The image of the little girl baby that I had been so sure I was carrying disappeared and I had to re-bond with two.'

RACHEL, 36, MOTHER OF NICK AND ELLA (4)

The birth itself may also be more 'medical' than you might like, as doctors will want to monitor the babies carefully, and you have a statistically higher chance of intervention. However, it's worth remembering that you are not ill, or stupid and that your preferences **still count**. You can negotiate about any proposed intervention and talk, in full, to your obstetrician about any issue that worries you. Finally, having a caesarean section is a real possibility (about half of all twin births are vaginal), so make sure you read Chapter 6: Surgical Birth.

The main advice for a twin or multiple pregnancy isn't terribly technical – it's SLOW DOWN. This pregnancy is going to put more strain on your body than a singleton pregnancy would. You will also gain more weight, and get significantly bigger, though twins are generally born earlier – on average around 37 weeks.

> **Where to go for help:**
> TAMBA (Twins and Multiple Births Association): 2 The Willows, Gardner Road Guildford, Surrey GU1 4PG. 0870 770 3305; information and listening service call Freephone 0800 138 0509, evenings and weekends. www.tamba.org.uk
> **Multiple Birth Foundation** 020 83833519 www.multiplebirths.org.uk
>
> **Further reading:**
> *Twins and Multiple Births: The Essential Parenting Guide from Pregnancy to Adulthood* by Carol Cooper (Vermilion, UK, 2004)
> *The Twins Handbook* by Elizabeth Friedrich and Cherry Rowland (Robson Books, UK, 1998)
> *Twins, Triplets and More* by Elizabeth M Bryan (Penguin, UK, 1992)

Multiple pregnancy tip:

Peggy Fitzgerald, a doula and mother of one-year-old triplets says, *'Expect to get big fast: buy maternity clothes early but not too many, because you will outgrow them and need to find bigger ones. (Even at 25 weeks, I outgrew most of the biggest maternity clothes I had – luckily I didn't have many – but still needed SOMETHING for doctor's visits....) Under the belly pants are more useful than ones that cover the belly – they just aren't made the shape you'll need. Also, make sure, early in pregnancy, that you stock up your freezer with meals: not just for the times when you can't cook (or the possibility that you'll be on bed-rest), but for your postpartum too.'*

A few other worries

Here are a few common worries and what to do with them. The list is potentially endless, so here's the rule: **ask your health professional if something is worrying you, no matter how silly and embarrassing it sounds**. They'll have heard it before and even if they haven't, they won't be shocked: they're here to help you.

WHAT YOU DRANK BEFORE YOU KNEW YOU WERE PREGNANT | Many of us drink too much alcohol in the early weeks of pregnancy before realizing there's a zygote in there. That Hen night you went on when two weeks pregnant, however, is not something to worry about. The real worry is if you can't stop now you know you're pregnant (see drinking advice below). Drinking too much alcohol throughout pregnancy can lead to fetal alcohol syndrome (where your baby is damaged because you are drinking 40–50 units of alcohol every week, or binge drinking). Get reassurance from your midwife and doctor about your early pregnancy behaviour, then move on to no more than two units (i.e. a couple of small glasses of wine) a week. This is the current UK government recommendation.

AIR TRAVEL | There is no evidence that holiday or business air travel will do you any harm whatsoever when pregnant. However, if you have pregnancy complications do consult your doctor before flying. The best time to travel is probably in your second trimester – in the middle three months. You will be less sick, more mobile, energetic and not yet the size of Free Willy. Take a large bottle of water, a bag of healthy snacks and move around a lot to avoid any chance of deep vein thrombosis (potentially fatal blood clots). Most airlines have a policy about pregnancy and air travel; most say you should not travel after a certain point in your pregnancy, usually 28–36 weeks. It may be hard to find this on a website, so try phoning the airline. Many will take your word as to how many weeks pregnant you are, though some may require a letter from your doctor. If you're considering stretching the truth, however, remember airline staff are generally not trained medical professionals. Giving birth 8,000 feet above the Atlantic would be less than ideal.

> **Where to go for help:**
> **About.com** has a list of airlines and their rules about pregnancy and flying: www.airtravel.about.com
> **The Royal College of Obstetrics and Gynaecology** also have guidelines for air travel safety on their website: www.rcog.org.uk

Air travel tip:
Obstetrician Lucy Chappell says, *'As a general rule, simply think about the health care system of the country you are going to and whether you would like to be in it, should any complications arise. Avoid islands – where you can't easily get to a hospital – and developing countries where possible.'*

VACCINATIONS | This is a legitimate worry. Some 'live' vaccines, like those against chickenpox are unwise to have when pregnant; others such as Hepatitis B, Hepatitis A, and tetanus are OK for pregnant women who are at risk of getting these diseases. Talk to your doctor about vaccinations if you've had them before you knew you were pregnant, or if you are thinking of having them before travelling.

AIR POLLUTION | Thousands of healthy babies are born each year in inner London, one of Europe's most polluted areas. Books will warn you about lead in traffic fumes, but really, if you live in an urban area, there's not much you can do about this short of ceasing to breathe or wearing a Michael Jackson mask. City life is not going to harm your unborn baby. If it did, half the babies in Hammersmith would have birth defects.

PESTICIDES IN FOOD | You will probably hear, at some point, that you should eat only organic food when pregnant or you will poison your unborn child with pesticides. Some women have the money to do this. Most of us, however, don't. The vast majority of us eat normal supermarket food when up the duff and our babies emerge just fine. According to the UK Government's 2002 Committee on Toxicity, pregnant or breastfeeding women are unlikely to be any more vulnerable to the 'cocktail' effect of low-level pesticides in food than anyone else. You should, however, wash fruit and vegetables thoroughly. If you peel fruit, by the way, you will reduce the vitamin and fibre content.

BENDING AND LIFTING | Your midwife or health visitor will be able to give you tips on how to avoid back strain, what you should and should not lift, and how to cope when you have to carry bigger children or toddlers. It's handy to pretend that you can't lift anything at all, so that your partner has to do all the supermarket shopping etc., but it is fine for a pregnant woman to lift moderate weights (i.e. a shopping bag or two) from the car to the house. The main problem is back strain, so bend from the knee rather than your back when lifting. Having said that, most mothers of more than one child have, at some point, been forced to wrestle a howling, kicking, 30lb toddler out of the toyshop/supermarket/playground while heavily pregnant with no bad consequences (other than to our mental health). The basic rule is: if it's heavy, try to avoid lifting it, and if you have to lift it, try to lift it with a good posture and try not to lift it above waist level. A physiotherapist-run class at your hospital will give you tips for bending and lifting. You can also divide your shopping into smaller, lighter bags: more trips, in general, are better than heavier bags.

HOT BATHS | The baby inside you does not have a temperature regulation of its own so if you get overheated your baby can't do anything about it. For this reason, hot tubs, saunas and Jacuzzis are not a good idea in pregnancy as they can raise your temperature too high for too long (above 39C/102F) which may affect your baby's heart rate. Normal baths (unless you go mad with the hot tap and sit there sweltering for hours) will do you and the baby no harm (and probably some good, as you'll relax).

Bath tip:
Keep a limb out of the water during your bath and lift your body out for a bit if you feel too hot or sweaty.

SEX | Unless you have a contra-indicating medical condition (for example, you have a low lying placenta, your waters have broken early or you have been warned by your doctor to abstain for any other reason) normal sexual intercourse will not harm your baby. Many women, particularly in mid-pregnancy, feel seriously sexy. Since most of us have a low sex drive after pregnancy (for up to a couple of years!)

make the most of any rampant phases you may have. Many men, paradoxically, can't look this gift horse in the mouth: the most common fear among male partners is that their penis's head will 'bump the baby'. Luckily no man – no matter how impressively large he is down there – is **that** well-endowed. He'd have to get through the vagina, mucus plug and cervix, into the uterus then through the amniotic sac before he could do any damage to your baby. **This is simply not going to happen**. It is, however, best to avoid really forceful or deep penetration – this can be uncomfortable, for a start. Nor will the weight of your partner squeeze the baby out (if only it did medical induction would be distinctly less common). The best tip is to experiment with positions: side-lying, your partner behind you, you on top of him – any angle really, once the missionary position gets tricky. Your orgasm will not make you miscarry (unless you are at risk of premature labour, in which case talk to your midwife). A vibrator is fine, too. There are no studies to show a vibrator cannot be used during pregnancy. But – brace yourself here if you're squeamish – introducing germs into the vagina during pregnancy is not a good idea, so clean your vibrator well and don't mix orifices.

Sex tips:
Don't insert foreign objects, air or water in your vagina during pregnancy.
If you bleed at any time after intercourse, contact your doctor/midwife straight away.

If, after orgasms, you experience a lot of uterine contractions, check with your doctor/midwife. Oxytocin, the 'love hormone' associated with orgasm, can also cause mild, clenching, harmless contractions in your womb after orgasms. (During labour oxytocin is actually the hormone that makes your womb contract to get the baby out.)

If you know you are at risk of premature labour, or if you have any other concerns, talk to your doctor/midwife about whether or not it's ok to have sex.

Sex can be genuinely beneficial (it tones the pelvic floor muscles, gets the circulation going, relieves tension) but it may feel a bit weird for you in your pregnant state. You have a greater blood supply to your vagina which can affect sensation (it may feel 'fuller' down there) and your clitoris may be extra sensitive. You may also feel either less or more lubricated (lubricants like KY Jelly can be helpful if sex becomes uncomfortable). You'll hear women boast about how rapacious they were throughout pregnancy but if your libido is paltry (or very variable) for nine months try not to feel cheated. You're swimming in hormones. You may be faintly distracted by the sight of your own body, even if your partner appears to be passionate about it. You may feel like your body has been 'taken over' by the baby, and you don't want to be assailed by anyone else. You may feel constantly sick, swell up like a balloon or have loony mood swings. You may simply be knackered. These things will not make you hot stuff in bed. And that's OK. Dr Petra Boynton, a psychologist specializing in sex and relationships at University College London says, *'What tends to disappear is not just the sex, but the communication, comfort, petting. If you're not feeling sexy you should at least be having rampant hand holding every night.'* We talk more about sex in pregnancy in Chapter 8: Blokes, Birth and Babies.

Dr Petra's sex tip:

'There is a bizarre idea that pregnant women are not supposed to be sexual. This is part Victorian hangover and part fear that sex is bad for the baby (it isn't). Sex toys can actually be a great bonus for pregnant women – they can be soothing as well as sexy. Go for vibrating toys designed for clitoral stimulation rather than penetration. I have had women tell me they used one of these in early labour to cope with low level pain. A colleague of mine, what's more, discovered that her silicon vibrator on a low, soothing, setting, wrapped in a towel and placed along her baby's back was a fantastic remedy for her baby's colic.'

> **Where to go for help:**
> You may have dropped this book in horror by now, but if you're still reading, or have always enjoyed this sort of thing anyway **www.nicesextoys.co.uk** might be worth a go (your guffaws will be fun for your baby anyway).

HAIR DYE | Except at your scalp, hair is dead tissue that cannot transmit toxins to your body. The hazard from hair dyes is therefore related to the amount of dye that can actually penetrate your scalp and enter your bloodstream while you're dying your hair, and from residues after you've finished. Some recent studies suggested a link between permanent hair dye and an increased risk of bladder cancer (yours, not your baby's), but no studies have found that dyeing your hair when pregnant will harm your baby. Most midwives will tell you that while the safest colour, when pregnant, is your natural one, dyes that involve minimal scalp touching, such as highlights, are extremely unlikely to damage your baby.

LOTIONS | No studies have found that lotions or make up cause birth defects or otherwise harm a fetus. If they did, there would be few healthy babies knocking around. However, many environmental groups have concerns about ingredients in cosmetics and lotions. This is an area of huge debate and there's no conclusive evidence either way. For more information try the Women's Environmental Network (WEN): 4 Pinchin Street, London E1. 020 7481 9004 www.wen.org.uk.

TOXIC SUBSTANCES | Watch out for things known to affect a fetus: cigarette smoke, drugs, large quantities of alcohol, lead (in water and paint – see below), carbon monoxide inhaled *in excess*, mercury, solvents, benzene and formaldehyde.

PAINT | Best get your partner to paint the nursery because certain types of paint and paint thinners may contain chemicals that aren't great for the developing fetus. I had a ludicrously strong 'nesting' urge towards the end of each of my pregnancies, and found myself uncontrollably painting wardrobes, cots, walls – indeed, anything I could get my hands on. My babies are fine but if I'd known about toxins in paint I might have taken up macramé instead.

Weight gain

Getting it into perspective

It's the infernally emotive topic: how fat will I get? Some admirable women simply don't care. They eat healthily and avoid the whole unnecessary issue. They are the minority. At the extreme end are those who quake over the scales, restrict their food intake and panic if they've gained an ounce more than the 'recommendations'. The rest of us, meanwhile, scoff cream cakes with gay abandon then whinge about how fat we are after the baby is born. Your weight in pregnancy should not be your prime concern. What matters is that you produce a healthy, well nourished baby. If you crash or fad diet during pregnancy you can severely damage your baby (inadequate nutrition can lead to low birth weight or premature babies who are at higher risk of complications and death[5]). So chuck out Atkins, the Zone, or whatever mad fad you're addicted to and feed yourself healthily for once (without beating yourself up, or getting paranoid). If your eating is genuinely out of control, or otherwise worrying you, it is essential that you find help and support so you can grow a healthy baby.

> **Where to go for help:**
> Your doctor/midwife is a good first base. You can also contact:
> **National Centre for Eating Disorders** They can refer you to specialist help in your area. 01372 469493 www.eating-disorders.org.uk
> **Eating Disorders Association** 01603 619090 Helpline 0845 634 1414 www.edauk.com

Weight charts and what to do with them

In the US, where I had Sam, my second baby, they stuck me on the scales at every antenatal appointment. At one point, I found myself apologizing to the nurse for my excessive bout of chocolate muffin-induced poundage. In Britain, doctors and midwives have realized that being constantly weighed has little medical benefit and causes many women undue anxiety and guilt. As obstetrician Lucy Chappell puts it: *'You don't weigh an oven to see if the cake is done.'* Your midwife usually asks your pre-pregnancy weight at your booking in appointment but is unlikely to weigh you after this unless there's a medical reason to do so. As a rough guide don't weigh yourself more than once a week.

How much weight you 'should' gain over the next nine months will depend on how fat or thin you are in your unimpregnated state. As a rough guide, if your pre-pregnancy Body Mass Index,[6] is in the 'ideal' range, you **might** gain about 25–35lb over the pregnancy. Very roughly this means a gain of about 3–6lb in first trimester, about 1lb a week in second and third. Loads of women gain far more than this, and lose it (albeit annoyingly slowly) afterwards. Do not succumb to the tyranny of weight charts: gain what is right for you. If you are already overweight doctors say you should gain slightly less than the average. If you are underweight, they say you should gain more. If you're worried about your rate of weight gain either way, talk to your doctor/midwife. For example, a really rapid weight gain (more than about 2lbs a week) could be an early sign of pre-eclampsia (pregnancy-related high blood pressure) if it is caused by fluid retention.

An experienced mother's weight tip:

'When I was pregnant first time around I weighed myself every morning. I avoided chocolate and anything fattening. I weighed out portions of food according to my pregnancy book's instructions. I panicked if I had put on more than I "should". I felt like I was on a radical diet. Once she was born, I lost the 6lb of 'baby fat' within a month. But I was exhausted all the time. With the other two I didn't care (too busy to care). I ate what I wanted, when I wanted – tried to make it healthy but didn't obsess. It was SO much more relaxing just to throw out all that weight worry for nine months. I was a stone heavier for a few months after the other two births, but it came off. And I had more energy with the second two babies. All my babies were healthy – and similar sizes – at birth. Looking back on it, that first time weight obsession was a ridiculous waste of time and energy.' Jules (40), mother of Chloe (7), Madeleine (4) and Daniel (1)

Fat fascism

Zoe, 33, was about three stone overweight at the start of her first pregnancy. *'Because I am fat, my GP treated me like a pariah. I was barely through the door on my first visit and he was talking about caesareans.'* In the end, Zoe gave birth to her 8lb daughter in water after a healthy pregnancy and eight hours of drug-free labour.

If you are overweight you may, like Zoe, experience confidence-sapping comments. The best advice is listen to the health professionals but get **facts** not opinions or knee jerk prejudices (ask, if necessary, for references so you can look yourself). Do not allow anyone to force you into believing that because you are overweight, you will necessarily have a complicated pregnancy and birth. Here are the basic things you should know about obesity and pregnancy.

Being clinically obese (two to three stone overweight, BMI over **35**), rather than just a bit chubby has the following documented risks:

1   **It can be harder for midwives and doctors to assess the pregnancy and labour** as it is harder to feel the baby and your womb. (Some health

professionals, by the way, can be offensive. *'I can't see baby, because of too much mummy,'* snapped one sonographer to a friend of mine, who, while plump and curvaceous is certainly not vastly overweight.)

2 **You will be, statistically, more prone to pregnancy complications** like hypertension, pre-eclampsia and oedema – where your body swells more because of fluid retention.

3 **You have a slightly higher risk of developing gestational diabetes** and consequently of having a larger than average baby.

4 **You have a slightly higher chance of having a caesarean section** (because of the baby's size, or your blood pressure).

5 **If you are obese and have a caesarean you have a slightly higher risk of some operative complications**.

Ask your doctor to refer you to a dietician for dietary advice and support during pregnancy if you are obese, and if any of the above worry you, discuss them in detail. Most overweight women have perfectly healthy babies.

Eating: the basics

Pregnancy eaters divide roughly into two extremes: neurotic self-abnegators, who take the books literally, cut out anything fun and start weighing out grams of fat and protein. And self-indulgers, who think 'Wey hey! Eating for two!' and start deep frying their Mars Bars. Ideally, you want to be somewhere in between the two. *'Before you close your mouth on a forkful of food,'* says the pregnancy book that tyrannized me the most in my first pregnancy, *'consider "is this the best bite I can give my baby?"…if it'll only benefit your sweet tooth or appease your appetite, put your fork down.'* Now, forgive my selfishness here, but satisfying my appetite, and even – gasp – my sweet tooth are, I believe, not an insignificant part of my overall well-being. This kind of nutritional fascism should really be outlawed by publishers of pregnancy books. You are pregnant. You are not on a diet. You are not sick. You are not going to harm your baby if you have the occasional bag of maltesers. However if you start eating in earnest for two, three or four, polishing off an entire tub of Haagen Dazs on the sofa, and generally throwing caution to the wind you will put on extra weight (just as you would if you weren't pregnant) and you might produce a slightly bigger baby. Being really too heavy will not help you feel good later in pregnancy, and of course it'll be harder to shift afterwards. Perhaps most important of all, you may not be giving yourself and your baby adequate nutrients if you're eating a lot of junk.

Most pregnancy books tell you that you only need to eat about an extra 300 calories per day when you are pregnant. This in itself is shocking news if you were expecting to be wolfing down the cream buns for the next nine months. Brace yourself now because many experts say the reality is *even harsher* than this. The most recent Department of Health guidelines conclude that (partly because of our reduced levels of activity, and partly because our metabolism alters) pregnant women **don't strictly need any extra calories whatsoever** in the first two trimesters of pregnancy. In the final trimester – hooray – we need about an extra 200 calories a day (a couple of large bananas).

Most of us, of course, eat loads more than this – because it's socially acceptable to do so when pregnant – and so we get a bit fat. This does us, and the baby, no harm. Most of us lose it afterwards if we eat sensibly and are reasonably active. (I put on 45lb with Sam largely as a result of moving to 'supersizing' America. My weight gain was technically 10lb or so 'too much'. I felt lardy afterwards, but the weight slowly came off and I was back to roughly my normal weight after maybe nine months.)

Verboten foods: what's the truth?

It's all horribly confusing. Can you eat that kind of cheese, or not? Can you drink that glass of wine, or not? One recent survey of British women by a baby formula manufacturer[7] found that most of us don't fully understand which foods to avoid when pregnant. Indeed, we often cut out foods that are beneficial, in the mistaken belief that they are somehow dangerous. Cottage cheese, for instance, is a good, low fat source of calcium. But many women avoid it in pregnancy thinking it's a 'soft' cheese, therefore verboten.

Our paranoia is understandable. For a start, the goalposts keep changing. When I was pregnant for the first time I stuffed myself with tuna, which I'd been told was an excellent source of fatty acids, protein and vitamins. Five years later, pregnant with number three, I was only allowed a couple of medium-sized cans a week. In the interim, studies had found that tuna may contain too much mercury and so harm a baby's developing nervous system if you eat too much of it in pregnancy (see guidelines on page 26). Swordfish, marlin and shark are now officially out, for the same reasons. And some reports have recently suggested that farmed salmon may contain unacceptable levels of toxins, though the Food Standards Agency says the benefits of eating salmon outweigh any potential harm as salmon is a fantastic source of protein, vitamin D and good fats that can help your baby grow. (If you're really worried you could try buying organic or wild salmon instead of cutting it out.)

There is, among all this confusion, some sensible evidence that certain foods should indeed be avoided during pregnancy. Mostly they are the ones that carry a very small risk of food poisoning such as listeria or salmonella, which studies have found may damage your fetus or cause miscarriage. Apart from this relatively short list of foods (see Pregnancy Eating Crib Sheet below), most doctors say you should eat basically as normal during pregnancy.

Why you should stop obsessing now

Phil Baker, Professor of fetal and maternal health at St Mary's hospital, Manchester says, *'I see so many women who are blaming themselves for a miscarriage or still birth when usually they could have done absolutely nothing to avoid it. It is important to have a basically balanced diet, which includes vegetables, protein, carbohydrate, fats and vitamins. If you are entirely starved it will have implications for the birth weight of your baby.'* Most of us do our best to eat more healthily when pregnant but even if we can't – because, for instance, we're throwing up – our bodies, says Professor Baker, should already contain good stores of certain nutrients which will get us through pregnancy. (This might explain why women with severe morning sickness, who can keep nothing down, can still produce miraculously healthy babies.)

Supplements

There is some debate over whether taking a general vitamin supplement in pregnancy is necessary or even helpful. (This does not include folic acid – see below – or iron supplements if you are anaemic.) I take a pregnancy vitamin pill each day when pregnant, but my attitude is that of the agnostic praying in times of duress: you don't want to rule anything out. *'You can look upon a general vitamin supplement as an insurance policy,'* says Dr Toni Steer, a nutritionist at MRC Human Nutrition Research in Cambridge, *'but make sure that your vitamin and mineral supplement doesn't exceed daily recommendations – don't take megadoses of one particular vitamin.'* Many nutritionists argue that it's the combination of nutrients in real food that produces benefits. And certainly, taking a daily dose of pregnancy vitamins, then eating crap all day is not the best option if you want a healthy baby.

Nutrition tip:

In summary, you will be fed a load of obsessive nonsense about what, how and when you should eat in pregnancy. Remember that a great many fetal and maternal health experts object to this kind of pressure – and the guilt, doubt and self-blame that result from it. Professor Baker says that most grown up women who 'use moderation in all aspects – who don't have particular food fanaticisms, or drink excessively' are doing all that is necessary – nutritionally speaking – to produce perfectly healthy babies. So, the best advice is just follow the basic safety advice and get on with your life.

Where to go for help:
Drinkline 0800 917 8282 www.alcoholconcern.org.uk
The Food Standards Agency guidelines (www.food.gov.uk) offer the most up-to-date, official advice.
The Eating for Pregnancy Helpline is useful for random panics ('Can I eat the prosciutto on this pizza?') 01142 424084

Otherwise, this crib sheet is the best place to start.

PREGNANCY EATING

Each day try to eat a variety of foods including:
- Plenty of fruit and vegetables
- Plenty of starchy foods (whole grains are best, such as whole meal bread, pasta and brown rice)
- Some protein (lean red meat, chicken, fish, eggs, pulses such as lentils are also good source of iron)
- Some low-fat dairy products (milk, cheese, yogurt all contain calcium)
- Drink lots of water

Foods you need for sure:
- Your diet needs to contain plenty of **iron** (good foods include: red meat, pulses, leafy green vegetables, fortified breakfast cereals, dried fruit). Vitamin C helps your body to absorb iron (drink orange juice when you eat iron-rich food). Both **calcium** (derived from milk, cheese and yoghurt) and iron are important for the baby's growth (anaemic mums may have low birth-weight babies).
- You should take 400 mcg **folic acid** a day in first three months (and three months before conception if at all possible). Folic acid can protect against neural tube defects, for example spina bifida, and may protect against the failure of the placenta to work well, which can lead to pre-eclampsia, still birth or growth problems.

Things to be cautious about:
- **Alcohol:** in the us pregnant women are told not to drink. In Britain, we are told to cut down to two to three units a week (that's about a glass and a half of wine). All doctors survey the same literature but draw different conclusions, so do not be panicked by signs in New York bars forbidding you to have a drink when pregnant. But do talk to your GP if you can't cut down.
- **Coffee:** there is no conclusive evidence linking caffeine and miscarriage, so there is no need to cut out the lattes entirely; cutting down to one or two a day may be sensible. The Food Standards Agency says limit your caffeine intake to no more than three caffeinated drinks a day (coke, pepsi and chocolate all contain caffeine). In the us women are advised to have no more than one cup of coffee a day.
- **Stop smoking** and don't take recreational drugs as they can damage your baby.

Foods doctors say you should avoid:

- **Soft mould-ripened cheese**, such as Camembert, Brie and blue-veined cheeses like Stilton. There is no risk of listeria from pasteurised hard cheeses (such as Cheddar), cottage cheese, processed cheese and yoghurt.
- **Pâté** (any type, including vegetable as it can contain salmonella).
- **Raw or partially-cooked eggs** (same reason) or foods containing raw eggs e.g. homemade mayonnaise. (Commercially produced mayonnaise in jars doesn't contain raw egg.)
- **Uncooked, or partially cooked meat, or ready prepared meals** Take particular care with sausages, minced meat, parma ham or other raw meats. These may contain toxoplasmosis (see below). Government guidelines say that eating cold meat and smoked fish is fine.
- **Unpasteurised milk or cheese.** Most cheeses you'll buy in British supermarkets are pasteurized except for Parmesan that is often unpasteurised.
- **Liver.** Don't eat it when pregnant. It contains too much **vitamin A** that can increase the risk of birth defects when eaten in large quantities.

Other words of warning:

- **Fish:** Don't eat more than two cans of tuna a week. No swordfish, shark and marlin (high mercury levels in these fish can damage the fetus' nervous system). Avoid sushi (it contains raw fish, a food poisoning risk). Oily fish like salmon, mackerel or sardines are considered to be great as they contain fatty acids known, amongst other things, to improve your baby's intelligence.
- **Shellfish:** only eat it if you know it's been thoroughly cooked.
- **Peanuts:** there is some evidence (though not conclusive) that eating them while pregnant can later cause an allergy for them in your child. If you have a family history of allergy generally (asthma, eczema, hayfever, food allergies) the possibility is greater but without such a history the risk is deemed very small.

Toxoplasmosis

To avoid catching toxoplasmosis (an infection that can cause disabilities in a baby) don't touch the cat litter because in the UK the bug is most commonly found in cat poo. If you do touch it, wash your hands thoroughly afterwards. Uncooked or partially cooked meat can also contain toxoplasmosis so never eat it 'rare' and always wash your hands carefully after handling it. Also, wash all fruit, vegetables and salad very carefully.

Where to go for help:
The Toxoplasmosis Trust, run by Tommy's The Baby Charity. Call their
pregnancy information line: 0870 777 30 60

PREGNANCY SUPERFOODS

Put a few of these on your shopping list
and try eating at least something each day:[8]

- bananas, oranges and other fresh fruit
- dried apricots and prunes
- broccoli and other green vegetables
- oily fish
- whole meal bread
- brown rice
- lean red meat
- chicken and turkey
- yoghurt
- pulses and lentils
- fortified breakfast cereals
- nuts (avoid peanuts) and seeds (e.g. sesame)

Superfeeding tips:
Take a snack bag to work of nuts, seeds and dried fruit. Chop fruit onto your
breakfast cereal. Make a load of lentil soup and freeze it in lunch-sized portions.

Business eaters

It's not easy, of course, to cook brown rice when you're flying business class to
New York. In work situations (meetings, planes, offices) you may find yourself
ravenous and devouring posh corporate cookies instead of lentil soup. Again, no
one is advocating a strict macrobiotic diet here but it might help to think and plan
more than you usually do.

1 **Think ahead:** take bags of dried fruit to work, or on business trips, as
   snacks. Grab some fruit from the hotel fruit bowl if travelling, to take with you
   as a snack during the day – don't fill up on the biscuits and pastries in the
   boardroom.

2 **Ask for healthy options:** in restaurants or hotels ask for the more
   nutritionally sound options: whole meal rolls, fruit or cheese instead of
   desserts.

3 **Avoid the constant 'treat mentality'.** If you do a lot of business travel it's
   tempting to go for the croissants at breakfast, the chocolate tart at dinner.
   This is fine in moderation, but if you travel a lot, you can't really do this (well
   you can, but it may not do you much good). Opt for the fruit salad at dinner at

least some of the time, eat whole meal toast and cereal for breakfast. Drink plenty of water and remember that the alcohol and caffeine restrictions are still relevant, even if you *are* in Paris.

A WORD ABOUT VEGETARIANS | If you are vegetarian you may need more iron, calcium and vitamin B12 (in dairy products and eggs) when pregnant, and you also need to get enough protein. Talk to your midwife. More information is also available from: **The Vegetarian Society** 0161 925 2000. And if you really want obsessive detail you can read *Your Vegetarian Pregnancy: a month by month guide to health and nutrition* by Holly Roberts but don't get too hung up here. If you're following the basic rules above, you are likely to be eating a perfectly healthy diet.

Exercise: the basics

Late for a book launch, about 37 weeks into my first pregnancy, I walked fast across central London in high heels, keeping up with my striding unpregnant colleagues. I ended up spending the last three weeks of that pregnancy immobilized on the sofa. I had strained my 'symphysis pubis' – the ligaments that hold your pubic bone together. I felt disabled and my confidence in my body was shaken. In my second pregnancy, through fear of a recurrence, I strained only to lift the box of Thorntons to my lap. This was not ideal either: I grew vast and tired.

The general advice out there on exercise in pregnancy tends to be outdated to say the least – I've lost count of how many times I've read 'light housework is OK'. You do have to be sensible about what you do during pregnancy. Strains like the one I had – particularly in later pregnancy and particularly in the pelvic region – are common because your body is swimming in a hormone called 'relaxin' which loosens the ligaments in preparation for birth. Indeed, physiotherapists say that nowadays, because we're all leaping around trying to be as thin as Hollywood starlets, 'diastasis symphysis pubis' (called DSP or SPD) – a strain in the joint at the front of your pelvis – is all the rage. This can be severe and even cause permanent damage but none of this means you should sit on your bum for nine months. Indeed, if you're the fitness type, this idea could really panic you. You don't have to put your exercise programme on hold while you gestate and indeed, if you're a couch potato, now is as good a time as any to put down the remote and go for a walk. You do, however, need to follow some basic rules, and remember that pregnancy is not a time to lose weight or become hell bent on shaping up.

> **Where to go for help:**
> **The National Childbirth Trust** offers help and advice on 'pelvic disfunctions' like SPD. 0870 770 3236 www.spd-uk.org

Reasons to exercise

Exercise that makes you warm and slightly out of breath is good for most pregnant women. It can strengthen your bones, give you more energy and help you sleep better.

- A basic level of fitness can help you cope with the marathon of childbirth.
- Exercise can keep you flexible, reduce aches and pains and help other pregnancy symptoms like constipation.
- Exercise can help lower your stress levels and lift your mood.

What types of exercise are good?

Low impact exercise, like walking (30–40 minutes, three times a week), yoga (an antenatal class) or swimming (aquanatal classes are good) are all generally safe to do, no matter how unfit you are in everyday life. If you've exercised or done certain sports before this pregnancy you should be able to keep going – **if it feels good** – but **DO** take the intensity down a notch and again, do set some reasonable parameters with your doctor. Avoid any exercise that is too jerky or has violent impact – such as high-impact aerobics – as this is more likely to strain you.

'I did spinning up until the last week of my pregnancy,' says Tiffany Lipelt, a certified health and fitness instructor with a BA in exercise physiology who is also a mother of two children under five, a long distance runner and yoga addict. *'I have had pregnant women in Tae-bo classes and lifting weights (all have to be modified eventually). It is important to keep your doctor updated and to know that it is not a "results-oriented" work out. It is just to keep you healthy and your mind clear as you get bigger and bigger. Your body and your baby will be your guide – if it doesn't feel good, it isn't! It is important to follow basic safety advice, but it is also important to remember that you are an individual and that if you work with your doctor you can come up with a middle ground that suits your exercise needs.'*

PELVIC FLOOR EXERCISE | This is one kind of exercise even couch potatoes can excel at. The pelvic floor is the cradle of muscles that keep your bladder and womb in the right place. Pregnancy stretches them. You may leak urine if they are weakened (see Incontinence, page 38). **What to do:** Stopping the flow of urine half way through peeing – or trying to – will help you work out what a pelvic floor exercise feels like. People will tell you different 'numbers' of exercises you should do, and it can get confusing. Just do some, as often as you can (about ten times a day is good).

Regularly during your day (at traffic lights, when washing up, waiting to cross the road etc.), tighten your pelvic floor, tighten some more, and then some more, as if going three floors up in a lift. Hold five seconds. Release in the same way. Repeat a few times.

Then do a squeeze, hold for a second, and release. Repeat this a few times (well, about ten times would be ideal).

At first this can be frustrating. You may feel you can't even find the muscles, let alone twitch them. Don't give up. Practise. Benefits include your long-term gynaecological health, improved sex life, protection against incontinence and, some say, a strong pelvic floor even helps you push the baby out.

General exercise safety rules

1   **Do not start anything new** (except antenatal classes). If you begin a sudden dramatic increase in your exercise routine on discovering you're pregnant, or start a new sport hoping to stave off the weight gain, it's possible you might harm your baby or yourself.

2   **Talk to your doctor** about any specific sports you do. If your temperature gets too high this can – theoretically – pose risks to the baby as its heart rate will speed up. The best way to gauge how hot is too hot, is to talk to your doctor about how high you should allow your heart rate to go when exercising. Get a heart-rate monitor and use it whenever you are exercising, to keep your heart rate at a level you have agreed with your doctor.

3   **Avoid exercises on your back (e.g. sit ups) after 12 weeks.** When you are on your back, the weight of the baby sits on the main blood supply from your legs to your heart. This can restrict the oxygen supply to the baby, whose heart rate could then become depressed.

4   **Modify your current fitness plan as your girth increases.** As your pregnancy progresses, you'll reach your maximum heart rate faster and your centre of gravity will change. Don't abandon your workout entirely (a recumbent bike or treadmill might replace an aerobics class for instance). And try not to be results oriented – remember you are not trying to achieve anything (except basic well-being) during pregnancy.

5   **Drink water.** Most pregnant women don't drink enough anyway and exercise makes this worse. Dehydration can lead to blood clots, and can also restrict the oxygen supply to your baby.

6   **Use common sense.** Some contact sports carry certain relatively minor risks. A severe blow to the abdomen, while unlikely, could damage the baby or cause you to miscarry. Ask your doctor if you are uncertain about the advisability of your chosen sport.

7   **Listen to your body.** If you have aches and pains, modify what you're doing quickly or stop and try something else.

Reasons to be extra cautious

A history of miscarriage – particularly in the second trimester – certain conditions like 'placenta praevia', where the placenta is over the neck of the womb, or an 'incompetent cervix', where the neck of the womb is weak, can all be reasons to be cautious. If your baby is not growing well, or if you are carrying twins (or more) you may also need to take it slow. As always, talk to your midwife or doctor if there are any concerns.

Danger signs: Stop, and tell your midwife or doctor if you have any unexplained bleeding, dizziness, heart palpitations, blurred vision, sharp pains in abdomen or chest, or contractions during exercise.

Impact tip:

If you're exercising at home (to a video, say) do so on a relatively soft surface, such as a yoga mat, to minimize the impact on your joints.

Falling down/being bumped in the belly: almost always the baby is fine when this happens. If, however, you feel the baby is moving less, or you are worried about pain or concussion, call your doctor/midwife.

PREGNANCY FITNESS

Specific forms of exercise

If you're doing a specific form of exercise already, it may be perfectly safe to continue though modifying it as the pregnancy progresses. But **always** discuss your exercise routine with your doctor as your pregnancy may have issues of its own that rule some things out.

- **Spinning** This can be great, but as your pregnancy progresses move from standing to sitting and don't crank up the knob up as much as you did. Talk to your doctor about maximum heart rates.

- **Running** Follow rules on intensity, watch the surface you are running on (not too hard or uneven) and beware your changing centre of gravity. If it hurts or feels uncomfortable, slow down. Walking may feel better.

- **Weight training** This should be fine if you did it before you were pregnant but you'll need to drop some weights as the pregnancy progresses (you're carrying weight already, don't forget). Avoid exercises that involve lying on your back after 12 weeks. Weightlifting with a partner who is looking out for you will keep your back straight and be another set of eyes keeping you safe. Always discuss your particular programme with your doctor.

- **Aerobics** As with any class, let your instructor know as soon as you know you are pregnant. Slow down, avoid high impact moves and watch your heart rate. If it starts to hurt, or you get any other danger signs, stop.

- **Yoga** Yoga is terrific in pregnancy. Drink lots of water and stop if you feel at all faint. If it's not specific antenatal yoga, tell your instructor you are pregnant.

- **Pilates** Great for pregnant women as long as you've got an experienced teacher. Most instructors will say it's not a good idea to begin Pilates when pregnant, but if you've done it before, it can help you stay toned in pregnancy, and bounce back more quickly. According to Jenny Miller, a certified Pilates instructor and mother of two: *'Pilates increases bone density, focuses on the ever-changing centre of gravity of a pregnant body and strengthens and maintains the muscles that support the growing belly.'*

Sports generally
A bad fall or strong impact to the belly – rather than your average bump against a chair, tumble or kick from a toddler – could harm the baby so make sure you've really thought through the risks and talk to your doctor before you continue.

A WORD ABOUT INSTRUCTION | Make sure the instructor is really knowledgeable and not just giving you her best guess. And always talk to your doctor about the specifics of your exercise programme first. Pilates instructor Jenny Miller says: *'In pregnancy the goals change from no limits to set limits. A good trainer will respect those limits. When a non-pregnant woman tells me she can't do a position, I may urge her to push through her pain and tiredness. When a pregnant woman says the same thing I back off entirely and we rest.'* That's the major difference with pregnant workouts: don't push through the pain – stop!

Tip for fitness fiends:
'See pregnancy for the temporary condition it is. If you are involved in an extreme sport or high impact fitness programme, consider doing something less risky for the few months you are pregnant.' Tiffany Lipelt, fitness fanatic and mother of two.

Online:
Start with the **Guild of Pregnancy and Postnatal exercise teachers** www.postnatalexercise.co.uk (click on 'information for mothers') for basic information, book and video recommendations and ways to find a qualified teacher.

Further reading:
The Pregnancy Exercise Book by Judy Difiore (Newleaf, UK, 2000) A good basic book.
Exercising Through Your Pregnancy by James F. Clapp (Addicus, US, 2002) One for the exercise enthusiast.
Yoga for Pregnancy, Birth and Beyond by Francoise Barbira Freedman (Dorling Kindersley, UK, 2004)
Preparing for Birth with Yoga: Empowering and Effective Exercise for Pregnancy and Childbirth by Janet Balaskas (Harper Collins, UK, 2003)

It could happen: specific pregnancy fears and what to do about them

Miscarriage

A survey carried out by The Miscarriage Association found that nearly half the women who miscarried said they didn't feel well informed about what was happening to them. Only 29 per cent felt well cared for emotionally. Many women who miscarry say books provided little or no information about it in advance. Many feel grief, depression, sadness, anger and loneliness after a miscarriage. This is why we're giving you some basic facts about miscarriage. It does not mean you should expect to have one. But it may help you to cope if you do (and also to be sensitive to women you know who have had one).

MISCARRIAGE: SOME BASIC FACTS

- More than one in five pregnancies end in miscarriage.
- Most women only miscarry once.
- Most miscarriages happen in the first 12 weeks of pregnancy, usually in the first eight weeks.
- Even when a baby stops developing at six or eight weeks, it may take some time before the physical process of miscarriage starts.
- Late miscarriage, where the baby stops developing after 12 weeks, is rare – it happens in about 2 per cent of pregnancies.
- The risk of miscarriage increases with the mother's age, with the greatest change after the age of 39.
- If you miscarry once, your chance of having a second miscarriage is not significantly greater than in your first pregnancy.
- Even women who have had five or more miscarriages will usually have a baby eventually.
- Smoking in pregnancy has been linked to an increased chance of miscarriage.

Many women feel bereft following a miscarriage, and say that they feel misunderstood and hurt when people say, 'Oh, you'll be fine next time' or 'It's nature's way' or 'At least you already have one child'. Many miscarriages are unexplained – indeed, about half of us never find out exactly why we miscarried. About half of all early miscarriages happen because of chance chromosome abnormalities, and there are certain hormonal and physical conditions that can lead to miscarriage. Often, in the absence of a medical explanation, we blame ourselves. While this is tempting and horribly common, it is usually completely unfounded.

WHAT IS A MISCARRIAGE LIKE? | What happens in a miscarriage can vary hugely from woman to woman and depends on how many weeks pregnant you are. Many women have heavy bleeding and cramps or even just blood spotting when miscarrying. Some describe it as being like a 'heavy period', others say their miscarriage was much more painful, and very shocking. Some women, however, have no symptoms at all and are appalled to discover during a routine scan that the baby has no heartbeat.

On a reassuring note: if you get blood spotting do not assume you're miscarrying. About 20 per cent of pregnant women have blood spotting in early pregnancy (I had it in all three of my pregnancies with no miscarriages). It's also tempting to worry if you feel a cramp or ache in your belly in early pregnancy. But cramps/aches/pains in the lower abdomen are a normal part of pregnancy (remember: your ligaments are stretching, your organs remodelling themselves around your swelling womb). Don't assume you are miscarrying if you get these symptoms. Do, however, call your doctor/midwife if you are at all concerned, and definitely call if you are spotting **and** cramping.

In some miscarriages, the womb empties itself completely. If not, you may be offered an operation (called an 'ERPC' or a 'D&C') or treatment with pills to empty your womb. You can, however, choose to wait and let the miscarriage happen naturally. Discuss this with your doctor.

PAST MISCARRIAGE | If you've miscarried in the past, early pregnancy can be one long anxiety-fuelled nightmare. *'Every time I go to the loo I am waiting to see blood in my knickers,'* says Sophie, who had four miscarriages before her son Jack's birth, has had one since and is pregnant again: *'Every time I get a twinge in my belly my heart plummets. Every scan or checkup I worry there won't be a heartbeat. I won't discuss baby names and with Jack I did not buy any baby equipment until a week before he was due. I have to protect myself, and this is how.'* Some women wrap themselves in cotton wool, fearing that doing anything will spark a miscarriage.

WAYS OF COPING WITH A MISCARRIAGE

1 Consult your doctor with a list of all your questions, and make sure you understand the answers.
2 Wait until you feel physically and emotionally ready before getting pregnant again. It is not a good idea to rush into another pregnancy before you have recovered.
3 Use the time before you get pregnant again to build yourself up physically. Eat as well as you can, start practising relaxation techniques, and get regular exercise.
4 Get emotional support and information from organizations that specialize in this (see below).
5 Join a support group for women who've been through it.
6 Remember that your partner may need support and information too.

7   Make sure you really trust your doctor – if you do not feel they take your fears seriously, consider changing doctors.

A WORD ABOUT A PREVIOUS TERMINATION | Roughly 17 per 1000 women aged 15–44 have a termination each year[9]. If you have had a previous termination (or more than one) it is extremely unlikely to affect this pregnancy. However, it is crucial that you tell your midwife, even if you find this difficult to do, as she needs to know your entire gynaecological history.

> **Where to go for help:**
> **The Miscarriage Association Helpline** can give you support and information. If you are worried about miscarriage – for whatever reason – even if you have not had one yourself, you can also contact them. 01924 200799
> www.miscarriageassociation.org.uk

Fear of having a big baby

It is common to be 'warned' by doctors or midwives at some time during pregnancy that your baby's a whopper. The first thing you should know is that all ways of estimating a baby's weight during pregnancy are just that – **estimates**. The technical term for a big baby is 'macrosomic' – that is, more than about 9lb at birth. Such information may be presented to you as 'fact' but it is usually nothing of the kind. Your midwife will measure the size of your belly and feel your uterus during each check up. But this 'manual palpitation' can be around 10 per cent wrong in either direction. The latest ultrasound technology can also be up to a couple of pounds out and is generally considered to be better at 'predicting' small babies than large ones.

There is some evidence that steep weight gain in the last trimester may be a 'contributing factor' in having a bigger baby. But do not beg for a caesarean if you find yourself gaining more than about 1lb a week: much weight gain in the final trimester can be fluid retention. You might, however, want to cut down on sugary foods if you're gaining very fast (as this may, possibly, affect your baby's weight). *'I was told by the hospital that my first baby was big,'* says Kaitlin, 36, mother of three. *'This panicked me completely – I was scared enough of the birth. It never occurred to me they might be wrong, they seemed so sure. In the end, I had an emergency caesarean because of failure to progress: she was 7lb2oz. I ignored all comments about baby size in my next two pregnancies.'*

Even if your baby does turn out to be big, your body will probably cope perfectly well with giving birth to it. Some women will have bigger babies but James Walker, Professor of obstetrics and gynaecology at the University of Leeds Medical School says: *'Plenty of women give birth to 10lb babies with absolutely no complications.'* He says, *'Shetland ponies have Shetland ponies'* (in less equine terms this means your baby is likely to be in proportion with you). *'Both my sons were nearly 10lb,'* says Sarah, who is 5ft 6in. *'And both births were great. With my second I did not even tear. What's more, I am not – despite my friends' jokes – the size of the Mersey Tunnel down there.'* Giving birth to a big baby can be tough, but so can giving birth to a 6lb one. So don't get hung up on your baby's size. Julia attended a birth where the mother, Grace, a nineteen year old, delivered a 10lb 5oz baby with no drugs. *'She was so young, and just hadn't heard all those dramatic birth stories – she just focused on giving birth. And it went just fine, partly I think, because nobody had told her she couldn't do it.'*

POSSIBLE BIG BABY COMPLICATIONS | With big babies there is a slightly higher risk of failure to progress during labour (i.e. when labour stalls or slows down). We talk more about this in Chapter 5: Your Options. There is also a slightly higher risk of shoulder dystocia (where the baby's shoulder gets stuck) at birth. Delivering your baby on your hands and knees, or in a kneeling position might help (see Chapter 5 for good positions for pushing). But the truth is complicated – births can happen to babies of any size. Risks, with big babies, tend to occur when a baby is particularly fat, not merely large. This mostly happens to diabetic women who can have fatter babies because of higher blood sugar levels during pregnancy. Head size (another myth shattered) is only very rarely a concern. Even big heads fold (normal, honestly: see Chapter 2) as the baby comes out of your vagina, and despite what many of us think about our brainy offspring, it is actually extremely rare for a baby to have a genuinely humungous head.

In other words, if you are told your baby is big (and you're not diabetic), have confidence in your body's ability to grow a baby it can cope with, prepare thoroughly for the birth and tell yourself size doesn't matter.

Your pregnant body and what it might do

Some odd things may happen to your body over the next nine months. Here are some of the most common ones and what to do about them. Reading sections like this can be alarming but do not obsess about them. You are not ill. Some women sail through pregnancy with barely a twinge. This list can't be comprehensive, of course, so the golden rule, again, is talk to your midwife if you're at all concerned. During pregnancy you may experience some of the following:

CARPAL TUNNEL SYNDROME | The carpal tunnel is the tube in your wrist through which run the nerves leading to your fingers. Extra fluid in this tube can cause numbness, tingling and pain in your fingers and sometimes up your arm. **What to do** Try wrist splints (from your GP). Or sweeping/moving your arm above your head to let fluids return to your heart. Call your midwife if this pain keeps you from sleeping or from your daily routine, and before taking any pain medications.

CONSTIPATION | Pregnancy hormones can bung you up, and if you are prescribed iron this may not help (the majority of women do not need iron tablets in pregnancy). **What to do** Drink lots of water, eat fibre-rich food (fruit, whole grain cereals, brown rice). Many women swear by a spoon of flaxseed on their breakfast cereal. Granny knew best when she put prunes on her All-bran. Four floz of pure juice a day can also help.

CRAVINGS | There are no definite statistics on this, but small studies and anecdotal evidence suggest that about 60 per cent of pregnant women crave certain foods when pregnant. I spent the first three months of my third pregnancy stuffing myself with beef-flavoured hula hoops (I'm a vegetarian). Julia's clients crave all sorts of weird things to eat but ice cubes, lemons, toothpaste and gherkins (with everything) come high on the list for many women. Cravings may be a response to unmet nutritional needs, but can also be linked to your emotions – a need for comfort, solace, treats (though where a muddy potato fits in here is anyone's guess). Craving for things that aren't food (e.g. coal, clay, chalk) is called 'pica' and is uncommon. Talk to your doctor/midwife if this happens or if you are craving anything particularly strongly. **What to do** Unless it's 'pica', indulge in moderation. You might also want to assess how balanced your diet is.

FEELING GENERALLY UNHINGED | Your hormones have gone haywire. You may feel genuinely unbalanced. Women, looking back on their pregnancy mood swings often use words like 'psycho' and 'loon'. It can feel like acid-fuelled PMT at times. **What to do** Talk to your midwife or GP. Make sure your partner understands it's down to chemicals and largely out of your control. Get counselling or other professional support if extreme. Try relaxation techniques, balanced eating, sleep and regular exercise. And remember it will pass.

HEADACHES | These are common, particularly in early pregnancy. **What to do** Eat small amounts regularly, drink plenty of water (at least eight tall glasses a day, more if possible), avoid caffeine, get fresh air. Try not to take any headache pills in first 12 weeks if possible. The safest over-the-counter remedy – in small amounts – is paracetamol. If headaches are severe talk to your midwife or doctor as this can be a sign of high blood pressure.

HEARTBURN | Pregnancy hormones make the valve at the top of your stomach relax, allowing acid to come up into your throat. **What to do** Small, frequent, low fat meals and avoiding coffee might help. Some women eat ginger biscuits or drink peppermint tea. An apple after a meal may also help. A doctor can prescribe antacids or liquids like gaviscon and some people say 'digestive enzymes', which you can buy at a health food shop, tackle the problem well. Though check with your midwife before you take anything like this.

INCONTINENCE | 'Stress' incontinence – leaking urine when you cough, jump, sneeze – and a certain lack of control, generally, over one's bladder is incredibly common in pregnancy, though you wouldn't think so by our buttoned lips on the subject. Indeed, about a third of us will still be experiencing some kind of urinary incontinence three months after childbirth. You are not, then, unique in your childlike ability to wet your pants: pregnancy incontinence is caused by the baby weight squashing your bladder, plus hormones which can have surprising effects on bladder control, plus (if you have given birth before) weaker pelvic floor muscles. Most pregnant women know – or find out the hard way – not to stray too far from a toilet. The more pregnancies you have, the worse this may get. **What do to** Do your pelvic floor exercises (see page 30), wear panty liners for mental comfort, and talk frankly to your midwife.

ITCHING | Your growing belly, breasts and sometimes the palms of your hands and soles of your feet might get itchy on and off in pregnancy. This is properly known as 'pregnancy pruritis' and happens as a result of your stretching skin and possibly your pregnancy hormones. Dry skin or eczema might also get worse. Severe itching during the second, or most usually during the third trimester, usually all over your body and sometimes – though not always – accompanied by nausea, vomiting, loss of appetite, fatigue, pale-coloured poos and jaundice, can be a sign of liver trouble. Called 'obstetric cholestasis', this affects about 0.7 per cent of pregnant women so call your midwife straightaway if the itching gets out of hand. **What to do** Avoid hot baths, use plenty of unscented moisturiser such as E45 cream, wear loose cotton clothing and avoid going out in the heat of the day.

> **Where to go for help:**
> **The British Liver Trust** 01425 463080 www.britishlivertrust.org
> **Itchy Moms** www.itchymoms.com (US website set up by an obstetric cholestasis sufferer)

LEG CRAMPS | These happen to most women during pregnancy, often in the second trimester, sometimes because of calcium deficiency. **What to do** Some women say a calcium/magnesium supplement stopped them. Tonic water, containing quinine, may also help.

MORNING SICKNESS | This can range from mild nausea to repeated vomiting throughout the day and, whatever level it is, can be depressing, embarrassing and tiring. As Julia remembers, *'I get a depression with that sickness that is scary. I'm otherwise not depressive at all, but the longer I can't make myself better, the more down I get. I had great difficulty caring for Keaton when first pregnant with Larson and only the understanding that it would get better helped me. You just have to wait it out and believe that it's worth it in the long run.'* **What to do** If extreme, get help from your GP (medication is sometimes available, and you may need extra fluids by IV). Otherwise, 'remedies' vary from ginger biscuits or ginger ale, to frequent savoury, starchy snacks like crackers, preferably with some protein, to small regular meals, travel sickness wrist bands, acupuncture, acupressure, drinking lots of water, meditating and smelling lemons. Some women swear by porridge.

Where to go for help:
Contact **Hyperemesis Education and Research Foundation (HER)** for help
with severe morning sickness www.hyperemesis.org

PILES (HAEMORRHOIDS) | These are varicose veins in your bottom. They can be
alarming when you first feel one bulging out, and can make pooing painful.
Sometimes made worse by pushing the baby out. These usually clear up soon
after pregnancy. **What to do** Eat a high fibre diet, drink lots of water, don't delay
if you need a poo, exercise. Talk to your doctor or midwife. Over-the-counter
creams such as Anusol are safe to use in pregnancy.

SKIN CHANGES | Skin tags, pigment changes, itchiness, dryness, spots, even
acne and warts are all common, hormonal skin changes in pregnancy. **What to
do** Try changing face products if you have facial acne; rub almond oil or similar
into itchy/dry skin. Talk to your midwife/doctor if severe and get any new or odd-
looking moles checked over. (See also Itching, page 39.)

SORE BREASTS | Tingling, aching, sharp pains, lumpiness, tender or sore nipples
– those girls have a life of their own right now. **What to do** Try hot baths,
showers or gentle massage, ditch your underwired bras, get fitted for a pregnancy
bra and wear it at night too if it helps. Some women say avoiding caffeine helps.
See your doctor/midwife if any lump, bump or sensation concerns you.

STRETCH MARKS | Generally considered to be a genetic thing, so spending
hundreds of pounds at the Clarins counter, while tempting, is probably futile.
They can look alarming at first (purple, red, raised), but usually fade after a few
months. If at all possible, decide to wear them with pride as the alternative is
futile, belly-focused self-loathing and money spent on creams that do nothing.
Cocoa butter and other lotions may help with any skin-stretch related itching.

SWOLLEN FEET AND ANKLES | Known as 'oedema', this is essentially excess
blood and water 'pooling' in your extremities. Don't be alarmed. It's common
and normal and will go away after you give birth. But it can be incredibly uncomfortable and inconvenient. Your shoes may not fit anymore, and you may feel
ungainly and bizarrely trapped in this new, inflatable body. **What to do** Elevate
your feet when possible (also keep a stool or pile of books under your desk); lie
on your left side when possible; put on waist-high support tights before you get
out of bed in the morning so blood has no chance to pool around your ankles;
drink plenty of water (surprisingly, keeping hydrated helps your body retain less
water); exercise regularly; avoid salty foods. **Word of warning** Sudden severe
swelling in your hands and face can be a sign of pre-eclampsia (see page 43), a
condition that is very serious. Call your midwife or doctor if this happens.

VARICOSE VEINS | Yes, sometimes we get these glamorous things in pregnancy, because of our increased blood volume. They are enlarged veins (blood vessels) close to your skin's surface and usually found in your legs and feet. They can ache, itch or throb, and they can look a bit grim. **What to do** Talk to your midwife if you have them/think you're getting them. She'll suggest keeping your feet elevated, wearing support tights, moving around a lot, avoiding certain sitting positions (crossed legs, thighs pressing on edge of chair), avoiding standing for long periods.

GROUP B STREP | This is a common bacteria, harmless to you and found in your vagina. If you have it, your baby can pick up an infection on its way out and can be damaged by it. You may be screened for this in pregnancy. There is more about this in Chapter 5: Your Options, page 163.

VAGINAL YEAST INFECTIONS (OR THRUSH) | This is very common in pregnancy because of hormonal shifts and appears as a frothy, yeasty discharge accompanied by intense vaginal itching. **What to do** Avoiding sugar may help and ask your GP or midwife about over-the-counter creams that are safe to use in pregnancy.

More serious health worries

There are, of course, endless rare, technical problems to do with pregnancy that we just can't cover in this book. We cover a few of the most common serious health worries below. If anything else crops up during your pregnancy, talk to your doctor, midwife or specialist: the basic advice is to become as informed about your particular issue as possible and get help from any support group you can find. The internet is always a good place to start, but ask at your hospital for recommendations too.

BED REST | If, for example, the baby looks likely to be born prematurely, you may be put on bed rest. This can range from literally not moving from the bed until the baby is born, to a low-key, temporary rest. **How to cope** Make sure you completely understand the reasons for your bed rest, and the extent of your limitations. Get specific information, such as how long can you stand in the shower everyday? Does this time include dressing? If allowed, sofa-rest may be more manageable (you'll feel more normal, less ill). Ask your doctor.

TIPS FOR BED REST SURVIVAL

- **Create your own space:** have the TV remote control, books, books on tape, drinks, wet wipes, toothbrush, chapstick, phone, pen and paper etc. all within reach.
- **Have something to look at** that will encourage you: the baby's scan picture, for instance.
- **Accept help** (laundry, food, with other children).

- **Network:** one of the best defences against depression is support from others in your circumstance (if you have a laptop it could be your cyberlifeline). Try http://fpb.cwru.edu/Bedrest.
- **Put on real clothes** if allowed to move. You aren't ill, so try and do the little things that will help you remember this.
- **Practise relaxation techniques** and do any doctor-approved stretches to keep your blood flowing.
- **This would be a great time to learn to knit** (yes, really: bizarre as this may seem to the non-knitter), or to address baby announcements, read War and Peace or do your Christmas cards (even in July). If you fancy having a go at knitting try: www.ethknits.co.uk, www.bust.com/knithappens
- **Bed rest may affect your finances.** Let your mortgage/loan officers and credit card companies know. Arrange new payment schedules if necessary that will keep you from lying there worrying.

BLEEDING IN PREGNANCY | Twenty per cent of us have early pregnancy 'blood spotting' or light bleeding. Dark red bleeding with tummy cramps can mean the start of a miscarriage, though not always. Call your GP/midwife if you experience bleeding – even if just for reassurance.

DIABETES | If you are a diabetic you need special care in pregnancy as you need to control your blood sugar carefully (there is an increased risk of miscarriage or complications with the pregnancy if it is poorly controlled). Discuss this with your doctor/midwife early in pregnancy.

GESTATIONAL DIABETES | About three to five per cent of pregnant women develop this kind of diabetes during pregnancy and it can usually be controlled by diet. It goes away afterwards. There may be no symptoms except sugar in your urine. There is an increased risk that you will have a big baby if you develop the condition. Policies on screening for gestational diabetes vary across the country. In many hospitals, your pee will be tested for sugar at your antenatal check-ups. Or you may be screened in your second trimester. Do talk to your midwife/doctor about screening, if you have any of the risk factors, or are worried about this. Risk factors include previous gestational diabetes, family history, a previous big baby, a previous stillbirth, obesity and certain medical conditions.

HIV | All health authorities in the UK have to offer you an HIV screening at your booking-in blood test. Treatment is available if you are HIV positive and there are important steps you can take to minimise the chances of passing on HIV to your baby (during pregnancy, birth and afterwards). Your doctor or midwife will give you more information and help. Or try the support organisation Positively Women: 020 7713 0444 (www.positivelywomen.org.uk).

INFECTIONS | Colds, flu and general tummy bugs will not harm the baby. Catching rubella or chickenpox, however, might. An early blood test at your booking in should assess your rubella immunity. For chickenpox, there are drugs that can reduce the effect of the virus so see your GP immediately if you think you're at risk (i.e. you have never had it, and have been exposed to someone with active chickenpox).

PRE-ECLAMPSIA | This is high blood pressure in the mother than can harm the baby. Mild pre-eclampsia affects about 10 per cent of pregnancies, but only 2 per cent of pregnancies severely (about three to five mothers in the UK die of it each year). There are no overt symptoms in the early stages but it can be detected by regular antenatal checks on your blood pressure and urine. It is curable only by having the baby, so some babies may have to be delivered – by caesarean – prematurely. You are more at risk if: you have had it before, are pregnant for the first time by a new partner, are over 40, overweight (BMI of 35 or more), suffering from other chronic medical problems, including hypertension, kidney problems, diabetes or are carrying twins or multiples. If you have a family history of pre-eclampsia, have had it before or have waited ten years or more since your last baby you are also at a slightly higher risk. For more information, ask your doctor/midwife or try Action on Pre-Eclampsia (APEC): Helpline: 020 8427 4217 www.apec.org.uk.

Busy woman's look at pregnancy stages

First trimester (1–12 weeks)

YOUR BODY | You may feel tired, nauseated, constipated, bloated, achy (pelvis and breasts). You may notice more vaginal discharge, more prominent veins, crave odd foods and have an acute sense of smell. Sickness usually peaks about Week 8. You may have fainting spells and headaches. Your waistband may feel tight as early as Week 4 (especially if this is not your first pregnancy, you may look five months pregnant at three months if you've stretched before). Your breasts may tingle, ache and the nipples may get darker and bigger. For most women, sickness abates around Week 12. You may be disconcerted that you 'just look fat', not pregnant. This won't last.

YOUR EMOTIONS | Mood swings can shock you and your partner but should level out around the end of the trimester. Erratic feelings are common: elation, anxiety, hope, panic, ambivalence, fear of miscarriage or gaining weight, depression. As you approach your second trimester your hormones calm down and you should think more clearly. First trimester may seem to drag on but enjoy the feel of a non-elasticated waistband while you can.

BIRTH PREPARATION | Think about your carers: change your GP if you are not happy with him/her, look at what options are available for antenatal care/birth in your area (see Chapter 5: Your Options). If you are booking an independent midwife, you can see her throughout all antenatal checks etc., so do this now. Otherwise, it is really too early to be obsessing on the birth itself. If you feel scared of the birth, write down all the things you fear: you'll deal with these later.

EXPERIENCED MOTHERS ADVISE | Give yourself a break. Go to bed at 7pm if you want to. Don't be afraid to whinge or cry. Take time off work if you need to. Let yourself be pampered (or pamper yourself if no one will do it for you).

YOUR BABY | **Month 1** The size of a little grain of rice. It's developing a spinal cord, nervous system, gastrointestinal system and heart and lungs. Your placenta is forming and creating the umbilical cord. You may spot a heartbeat on an ultrasound, but it could be too soon even for this. **Month 2** Less than one inch long. Her face is forming with tiny eyes, ears, mouth and tooth buds. Her arms and legs are moving (you won't feel them yet). Her brain is forming and you can see her heartbeat on a scan. **Month 3** Three inches long and 1 oz, with wiggling fingers and toes and even tiny fingerprints. She can even pee. Unbelievably, scans can show smiles, frowns, swallows and sucking.

Second trimester (13–25 weeks)

YOUR BODY | Risk of miscarriage drops considerably, nausea usually lessens and you may be lucky enough to get an energy surge. Abdominal pains and twinges (your ligaments are stretching), tender breasts, heartburn, bleeding gums, cramps, a dark line down middle of belly (linea negra), food cravings, nasal congestion, leg cramps, occasional nosebleeds and constipation are all normal. If this is not your first pregnancy you may feel the baby move as early as the start of the trimester.

YOUR EMOTIONS | Placenta Brain starts creeping in: forgetfulness and disorganization are common, as are creativity and insanely vivid dreams. Your belly should finally start looking like a pregnancy not a surfeit of pies. Start talking to your partner about how a baby might affect your relationship, budget, lifestyle: big issues need to be dealt with. Also talk about how your new girth is affecting your sex life (many men can be scared of hurting the baby and need reassurance).

BIRTH PREPARATION | Book maternity leave. Start to focus on your feelings about the birth, beginning to resolve past birth experiences if this isn't your first; work out what preconceptions you have about birth, from family, friends, media images. Read Chapter 5 carefully: visit your hospital and other birth-place options in your area. Consider hiring a doula (see Chapter 9). By end of trimester: register for childbirth classes.

EXPERIENCED MOTHERS ADVISE | Wear tight clothes to show off your belly (tents will just make you look fat). Hide bathroom scales. Take advantage of energy if you have it. Start dealing with emotional issues around childbirth: it can be a long haul.

YOUR BABY | **Month 4** About five inches long and 4 oz, strong heartbeat, thin transparent skin, soft hair over body. Little finger- and toenails are forming and he's moving well in an increasing amount of amniotic fluid. **Month 5** Ten to 12 inches, with hair, eyelashes, eyebrows and even the occasional hiccup. He can hear your voice and you will probably start feeling him move (about 18–22 weeks). A scan around 20 weeks can tell you the baby's sex. **Month 6** Eleven to 14 inches, about 1lb, his eyes are open. Pruny skin covered in 'vernix'. Now looks like a small, very real baby. Ten to 20 per cent of babies if born now will survive.

Third trimester (26–40 weeks)

YOUR BODY | Interrupted sleep, nasal congestion, shortness of breath, heartburn, itchy skin (it's stretching), stretchmarks, abdominal aches, backache, varicose veins, feeling hotter, bleeding gums, swollen ankles and feet and haemorrhoids: it's a laugh a minute. Then again you may feel on top of the world. 'Braxton hicks' contractions can start now (a tightening feeling in belly: just practice contractions that are not labour). Your sex drive may evaporate or accelerate. Incontinence and frequent peeing are common. Do your pelvic floor exercises (see page 30).

YOUR EMOTIONS | Anxiety about birth is normal. But really get on top of your fears. Keep talking to your partner about all of this. You may feel more vulnerable (or, conversely, powerful). You'll probably get increasingly tired. If you have other children, start preparing them now for their sibling's arrival. You may start 'nesting' furiously towards the end and everyone will think you've gone mad.

BIRTH PREPARATION | Start childbirth classes. Start work on your Blooming Birth Plan (Chapter 7). As you near the birth make sure you are happy with your choices (you can still swap – even late in the day), really deal with your fears and worries about birth (get professional help if you are bogged down), and solidify your plans about how you'll cope with pain etc. Make practical plans regarding other children and the birth/work handover/finances. Work on your confidence: you can do it, you **will** cope.

EXPERIENCED WOMEN ADVISE | Celebrate your hugeness: get a photographer to take pics of you or an artist to sketch you, don't try and hide your belly (it's futile and you'll end up looking like Hattie Jacques). Ask people for a seat on the tube or bus (they may not offer but don't suffer in silence). Sort yourself out about the birth and talk to your midwife about all worries. A doula can be invaluable at this stage. Pack hospital bag two weeks early and buy baby clothes/cot/nappies etc. by 38 weeks.

YOUR BABY | **Month 7** Fourteen to 17 inches long, 2–3lbs, she's putting on much needed body fat and her lungs are developing. **Month 8** Sixteen to 18 inches, 4–5lb, she wakes and sleeps, can respond to sounds and knows your voice. Her bones are soft and flexible and she's starting to get into position for birth. **Month 9** About 19 inches and 6+lb, she has less room to kick and wriggle, her vernix covered skin is plumped out, the fine hairs covering her body are almost gone: she's getting ready to be born.

Overdue (41 weeks +)
This affects around 5 per cent of us. See Chapter 5: Your Options for ways to deal with this.

YOUR BODY | You may be feeling knackered and uncomfortable with all the symptoms continuing as before, possibly even more noticeably.

YOUR EMOTIONS | If you've prepared yourself for how common it is to go past the due date, you might be coping well (if slightly nervously or impatiently). If, however, you're getting ten calls a day asking where the baby is, and you were convinced that by now you'd have him in your arms, you may be in despair. Fear of induction is a biggie (see Chapter 5). Know the facts about overdue babies, understand your rights and your choices and induction can be totally manageable.

BIRTH PREPARATION | Keep working on your confidence and relaxation. Rest, and work through lingering worries. Have a good induction plan.

EXPERIENCED WOMEN ADVISE | Sex (go on, force yourself), vigorous uphill walking, acupressure, acupuncture, ensuring all emotions and fears are sorted out, patience and distractions (salon appointments for manicures, pedicures, hair are one strategy to make you feel pampered when you really need it).

YOUR BABY | May be 20 inches long, and around 8lb. Regular checks by your midwife will ensure he's safe and well. You may get some pressure to have an induction. Inform yourself fully before you make any decisions on this one.

Interestingly, blaming your partner may be legitimate at this point: Danish research published in the *British Medical Journal*, November 2003, suggests that a father's genes play a major part in deciding the timing of the birth, and your chance of having a 'prolonged pregnancy'.

Where to go for help:
For fetal development in more detail try *Your Pregnancy Week by Week* by Dr Glade B.
Curtis and Judith Schuler (Da Capo Press, us, 2004)

Antenatal checks and tests

How many visits?

The National Institute of Clinical Excellence (NICE) guidelines say low risk
pregnant women should have an antenatal appointment (with the midwife) at
about ten weeks (to be booked in), then at 16 weeks, then 19–21 weeks (for a
scan), then every three weeks until you are 36 weeks pregnant, then every two
weeks until you are 40 weeks pregnant, then weekly until you deliver.

At each visit your urine will be tested for protein (sign of pre-eclampsia) and
sugar (diabetes). Your blood is pressure taken. The midwife will feel and measure
your uterus (from the outside!) and check the baby's heartbeat. Use these visits to
get to know the midwife, and talk over your worries/concerns/options generally.

Initial 'booking' visit

At about ten weeks: Your medical history and general health: weight, height,
heart, lungs. Test for sugar and protein in urine. Blood pressure. First blood test
(see below).

Ultrasound scans

These are the most common scans, though they are not offered by every hospital:

- **Dating:** 8–12 weeks. To assess when baby due.

- **Nuchal fold:** 11–13 weeks. Looks at thickness at back of baby's neck. Gives a
  'risk' of Down's syndrome, from which you can decide if you want to take
  further tests (see below). About 80 per cent of Down's babies are detected in
  this way.

- **Anomaly scan:** 19–21 weeks. To assess baby's overall development. Looks
  specifically at the development of the palate, brain, spine, bladder, kidneys
  and stomach.

Blood tests

- **First blood test:** taken at booking-in visit at around 8 weeks. Determines
  your blood group and whether you are rhesus negative or positive (can affect
  your body's response to your baby). Also checks for: anaemia (supplements
  may be needed), immunity to rubella (German measles – can damage the baby
  if you catch it in pregnancy), syphilis, hepatitis B, HIV and genetic conditions
  such as sickle cell and thalassaemia. These are inherited blood disorders.

In Britain, sickle cell disorders are found mainly in those of African/Caribbean descent and thalassaemia is most common in people from Mediterranean, Asian and Middle Eastern ancestry.

- **'Triple screen'**: about 16-18 weeks. Screens principally for Down's syndrome and also for spina bifida. Only 65 per cent of these conditions are detected. Do not panic if you get a 'high risk' result (see below).

- **Anaemia:** usually at around 28 and sometimes at 36 weeks too.

Invasive diagnostic tests

These are usually offered, with a local anaesthetic, if other tests show you are at a slightly higher-than-average risk of having a baby with chromosomal abnormalities or neural tube defects.

- **Chorion Villus Sampling** (cvs): | done after 11 weeks. Needle inserted through your abdomen takes a sample of placenta. One to two per cent risk of miscarriage.

- **Amniocentesis:** | done after 15 weeks. Very fine needle inserted through your abdomen takes a sample of amniotic fluid. One per cent risk of miscarriage.

Decoding Results

Many of these tests, with their talk of statistics and probabilities, put the fear of God in you and many hospitals don't offer adequate counselling. **Most women who have 'high risk' results go on to have perfectly healthy babies.** Do not let these tests panic you. If you are at all unclear or confused by any test result ask the hospital if there is anyone who can sit with you and talk over the results. And/or call: **Antenatal Results and Choices (ARC)** 020 7631 0285 www.arc-uk.org.

Where to go for help:
Sickle Cell Society 54 Station Road London NW10 4UA. 020 8961 7795 info@sicklecellsociety.org www.sicklecellsociety.org.
UK Thalassaemia Society 19 The Broadway, Southgate Circus, London, N14 6PH. Freephone advice line: 0800 7311109 www.ukts.org.
Association for Spina Bifida and Hydrocephalus (ASBAH) ASBAH House, 42 Park Road, Peterborough PE1 2UQ. 01733 555988 (9am-5pm) www.asbah.org
Down's Syndrome Association Two babies with Down's syndrome are born every day in the UK. Around one in every 1,000 babies born will have Down's syndrome. Many (but not all) parents will know this, in advance, from screening tests done in pregnancy. Langdon Down Centre, 2a Langdon Park, Teddington TW11 9PS. 0845 230 0372 www.downs-syndrome.org.uk
HIV: Positively Women 347-349 City Road, London EC1V 1LR. Administration tel: 020 7713 0444 (9:30am-5pm Monday to Friday) Helpline staffed by HIV positive women: 020 7713 0222 (10am-4pm Monday to Friday) www.positivelywomen.org.uk.

Resources

Maternity shopping from your desk

FOUR PLACES TO BUY BASICS

Next www.next.co.uk

Mothercare www.mothercare.co.uk

JoJo MamanBebe www.jojomamanbebe.com

Blooming Marvellous www.bloomingmarvellous.co.uk

FOUR PLACES TO FIND A SPECIAL OUTFIT

Isabella Oliver small collection of stylish basics 0870 240 7612
www.isabellaoliver.com

Seraphine designer-y range www.seraphine.com

Small but trendy range of genuinely nice clothes www.serendipity-online.com

Formes expensive but fantastically cut French clothes www.formes.com

MATERNITY BRAS

This website has a great rundown of what to look for, and bras tested.
It's a great place to start:
www.midwivesonline.com/centreofexcellence_breastfeedingbras.htm

Maternity Rights

Department of Trade and Industry regulations You can get leaflets on all
aspects of maternity/paternity pay and rights direct from here. Working Parents
helpline 08457 47 47 47 www.dti.gov.uk/er/workingparents.htm

The Maternity Alliance National charity working to improve rights and
services for pregnant women, new parents and their families. This is absolutely
the best place to go to decode your rights to maternity (and paternity) leave and
pay. The website is particularly helpful if you want to work out what you're
entitled to. Third Floor West, 2-6 Northburgh Street London EC1V 0AY. E-mail:
office@maternityalliance.org.uk. Information Line: 020 7490 7638
www.maternityalliance.org.uk

Further reading

Two good books to start with

Birth and Beyond: Pregnancy, birth, your baby and family – the definitive guide by Yehudi Gordon (Vermilion, UK, 2002). Gordon is obstetrician to the stars – the ones in North London who aren't 'too posh to push' that is. He's into holistic care, and this book is packed with excellent medical stuff as well as some more 'alternative' angles (he'll tell you about homeopathic remedies and yoga poses as well as giving you obstetric facts).

The New Pregnancy and Childbirth by Sheila Kitzinger (Penguin, UK, 1997) Kitzinger's life work has been to empower women about birth: this includes helping you to avoid unnecessary medical interventions.

Solid advice for first timers

Conception, Pregnancy and Birth by Dr Miriam Stoppard (Dorling Kindersley, UK, 2000)

The National Childbirth Trust Complete Book of Pregnancy by Daphne Metland (Thorsons, UK, 2000)

Books about fetal development

From Conception To Birth: A Life Unfolds by Alexander Tsiaras and Barry Werth (Doubleday, US, 2002)

What's Going on in There?: How the Brain and Mind Develop in the First Five Years of Life by Lise Eliot (Bantam, US, 2000)

Online

Mumsnet online chat, information, bonding for mothers-to-be and mothers who've been there www.mumsnet.co.uk

Baby World includes a 'pregnancy complications' section with 'click on your complication' function (!) www.babyworld.co.uk

Baby Centre endless resources on pregnancy, birth and babies including a function that sends you weekly 'updates' on your fetus's development. www.babycentre.co.uk

Glossary

Amenorrhoea absence of menstrual periods

Amniotic fluid the 'bag of waters' that surrounds your baby in the womb. This usually breaks before or during labour, letting the water rush out via your vagina – the 'breaking of the waters'.

Antenatal before the birth

Cervix the neck, or opening, of your womb.

Fundal height The distance between the top part of the uterus (the fundus) and the top of the symphysis pubis (the junction between the pubic bones). Midwife measures this to check that the womb is growing as expected in pregnancy, shrinking as expected afterwards.

Oedema swelling during pregnancy.

Postnatal (or postpartum) the period after the baby is born – usually the first 12 weeks.

Quickening First point at which you recognize the baby's movements in early pregnancy. Can feel like butterflies in your lower abdomen. Or wind.

Trimester three months. Hence pregnancy is divided into 1st, 2nd, 3rd trimesters.

Chapter Two:
Birthing for beginners

'When I think back to Lorelei's birth, I think of it as the time in my life that I was the strongest I've ever been. Contraction after contraction came, and I made it through each one. Each contraction felt like nothing I had ever known, but the feeling of coming through each one was exhilarating.'

SUSAN, 34, MOTHER OF LORELEI (3)

1 **Labour is finite** and at the end of it, you'll have a baby.
2 **In labour you have choices:** you are giving birth at a time when your choices for how, when and where you labour have never been taken more seriously by the medical establishment.
3 **In labour, you will cope:** you bought this book – you are therefore well on the way to working out how to handle giving birth, **whatever happens**.
4 **You can now hire someone to support you in labour:** doulas are specifically trained to give you and your partner unconditional encouragement, information and support in labour – all without resentment or hidden agendas. (See Chapter 9: The Love of a Good Woman.)
5 **In labour, social niceties don't matter:** uniquely, this is a day when demanding drugs and/or pooing in front of strangers will be perceived as neither insane nor illegal, and may even be greeted with genuine excitement and pleasure.
6 **In labour, you can be rude:** you can shout obscenities at your partner (or sister, or mother-in-law) safe in the knowledge that none of them can hold it against you or answer back.

Losing control and why it can be helpful

My experiences of childbirth were so different that it's hard to imagine they involved the same body. From Izzie's caesarean to Sam's vaginal birth and Ted's homebirth, my labours were virtually unrecognizable to me each time. Midwife Jenny Smith likes to remind women that this is because *'there are three of you – you, your partner and your baby – and you're in this together.'* There's a lot you can do to influence this dynamic, but ultimately if your baby decides sometime during labour (or even before) that she's unhappy, there is little you can do but accept it and change your plans accordingly. As Jenny Smith puts it, *'Your baby's brain, and the rest of her life, is more important than your birth plan.'*

Perhaps the first thing to accept then, about childbirth, is that there are certain things you cannot completely control:

- When labour will start
- What position your baby will be in
- Whether you, or your baby, will develop an unforeseen medical complication
- Whether you will need medical intervention or drugs.

Even the most straightforward birth involves an unprecedented relinquishing of bodily control. Unlike most things in life there's no going back if you decide labour has all been a terrible error. You can't stop the contractions because you don't like them, there are no guarantees that your efforts will lead you exactly where you want to go, and there are no meaningful 'standards' by which to measure yourself.

This is worth embracing if you possibly can: *actively* losing control – at least of your conscious, rational brain – can be a **good thing** in childbirth. It allows your body to really get on with giving birth. In the final stages of producing Ted, my third baby, I felt like there was some huge force field coursing through my body, ushering him out of me. I just had to surrender to it. This kind of experience, if you're used to calling the shots, can be unsettling to say the least – and deeply shocking if you're not prepared for it.

This loss of control turns many sorted, empowered women into fatalistic loons when it comes to childbirth. You'll hear women who mastermind multi-million pound deals, fire and hire staff, make momentous professional decisions and run their families like clockwork, tell you that birth is all about 'luck' and there's nothing you can do with the 'cards you're dealt'.

This is not wholly true. Yes, certain **aspects** of birth cannot be controlled. And yes, your options are limited somewhat if your baby really does want to enter the world bottom first; or if you develop pre-eclampsia or some other medical complication. But you can exert a **vast** amount of influence over the hundreds of variables that will make up your so-called 'birth experience'. Your willpower, endurance, courage, confidence and determination can make a huge difference not just to what happens during childbirth, but how you handle the more unforeseen aspects of it. The choices you make – in advance and while giving birth – the fears you master, the facts you learn, will also make an enormous difference to the outcome. We've become deeply disempowered about birth and it's time to wake up to this. Instead of thinking 'there's nothing I can do', you should be preparing for childbirth as if it's the expedition of your life. The sum of these preparations is what will make your birth acceptable, bearable – and maybe even fantastic. The birth you want, in short, is one you're coping brilliantly with. And you're more likely to cope brilliantly if you understand the basics about what is happening to you.

Wot no textbook?

The first, perhaps most important, step in preparing to give birth is to understand what childbirth, in its raw state, can really be like. We're going to give you a realistic picture in this chapter of **birth in the real world** – a picture that goes beyond the textbook version of what birth **should be like.** If you want to know more about birth in nice safe clinical stages (and it's a good idea to be well-informed), pick up any one of the medically orientated childbirth books you probably own already (see Further reading, page 82) or see below. Our aim, in this chapter, is to stop you becoming freaked out during labour by helping you to understand what can actually happen when it's going well; your emotions, the smells, sight, feel and occasionally the sheer extremity of the whole endeavour. This chapter, then, will reach the parts that the other books don't touch.

But it's worth getting to grips with the text book facts first. These are the nuts and bolts of birth. Knowing them will help you understand the terms and assumptions that will be used about your body and baby when you are in labour. They'll help you navigate labour when you're in it – providing you understand the other possibilities too.

A WORD ABOUT 'HIGH RISK' PREGNANCIES | There is no formal, or universally accepted, definition of a 'high-risk' pregnancy. At its most general, it means that you or the baby is more likely to become ill or die than usual, or that complications before or after delivery are more likely to occur than usual. Doctors will identify 'risk factors' which roughly fall into these categories:

1   Whether you have a significant medical condition before your pregnancy, such as diabetes
2   Whether you have developed a significant disease during the pregnancy, for example pre-eclampsia
3   Whether there is a problem with the baby, such as growth restriction
4   Whether you have a history of a previous problem with a baby, for example a previous premature labour

They use a scoring system to determine your degree of risk. If you're classified 'high risk', you'll need extra medical attention during pregnancy and birth.

This is not a diagnosis that should be given lightly, or received casually. Nor is it a status given by any past doctor making a prediction about your future or by self-diagnosis. So, if your midwife or doctor mentions the words 'high risk', ask the following questions, and feel free to get a second opinion:

- Define high risk
- Explain why you classify me in this group. What has lead to this?
- Explain what this means to my current pregnancy and my everyday activities?
- How will this affect my birth plan?
- Is there anything I can do to improve my status or to get myself removed from this classification?
- What are the risks to me and my baby in regard to my 'high risk' status during pregnancy, labour and postpartum?

If necessary, get them to write things down for you. It is really important to be totally clear about any 'high risk' label. If you are having twins, or multiples, you may be classified as 'high risk'. This, for many mothers, is demoralising. But there are still choices you can make, and things you can do to have a better birth. Keep reading.

High risk tip:
'High risk' does not necessarily mean you lose all control over this birth. Midwife Jenny Smith believes it's important for medical teams to work with the woman,

when it comes to high risk births: *'One mother I looked after was 45 years old, and pregnant from IVF. She had "white coat hypertension" – in other words, a fear of doctors – and her blood pressure would shoot up when monitored. She also had fibroids, but wanted a normal birth. Following a full check that she did not have pre-eclampsia (a high blood pressure condition that can be fatal for mother or baby), she went on to have a labour in a dimly lit room on the floor with beanbags and mats and delivered on the birthstool. We carefully prepared, with all the equipment ready, in case she should have a haemorrhage. I believe managing high risk is all about being realistic about the risk, thinking individually about every woman, listening to her and discussing her individual potential risks very fully with her before making an appropriate plan for labour that all carers are aware of.'*

LABOUR AT A GLANCE: THE TEXTBOOK VERSION

- **First stage** This stage begins when your cervix starts to open and ends when it is 10 cm or fully dilated. Often begins with a 'bloody show' or 'loss of mucous plug'.
- **Early phase** Also known as 'latent labour', 'pre-labour' and sometimes, rather tactlessly, 'false' labour. It can take one to 12 hours for the cervix to dilate to 3 cm and the beginnings of effacement. Mild contractions begin at 15–20 minutes apart and last 60–90 seconds. Contractions then become more regular, until they are less than five minutes apart.
- **Active phase** The cervix dilates from about 4–10 cm. Contractions become stronger and progress to about three minutes apart, lasting about 45 seconds. Takes one to six hours.
- **Transition phase** The cervix reaches full dilation (or about 9 cm) before there is an urge to push. Contractions happen two to three minutes apart and last about 60 seconds. Takes five minutes to two hours.
- **Second stage** With a fully dilated cervix (10 cm), you start to push the baby out. This phase may last five minutes to an hour (or longer). Contractions may slow to two to five minutes apart and last 60–90 seconds.
- **Third stage** This last stage of childbirth begins once the baby is born and ends with the delivery of the placenta and membranes. Usually happens within 15–30 minutes of the baby's delivery. It is a short stage lasting 15 minutes or less. Contractions are closer together and may be less painful. The placenta separates from the uterine wall and is delivered.

Wot no drugs?

You will not find descriptions of drugs, implements and surgical procedures in this chapter. This is not because we're trying to encourage you to give birth in a field, gnaw through your own umbilical cord and evoke only the goddess Kali for relief. We know (we've been there) that you may need, want, or have to have drugs or interventions at any stage of childbirth. We cover medical interventions, pain relief, and other common eventualities in Chapter 5: Your Options. However, normal birth can frankly feel anything but normal (shifting an 8lb object through your pelvis and vagina is hardly an everyday event after all). Birth can be outrageous and amazing. If you know this in advance you're less likely to lose it when you encounter some of the weirder, less publicised 'stages' of childbirth.

A note to second timers

You may have been there once already but don't think you can get away with skipping this chapter. You may experience different things this time (if you had a difficult first birth, we're here to make sure you will have a better one this time). It's possible you will not need the intervention you had last time, and things may be quicker or slower, or feel utterly different. So read this chapter.

A WORD ABOUT CHILDBIRTH CLASSES | Childbirth classes can be extremely useful, and it's definitely worth enrolling in one if this is your first baby (see different classes in Chapter 5: Your Options, page 179). But be aware that some classes may give you the impression that the birth will follow a pre-arranged, easily identifiable pattern of three distinct 'stages' (see above). Most of us, before giving birth, actually learn little more than what really *ought* to happen on a good day. This, of course, is immensely seductive to your average squeamish worrier. We all want nice, manageable, safe facts to cling to when facing an abyss of bodily lunacy. And once a week, as our bellies swell to alarming proportions, this is exactly what we get. We learn nice round facts about drugs, plugs and pushing. We look at neat diagrams. And if we're lucky we learn some useful relaxation techniques.

'*After I gave birth the first time, I realised my childbirth class had been useless,*' says Saadia, 35, mother of Imaan (4) and Zahra (2 months). 'The birth was nothing like what I'd been taught it should be – I ended up with an emergency caesarean and I was totally shocked by it.' Second time around, Saadia took a very different approach. 'I read tons, I did a prenatal yoga class, built up an honest picture of birth, hired a doula, worked on my emotions and fears, made conscious choices about my care and ended up having faith in my body. Zahra's birth was phenomenal.'

My own experience was a lot like Saadia's. I remember that in my first antenatal classes there seemed to be no doubt in anyone's mind that, around my due date, labour would begin spontaneously. I'd have a 'bloody show' in my knickers, move seamlessly into 'pre-labour' experiencing manageable, erratic, early contractions which would, after a bit, settle into a regular pattern of painful contractions (known as *Stage One*, see page 57 above). I'd then go to hospital with my beanbag and CD player. My cervix would proceed to dilate at 1 cm per hour. My waters, at some point (probably early on), would break and labour would speed up. I might choose analgesia. And after a tricky period of 'transition' (during which I might – good Lord – swear and be sick), I would push my baby out of my vagina (*Stage Two*), preferably standing and making grunting noises, possibly sustaining a tear to the perineum (the skin between your vagina and anus). I would then, about 20 minutes later, push out a placenta, thereby completing *Stage Three*.

What really happened bore little relation to this. No one talked about emergency caesarean in our antenatal class. Half the class, including me, ended up with one. My experience – the 'failure to progress', the drugs, hormone drips, monitors and interventions – is a surprisingly common one for first time mothers. It's really not that normal, first time round, to have a straightforward, nicely timed birth. In Julia's 14 years as a doula, she's only attended a couple of births that followed this neat, regular childbirth-education pattern. So, use your childbirth class as a starting point: follow up issues raised with reading, research and discussions. Your teacher, if she's good, will be able to help you with this.

A WORD ABOUT HOSPITALS | Many of us have never stayed in a hospital before. If we have, chances are it was because something rather unpleasant was happening. Hospitals can smell, look and feel intimidating. Taking a tour of your hospital is a good idea because you do not want the surroundings to panic you when you come in to give birth. On the tour, they will show you the clinical equipment in the labour room. This can be worrying, particularly if you're scared of hospitals. I remember going home from my first hospital tour in tears: I found all the medical paraphernalia deeply scary. I couldn't help but picture myself in the midst of a medical crisis. I'm slightly hysterical about this sort of thing, but even if you're not, it's better to look at the hospital in advance. Being somewhat familiar with your surroundings will help you feel safer, and more confident. (See Chapter 5: Your Options for tips for hospital tours, page 142.)

Labour: the real woman's version

So, you've had the official version of birth. And we hope you will end up with one. But it is equally likely that your labour will have quirks and kinks all of its own. Many of the women we spoke to for this book used words like 'panic' 'excitement', 'confusion', 'fear' or even 'demoralisation' when talking about their first experiences of labour. Most said that much of what they learned in their childbirth classes seemed inadequate on the day. They felt they'd not been 'warned' in advance of how painful, difficult and confusing labour could be, or how it could deviate from the 'safe' pattern they'd memorised. So here goes.

Nesting
This is your inner cavewoman speaking to you: you get a primal urge to make your 'nest' clean, safe and warm for the baby. This usually happens in the last

weeks of the pregnancy, escalating just before you go into labour. It can take many forms but it usually involves you doing something domestic that is completely out of character. Before Izzie, my first baby, was born, I sewed curtains, something I'd now rather die than attempt. A friend of mine who can't cook a boiled egg found herself trying to prepare elaborate meals involving tons of obscure ingredients. *'I'm not into excessive cleaning,'* says midwife Jenny Smith, *'but before Oliver, my first baby, was born, I decided to clean the outdoor step. This took all day and involved a multitude of cleansing preparations and an old type of scrubbing brush. I remember showing my husband the step at 10 p.m. I slept deeply to be woken at 6 a.m. with contractions.'* You may not nest at all. Or you may behave like a deranged Mrs Beeton. If you do, you'll think it's normal. Everyone who knows you will, of course, know you're crazed.

In the beginning: labour kicks off

WHEN TO CALL YOUR MIDWIFE

- You feel firm, fairly regular contractions (e.g. contractions that come three to four minutes apart, lasting about a minute each, over the course of an hour).
- You are leaking fluid from your vagina (with or without contractions).
- You have any vaginal bleeding.
- You have had a bloody show in your knickers (can be pinkish, brown, yellowy-green).
- You feel headachy, dizzy or your vision is blurred.
- You feel burning or stinging when you pee, or feel a frequent urge to pee.
- You feel abdominal pain.
- You have diarrhoea or backache that may come and go.
- You have a slight fever.
- You feel anything unusual to you – any sensations that concern you. Labour comes in different packages, so don't be afraid to call.

'Latent labour'

Your labour may not begin with thunderclaps, a strike-me-down contraction, and the gushing of broken waters. And it may not begin when you think it should. Roughly three out of ten babies come before their due date, and seven out of ten are born after it.

How the earliest bit of labour feels and how long it takes varies greatly from woman to woman and from pregnancy to pregnancy. Your labour may actually have begun days before you realise it. You can be watching a movie, going to the hairdressers, cleaning your loo, and all the while your cervix is slowly opening – without a twinge. If only this pattern went on until it was time to push, you'd have no need for a book like this. But things do hot up – eventually.

VAGINAL CHECK-UPS | Some women ask for a vaginal exam around their 'due date', so that they have something to report. This may not be helpful. First of all, the fewer checks you have the lower your risk of infection, and secondly, the numbers at this stage really don't mean much in an average pregnancy. You can dilate rapidly or slowly no matter when the process begins. Latent labour may take a couple of hours or it may go on – literally – for days. It may be unnoticeable at first, or really quite painful. There are, however, a few signs that indicate some action:

BLOODY SHOW | The 'mucous plug' which blocks your cervix, keeping it sealed, falls out when the cervix starts to stretch. This appears in your knickers (painlessly) as brownish discharge. If you see red, or fresh blood, call your midwife straight away (but do not panic, it may be perfectly fine). Do not, however, assume you're about to be instantly ravaged by contractions if you see your 'show'. Many women have 'a show' up to two or three weeks before they go into labour. For some it's a matter of hours.

WATERS BREAKING | *'When my waters broke with my first baby I was shocked,'* says Sandy, 33, and 5 months pregnant with her second baby, *'I had no idea that one cup or more of clear fluid would pop out of me.'* Your waters may break suddenly to be followed swiftly by contractions and a baby. This can be a surprising (though not painful) moment, particularly if it's earlier than you'd expected: *'Celeste came three weeks early,'* says Mary, mother of Celeste and Nell. *'My waters broke at four in the morning and I felt all this water just gushing and gushing out – I was certainly not prepared for that.'* But the breaking of waters is not the Biblical sign of labour's onset that popular myth implies. Many women's waters break ages before they feel any contractions. *'My waters broke at 11 p.m. and I couldn't sleep all night, out of excitement and fear,'* says Jennie, 28, mother of Poppy, 3. *'I was beside myself when nothing had happened by the morning. Eventually, my labour was induced – 24 hours later.'* About nine out of ten women go into labour naturally within 24–48 hours of their waters breaking. If your waters break and labour doesn't begin, you should call your midwife. The hospital will want to assess you and the baby for any signs of infection if labour doesn't start soon. They'll check whether your waters were clear (i.e. there were no signs of 'meconium' or baby's first poo. This makes the waters look green or brownish and can signal that the baby is in distress). They'll also check the baby's heart rate and whether you have any temperature, and they'll do a vaginal swab. The official government guidelines are that if you are having a healthy pregnancy and are 'at term' (i.e. your waters have not broken prematurely) you can be monitored like this for up to 72 hours (at which point, they will have to induce labour as the risk of infection rises).

For other women, the waters don't break until they are well into established labour. Once in a while babies can even be born with the bag of waters intact.

Word of caution: if you think at any time in pregnancy that fluid is coming out of you (even if it's just a dribble) then call your midwife. It might be a little leaking pee, but it needs to be checked.

IT COULD BE LABOUR IF:

- You have been pregnant for at least 38 weeks
- You have an increased backache or feel pressure in your pelvis or bottom
- Your nesting urge skyrockets
- You have soft poos, or diarrhoea
- You have a bloody show
- Your vaginal discharge changes (more thick and mucous like)
- You feel a manageable, but slightly painful tightening in your abdomen that may not be an intermittent Braxton Hicks contraction
- You are restless and feel fluey or have much pinker cheeks than usual (!).

Real birth tip:

Don't assume you're in labour just because you feel you should be. Sticking rigidly to a preconceived idea about when and how your labour will kick off may be hard to handle, emotionally. Julia had one client, Tia, who insisted (at just 37 weeks) that she was overdue.

'Her doctor had ventured a guess months before that this small-boned woman would deliver early, and so Tia just moved her due date. By the time her real due date came, she was telling everyone she was two weeks overdue. Eventually her somewhat harassed doctor checked her: her cervix was tight and there was no effacement. Tia was absolutely devastated. Days later, her labour gently and normally began but she would not distract herself and went straight to the hospital, soon becoming frantic about her 'failure to progress' (she said this, not her doctor). She relied so much on a perceived timescale for her own labour, that she let it rule her birth.'

WAYS TO HANDLE LATENT LABOUR | Managing latent labour is a key part to managing the birth as a whole. Strangely, though, this crucial stage is often ignored in discussions about childbirth. When you feel the first intermittent contractions, or have a 'show', you might feel a rush of adrenalin, excitement or even fear. If you're overcome with thrills or worries, and have a doula, she'll be a good person to talk to now. Call your midwife, too, so that the maternity ward knows to expect you at some point. She'll ask you a few questions and reassure you about when to come into hospital. Talking things through at this stage can be very calming.

This part of labour is all about **distraction** and **rest**. The last thing most of us should do, on feeling the first few mild, clenching contractions is fling our bags into the car and speed to A & E. But – especially if it's your first baby – it's virtually impossible to say to yourself 'ho, hum my first contraction: I think I'll wax the car'. When my contractions with my first baby started, I had my husband massaging my back in a flash, I took each twinge deeply seriously, switched off all the phones, refused to sleep and paced the house. I was convinced I'd meet my baby very soon (and terrified at what it was going to take to get to meet her). Twenty-four hours later I was still in labour. My back was rubbed raw. My cervix was still at 3 cm.

Of course, it can take a certain lack of imagination to put your feet up with a good book when labour arrives. But this is exactly what you should be doing. Your latent labour could go on for **a very long time**. It's worth preparing yourself for this possibility: *'My first was a long labour with regular painful contractions and no dilation at all for first 30 hours,'* says Astrid, 36, mother of Levi (5) and Lilly (3). *'This was devastating psychologically. I was prepared for a long labour but not for such lack of progress.'* If you lose too much sleep at this stage, you could, if it does turn out to be a long haul (and many first labours are), end up with a sleep deficit of two or three nights. This can make you utterly exhausted when you most need energy (i.e. when you are in hard labour and then have to push that baby out).

One of Julia's clients was scared that if she slept she'd 'miss' this part of her labour. Real, active labour, like a screaming newborn, will WAKE YOU UP. Your real labour contractions will not stop if you lie down or drink too much water (a worry bizarrely common to many first-time birthers). So, take this stage of labour seriously: it is your chance to gather your strength, which you will need as you are going to give birth. Maybe not today, maybe not tomorrow, but soon.....

Early labour tip:
Midwife Kim Kelly has this motto: *'Deny labour until you can't any longer.'*

Proviso: If you have a history of precipitous (i.e. very swift) labour, or some other medical condition that can affect this birth, you will have prepared in advance by going over your latent labour routine with your midwife (see When to call your Midwife, above). And if your contractions start strongly, very painfully, and close together, call your midwife right away. **Trust your instincts, and call your midwife if you think labour is beginning.**

This is how Julia handled her own latent labour:

"I called my midwife who thought I'd have a fast labour this time (I didn't) then called my doula. It was 5 a.m. My family was up and excited – my son stayed home from school and the house became very active. I took a walk alone and by the time I got back, my home was packed: a friend to watch my four year old, my midwife and her assistant, the birth tub woman, the photographer and her equipment and my neighbours. I started to feel like the proverbial watched pot. So I cooked. My contractions were still not strong. Hours passed and I became frustrated. We sent everyone home. I took a nap, woke up and stomped on my treadmill for a bit, took a

long shower, called my mother, went to lunch, and then, despite knowing better,
began to panic that my early labour was taking too long. Having a hysterical sob (to
my midwife on the phone) finally started my (active) labour. I let it all go; the worry
and the expectation. Through those surprisingly strong sobs my active labour quickly
began. Larson was born four hours later.'

YOUR PARTNER AND LATENT LABOUR | Your partner may leap into a whirling
state of anxiety at the first sign that his progeny is on the way. He's been waiting
nine months too. And he's probably worried about you. He may show this in odd
ways. Many men take a sudden interest in mechanics: the camera, the PC, the
camcorder, setting the video to record the big match while you're gone. He may
suddenly need to call a relative or mate, balance his online account or pay some
bills. Julia has attended many births with very long early labours. In one, the
husband sat at the computer the whole time buying and selling stocks. It worked
well for this couple, as he was calm and distracted and not bugging his wife,
who was happy to get on with her side of things.

It is important that your partner eats and rests too so that he can be there
for you over the course of this birth. If you don't need him, and he feels that
organising his fantasy football team is a necessity at this point, it may be for
the best.

TEN WAYS TO HANDLE LATENT LABOUR

1 **Think in terms of your 'birth month' rather than due date**
   (i.e. two weeks, roughly, either side of the due date). This way you will
   not become obsessed when your labour is 'supposed' to start. And
   remember latent labour can go on for days.

2 **Sleep:** you'll need all the sleep you can get so if you can possibly kip,
   do so now.

3 **Distract yourself:** if sleep isn't an option listen to music/walk your
   dog/ bake a cake/watch a movie/make some phone calls/put photos in
   the album/knit/organise your files and try not to think about what's
   ahead: it'll only make you tense.

4 **If you can't stop thinking about it,** talk to your midwife/birth
   partner. Go through your birth plan and your list of fears and what
   you're going to do about them. (See Chapter 4: Fear and Pain, page 126
   and Chapter 7: Expect the Unexpected, page 216).

5 **Practise** your relaxation and visualisation techniques (see Chapter 4,
   page 108).

6 **Refuel:** eat a healthy protein-filled meal, preferably with whole grains
   for sustained energy. Julia recommends quinoa – a grain you can buy in
   health food shops; it's high protein, quick to make and easy on the
   tummy (you can eat it like a salad, with chopped tomato and cucumber,
   and French dressing, or hot, like rice).

7 **Call your female birth partner:** for moral support as well as to give her some warning. (See Chapter 9: The Love of a Good Woman for ways a friend, doula or other female companion can help you in labour.)

8 **Before you phone the world** to tell them you're in labour, consider whether you really want your mother barking orders/threatening to call an ambulance for you or friends calling every few hours to see if the baby's 'out' yet.

9 **Let your partner do his own thing if he wants.** Encourage him to stay calm and distracted, and to eat and rest. Get him to re-read Chapters 8 & 9 of this book to remind him of his role.

10 **If you are obsessively thinking about the birth,** re-read sections of this book that you found the most comforting and relevant.

Getting going: labour by numbers

For most of us labour quickly becomes a numbers game. Rates of dilation, effacement, station, blood pressure, time, body temperature, contraction counts, fetal heart rates and IV infusions may zip around the room while you're trying to have productive contractions. Sometimes these stark facts can be reassuring (10 cm! you're doing brilliantly – you're ready to push). But most of the time, they'll just make you anxious and demoralised (only 5 cm – how will you go on?), not to mention distracted from your 'real' job.

'When I found out I was only 5 cm dilated, after what seemed to me hours of really strong contractions, I started to despair,' says Emily, 34, about her second birth. *'I couldn't believe it as I assumed I'd be at 8 or 9 cm by that time. It really shook me. I went on for another hour, but when I was still only at 7 cm, I kind of lost it, mentally. I now think if I hadn't become so obsessed with how dilated I was and how long it was taking me, I'd have coped much better. I had a fixed idea in my mind of how I should be progressing, and hearing the discouraging numbers dented my confidence.'*

The same can be said for your partner. *'I was reading the electronic fetal monitor print out,'* says James, 29, a first time father. *'I could see the baby's heart rate dipping, and I became obsessed by that print out, watching it spew out of the machine – noting every little deviation in the figures. I almost forgot Kat was there.'* If your partner is doing frantic mental arithmetic, one eye on the machine, he is unlikely to be the fully reassuring presence you need.

When I had my first baby I was hooked up, or so it seemed, to every mechanical device available to modern obstetrics. At any given moment I could probably have told you exactly how many minutes I'd been in labour for and the exact dilation, or lack of it, of my cervix. Midwives and doctors came and went, barking stats, checking and rechecking print outs, monitors, IVs. I felt increasingly inhuman and irrelevant and slowly it dawned on me that I'd never be able to push a baby out like this.

When I was having Sam, my second baby, Julia encouraged me (and my midwives supported this) to approach the whole thing differently. I asked to have as few vaginal exams as possible while in labour. I asked not to be told how dilated my cervix was. I didn't want anything to do with a clock or a watch. I negotiated so that no abstract time restrictions would be placed on how long I could labour for - unless there was a pressing medical reason for them. This allowed me just to get on with giving birth. The whole experience was radically different. The only time I heard a fact was when my midwife told me I was fully dilated and ready to push. Consequently, my confidence that I could give birth to Sam never wavered. The same happened when I gave birth to Ted, my third baby, at home. My midwife Penny knew I didn't want any 'interference'. I had no vaginal exams, no sense of time, or progress, and just got Ted out my way (with Penny monitoring his heart rate frequently, and unobtrusively, the whole time).

When Julia had Larson, this strategy really came into its own. She'd agreed in advance with her midwife, Kim, that they wouldn't 'talk numbers'. After she'd been in hard labour for a few hours, Kim checked her cervix and reassured her that she was progressing well. I noticed a fleeting look of concern on Kim's face as she turned to her notes and Julia was clearly in a lot of pain. I peered at what Kim had written - she was only 5 cm dilated. I had assumed Julia must be almost there (10 cm), and began to worry that she'd never make it through the long hours it would take her to dilate another 5 cm. Over the next 20 minutes, and a few massive contractions, Julia's cervix dilated to 10 cm. Julia says not knowing the numbers was crucial. *'Regardless of my experiences as a doula and my strong belief that labour happens in its own time, I know I would have succumbed to the pressure if I'd known I was only 5 cm at that point. I was in a lot of pain and I would have felt utterly defeated. Instead, I trusted both my midwife and my husband to keep me safe and I was able to labour without my brain undermining me.'*

Progress tip:

Real labours can progress in spurts. Sharon, 28, mother of Joshua (2) and Maria (6 months) says, *'With Maria I'd been in painful labour for several hours, with regular contractions and when I was told I was only 1 to 2 cm dilated I was distraught... I kept labouring but increasingly I felt that my pain wasn't being acknowledged. I couldn't breathe through the contractions anymore. I wanted out. The midwife gave me some pethidene [an injected drug for pain management] to calm me down (I was hyperventilating) then went out to find the doctor. But then I felt I needed to push. She said that was ridiculous as it had only been half an hour since I was 1 to 2 cm but she examined me and could actually see the head. So I pushed and pushed and my baby was born at 10.16 p.m.!!! No extra help, no major tears. My first words this time were "I did it!"'*

Midwife Jenny Smith says, *'It helps to remember that labour progress is multifactorial - it's not just about cervical dilation, it's about contractions building up, the head descending, the cervix thinning.'* You can, then, decide to ditch the maths. This is not something many of us think about – or many midwives are asked to do – but this strategy, laid out in your birth plan and reinforced during labour by your birth partner, can be immensely helpful. A great many experienced doulas encourage their clients to do this. Your midwife may be taken aback when you ask her to do this, but explain your reasoning to her and she should respect your wishes.

EIGHT TIPS FOR A NUMBERS-FREE LABOUR

1 **Do not assume** your labour – or any stage of it – will last for any particular length of time. (A favourite doula adage: *'Prepare for a long labour, hope for a short one'.*)

2 **Cover the clocks** (literally) – at home and in the hospital room.

3 **Ask people not to discuss time with you** during labour – how long you've been at it, how long you may have to go on for.

4 **Eat, drink, pee, sleep when you want** – your body knows best.

5 **Do not accept medical intervention** to speed things up unless there is a good clinical (or personal) reason to do so.

6 **Negotiate about your hospital's imposed time restraints** on the stages of labour unless there is a good clinical reason to stick to them.

7 **Ask the midwife to do as few vaginal exams as possible:** they can be distracting and uncomfortable.

8 **Ask the midwife not to tell you how dilated you are** unless there is a good medical reason to do so.

Vaginal exam coping tip:
No one tells you, but vaginal exams done by the midwife when you are in labour can be painful. If it's a routine check of your progress ask her to wait until you are ready and can catch your breath. Then prepare as if for a big contraction – use whatever was just working for you. Arching your back slightly might relieve the pressure you feel from her fingers, but the best defence is to breathe and get through it. Most midwives will be gentle and as quick as possible.

Now that's what I call real labour
When labour hots up you'll become very serious about your contractions which will probably be longer and more regular than before. This kind of contraction can feel overpowering. Women talk of 'sledgehammer' contractions, 'fierce' ones, feeling pain around their middle, in their back and sometimes up and down their thighs. This sounds scary, but when it is happening, if all is well and you feel safe, your body will somehow be coping. You will soon be unable to talk through this kind of contraction and you'll have to focus on breathing and making noises. Remember, too, that each contraction lasts less than a minute and there are breaks between them for you to 'regroup' mentally. By this time, if you're having

a hospital birth, you are either in your delivery room or on your way there. Your partner may be baffled if you were cracking jokes before, and have now gone silent, concentrated or snappy. (Partners should remember to follow your lead – if you've gone all introverted and they're still jesting, they're not going to be helping you much.)

Another progress tip:
Regular contractions don't happen in every birth, so try not to attach yourself to timing them rigidly. The Signs of Progress list (below) is also a good way to tell how you are doing.

SOME GOOD SIGNS THAT YOUR LABOUR IS PROGRESSING

- Frequent contractions
- Backache
- Deep pelvic pain
- Waters breaking
- More bloody show
- Breathing changes
- Tender belly or back
- Curling toes
- Making animalistic noises
- Perspiration, shaking legs, chattering teeth
- Thirst
- Loss of appetite, nausea, vomiting
- Hiccups/burping
- Intense concentration on contractions
- Not wanting to be touched
- Not wanting to be left alone
- Tiredness
- Asking for medication/help

  Emotional signs:
- Anger/frustration/demoralisation
- Confusion or apprehension
- Surprising lack of modesty
- Obsession with ritual
- General irritability
- Amnesia between contractions
- Restlessness

'Hard' labour is usually shorter than early labour, thank goodness. If you don't have drugs or clocks you may not have any idea of how long it lasts. You may get into a trance-like state, needing weird rituals or objects. This is when you really rely on your birth partner(s) and midwife: they'll help you with positions, find ways with you to keep the labour progressing, and will keep you confident and calm. You might sound odd at this point. During the hardest part of Ted's birth my husband John says I sounded like an old drunkard. I'd be moaning 'Penny, is 'e ok?' and Penny (my midwife) would say 'Yes, he's doing very well. He's fine.' And two minutes later I'd slur, 'Is 'e ok Penny?' Lucky midwives are so patient.

Your waters might break (if they haven't already) during this phase. This can help your labour to progress. This is why sometimes your midwife might want to break your waters for you – 'artificial rupture of membranes' – to help the birth along. You may become irritable or even angry between contractions. *'Many of my clients are totally bitchy here,'* says Julia *'and I'm usually relieved – it's a sign that they are moving to the next part of labour. Most also tear at their clothes and become naked as this part of labour goes on.'* If you're shy about nudity, wear a sports bra. Do not let incidental worries like baring your boobs stand in the way of this birth.

Many women begin to lose touch with what is going on around them during hard labour. This sounds scary for the control freaks among us, but it can be strangely liberating. With Sam, I was extremely concerned not to go to the hospital too soon (as I did in my first labour). It took John nearly two hours to get me from the bathroom in our house to the hospital car park (a five minute car ride away). Julia watched through the hospital window as it took me another 20 minutes to get from the car to the door of the hospital. I arrived on the labour ward in the lift on hands and knees, baying like a cow. If you find this disturbing remember: the midwives, doctors and nurses (and, presumably your husband) have seen it all before. They do not care what parts of your anatomy are showing or what noises you are making.

Hard labour tip:

'Labour hurts,' says Chari, 30, mother of two. 'Why don't women speak realistically about that? My mother said it felt like menstrual cramps – but if that's what her cramps felt like, she should have had a hysterectomy. I had trouble catching my breath; they started with BAM! one on top of the other, and all my natural childbirth plans flew out the window. Labour hurts but it doesn't have to be scary, that's what I tell my friends.'

TEN WAYS TO COPE WITH HARD LABOUR

1 **Move around and change positions often.** You can walk around then stop and lean against someone when the next contraction comes.
2 **Don't lie on your back.** This can slow things up and lead to other interventions.
3 **See each contraction as a separate entity** – not as part of a chain. This can stop you getting too demoralised.
4 **Try every comfort measure** you can, and do what works, while it works.

5 **Relax between contractions:** try not to stay braced for the next one as this can really tire you out.

6 **Drink and pee regularly.** Sometimes just moving to the loo can move things along.

7 **Wear something you are comfortable in** – if you're shy about showing your bottom, wear a longer nightie or robe. Your knickers will be lost at some point. Make your 'outfit' something you don't mind ruining.

8 **Make sure your partner knows you may yell** at him and other people so you can just do it if you feel the need.

9 **Do not be afraid** to make a lot of noise if it helps.

10 **Do not be afraid** to be quiet either, if that helps.

GETTING YOUR HEAD AROUND HARD LABOUR | One of the most important aspects of hard labour is your head. Women in hard labour often say things like 'I can't go on', 'How will I do this?', 'Make it stop'. This may sound a bit scary when you're sitting reading this in the real world. Indeed, the immediate injection of large quantities of narcotics might seem like the obvious answer. This is usually an option. But many women say that they knew they were coping, internally, at the time they said these things and were glad no one gave them the epidural so late in the day. I know that when I was in the peak of labour with Ted, a small part of my logical brain was still up there, calmly narrating events to myself. At one point I heard the noises I was making turn from high pitched squealing to low grunts. I'd been working on this chapter before Ted's birth, and the little logical narrator in me said, 'Right, good – a sign that you're ready to push.' Weird, this split personality thing, but it shows that even when you are in the height of labour, it is possible also to feel you are on top of things.

Most experienced midwives will look on your yells and demands, in the later stages of labour, as excellent signs. But don't panic – any request for drugs at this stage will not go unheeded; if you are clear about your needs, and have good support, you will end up with what you want. (See Chapters 5 and 9.) **Support** is crucial here. Your midwife and birth partner should have techniques for helping your body and your head get through this part of labour. But you – and your partner – need to know that expressing doubts and despair are **totally normal** and in fact **a good sign** at this stage. Hard labour is hard. But the good thing about it is that your baby is **really** on its way.

YOUR PARTNER AND HARD LABOUR | When your cries meet your partner's high emotions head on it can be a powerful cocktail. He wants you out of pain, and now, finally you're asking to be. There is one crucial thing he needs to know and remember: comfort is essential in the early stages of labour but sometimes pain, towards the end, can turn labour into motherhood. Drugs can actually slow and complicate things, so they're not always your best policy if labour is progressing well (see Chapter 5: Your Options).

Dilated, effaced and ready to push

POOS AND WHY THEY ARE GOOD | Your cervix is now fully dilated (which means it is 10 cm open, ready to have a baby pass through it). Your mood may be dramatic; you could be laughing, sobbing or both. Some women throw up, or start to shake or suddenly need to poo. This is your body's way of getting rid of anything that may hinder the baby's progress. **Poo is progress**. Sometimes moving to the loo helps – it's a place where we are used to pushing and you can totally empty your bladder and bowels before the birth. You may, however, poo without being able to stop yourself. For many women this can be a traumatic thought. Mary, who gave birth in Belgium says, *'I sat on a birthing chair and kept saying "je ne veux pas faire kaka" because for me that would have been so embarrassing. They thought I didn't want the baby to be born, but really it was the idea that I'd crap myself in public!'* You have to get past this one. Pooing happens at some point in virtually every birth. Your midwife will have seen women pooing several times a day, virtually every day of her career. The amount of poo is usually very small, she'll be ready for it, and she'll whisk it away without a second thought. Indeed, uniquely, she'll probably be pleased you've done it: pooing is a fantastic and normal sign that you're finally ready to get that baby out.

'I CAN'T COPE' AND HOW YOU WILL | You are probably tired or restless now, and you may doubt your ability to cope. *'I couldn't believe I still had the baby in there,'* says Sophia, 29, of her first birth. *'I'd been in labour for nearly 36 hours and I was exhausted. I cried for a bit and asked if I needed a caesarean (I didn't). With my second baby, also a long birth, I recognised that "downtime" and used it: I actually fell asleep for 5 or 10 minutes and woke up with some energy to push.'*

This is a fairly common experience – your body may have a natural 'rest'. (Though make no assumptions here either: you may well continue with the normal pattern of contractions with no break.) Take advantage of this 'rest' if you get one: many women panic thinking their labour has stalled and that they're going to need intervention to get the baby out. *'The midwife and her student wouldn't leave me alone, insisting I start pushing, while all I wanted to do was sleep and wait for the urge to push,'* says Clare (28), mother of Siri (2). Your midwife should be monitoring you and the baby closely, but unless there is cause for concern, she should not be pressurising you to push, if your body is saying sleep. Julia attended one birth where the rest period was freakishly long but *'Everything was just fine with Ana and the baby – she peed, ate, sang and laughed. When it came, her pushing stage was relatively short and she had plenty of energy for it, despite a long previous dilating stage.'*

ABNORMAL FEELINGS AND WHY THEY'RE NORMAL | Some women, at this time in labour, feel surprisingly serene. Others feel relieved and suddenly more human. You may start joking with your partner, who will then wonder if you've become delusional, having got used to you incoherent, grumpy or focused. There may be downsides to this renewed lucidity: worries about how you are going to achieve the unthinkable next bit can flood in. You may simultaneously worry that you don't feel normal. You are not normal – a large baby is about to come out of your vagina. There is, and should be, a phenomenal amount of lower pressure on your back and pelvis (though this may – honestly – not feel painful). If you can, at this point, shove aside your worries and rational thought. Focus on the fact that you're about to meet your baby. The only way out is THROUGH. And you can do it.

PUSHING YOUR BABY OUT | Your cervix is fully effaced and dilated. Your body is ready to start active pushing. Many midwives now encourage women to give birth on hands and knees, or squatting – gravity can work in our favour this way.

Loads of us have preconceived ideas about the length of time we'll push for. You may only push once or twice. Then again, it may take you much longer to get the baby out. If your body and baby are coping well, being closely monitored, and you are not obsessed with the clock this might not feel particularly relevant. Sometimes it just takes a while to get the hang of pushing. It is worth checking with your hospital, in advance, whether they have policies about how long you are 'allowed' to push for (see Chapter 5: Your Options, page 143). Most midwives will start to keep track of time when you start active pushing (that is, giving hard pushes during every contraction). The general policy is to let you push like this for about an hour. If you're in a good pushing position, have waited until you get the urge to push before you start pushing, and have got the hang of how to do it, this should be fine. If you are still pushing like this after an hour the midwife will examine you to see how well the baby's head is descending, to check what position the baby is in and to assess how you are both coping. If there are not enough signs of progress, she may suggest that you need some interventions to deliver the baby (see Chapter 5: Your Options, page 164). Though you've grown up hearing comparison jokes about pooing watermelons many women say the pushing part of labour was actually the least painful. It can actually feel empowering or productive to be doing something this active. This isn't to say it won't hurt. But the key thing about this stage is that you're **almost there**.

THE MYSTERIOUS URGE TO PUSH | *'I was told I'd experience an "overwhelming" urge to push,'* says Fay, 29, mother of Mia (4) and Claudie (1). *'I never felt any urge to push whatsoever, with either of my babies. This panicked me the first time. I had to be 'coached' by my midwife the whole way through the second stage.'* Fay's experience is quite common. *'Mostly women who have had a vaginal birth before don't need to be told how to push – they do it automatically,'* says midwife Jenny Smith. *'But first time mothers often need lots of support and encouragement that they are doing well, and upright positions are essential.'*

Pushing can feel like the greatest feat of physical endurance you'll ever encounter. I remember using every single ounce of strength in my entire being to push Sam out. I was aware that I'd never done anything remotely strenuous before this point in my life. Getting a mirror and actually looking at your baby's head appearing as you push may sound like something from a 1970s feminist workshop, but many women say it's surprisingly helpful. It can seem unfeasible to you that your gargantuan efforts will actually make a baby emerge. And it is easy to lose heart if your baby does not pop out straight away. Seeing (or touching) a tuft of wet hair can be a shocking experience – one that helps you realise you're really producing a baby. And – yes – it's genuinely going to come out that way – soon.

This is what pushing may look like if you see it in a mirror: your vulva gently opens with each push and fluids trickle out. Your pubic hair blends in with the hair of your baby. (Many husbands need to have this pointed out to them. They then become very moved to see their baby's hair coming out and disappearing in what can be a hide and seek game.) The smells may be very strong now – acrid and pungent. In a hospital the smells of birth combine with clean, medicinal smells as well.

Pushing tip:
'Ask to use the birth stool if there is one, or sit on the loo at the beginning, when you are learning how to push properly – particularly in a first birth,' says midwife Jenny Smith. 'This helps you to feel the urge to push in the correct place, and can reduce the length of the pushing phase. You can come off the loo once you've got the hang of pushing so there's no worry about your baby being born into it!'

OH, WHAT AN ATMOSPHERE | The room may feel busy as the midwife prepares to 'catch' and care for your baby. If there are any concerns for you or the baby another midwife, or a doctor, will be called in. The bustle can make you lose focus. Many of us, seeing all this action, get scared that something is wrong. In fact, activity, at this point, is normal, and a doctor can be called in as an extra safeguard. Touching your baby's head can help you focus in again. It will feel a bit spongy and slimy.

YOUR PARTNER AND PUSHING | He can see his baby, along with a certain amount of blood and fluid, if he peers down there. If he has read Chapter 8 he should, at this point, not crash to the floor (he'll be hydrated, fed and mentally prepared). You might have planned to video or photograph the actual birth. If your partner is overwhelmed (and he will be) he'll probably forget about things like cameras. If you have another birth partner with you, arrange in advance that it'll be her job to take a photo or two.

A WORD ABOUT THE 'RING OF FIRE' | When Julia asks clients to break down the fear they have about labour, about 40 per cent of the time they point to this – the moment when the baby's head comes out (crowns) and the perineum is stretched to its limit. Just thinking about this moment could bring a non-pregnant woman to her knees. But most of us cope perfectly because it brings the baby. It's not always bad. Julia has an amazing photo of a client laughing as the baby crowns. Having said this, when I gave birth to Sam I do not remember crowning as being particularly amusing: in fact, it was exquisite agony – but it was fleeting and was instantly outclassed by the big baby boy who shot out. This, I have to say, is one of the greatest miracles of motherhood: our ability to forgive and forget. Julia's water birth experience was very different: *'I did not feel the ring of fire at all,'* she says. *'I gave birth under the water, which is known to significantly lessen the pain of this stretching.'*

YOUR PARTNER AND YOUR PERINEUM | Sometimes men find the moment at which the next generation appears through their loved one's holied vagina utterly mind-blowing. If your man removes himself from the room, sits down or sobs, it really is not a sign that he won't be a good father, or that he's abandoning you. Frankly he could be swinging from the rafters in a tutu as your baby crowns and you probably wouldn't bat an eyelid. He's better off outside, gathering his emotions for fatherhood, than he would be screaming, fainting or openly panicking next to you. Men can also become uncharacteristically emotional when their baby emerges. Julia's husband Buckley sobbed so much at their second child's birth that before the cord was cut Kim, the midwife, roused Julia to see if he was OK. *'It's all the emotions of life, in just a few seconds,'* says Buckley. *'It all rushed out of me in sobs of joy and relief.'*

BABY!

Actually producing a real baby can be totally surreal. You've been planning and obsessing about this for months, and here it is. And it was inside you. You grew it. Seeing this large, slippery, funny coloured, funny smelling, actual baby – before it has even taken a breath – can feel overwhelmingly weird.

WHAT IS GOING ON | *'There is a moment, after a birth, when the room may be silent or loud, but the energy shifts,'* says Julia. *'All that fear and anticipation is released and is hanging there in the seconds before the baby cries.'* Julia has had so many clients (men especially) tell her that they thought something was badly wrong at this point. When I watched Julia give birth, I certainly wasn't prepared for this moment. The time before Larson cried – it must have been 30 seconds or less – felt like infinity. *'The whole thing is a disaster,'* I thought lucidly. *'They will never recover from this.'* Larson yowled loudly a moment later: he was fine. Julia remembers this moment differently – the midwife rubbing her son, her sharp voice as she asked her assistant for the bulb to suction the mucous from his nose and mouth. She remembers a fleeting moment of concern, then her baby's voice. At this point, the trance-like hormones of labour can be a real advantage.

Fathers don't have these hormones. Victor, a first time dad, was calm throughout the birth but when his daughter Elizabeth emerged, he became certain something was wrong: *'My heart was pounding out of my body. I looked at the midwife, the nurse and then the doula – and saw they were all calm, though excited. I tried to stay calm too. None of the women in the room were even aware of the time before Elizabeth took her first breath but for me it felt like forever.'*

Most babies just need a rub from a towel. They aren't hung upside down, or smacked on the bottom, like they once were (thank God). Some babies may need oxygen, or occasionally have the mucous suctioned from their nose and mouth with a bulb syringe. Your baby may be taken off to a different part of the room, after the cord has stopped pulsing and is cut (no, you cannot feel this) so that the midwife can check her over. Some men ask to cut the cord themselves (it feels, apparently, like cutting a piece of chicken and it has no nerves, so don't worry). Even after the birth the placenta gives your baby healthy blood and oxygen for up to 20 minutes – this is why many women decide to ask the midwife not to cut the cord until it has 'stopped pulsing'. Your baby's vital signs will then be checked and she'll be given something called an 'APGAR' score (see below).

BABY CHECK-UPS

1   The midwife checks your baby at the birth and he is given an **APGAR** score out of ten (ten being the optimal number), based on the following:
    - **Activity/muscle tone** (limp/no response to active/taut arms and legs)
    - **Pulse/heart rate** (absent to >100bpm)
    - **Grimace** (first breath response none to sneeze or cough)
    - **Appearance** (colour – white/blue/gray to pink all over)
    - **Respiration** (absent to good/cry at one, five, and sometimes ten minutes)

2   Usually, your baby will also be thoroughly checked by a paediatrician the day after the birth (before you leave the hospital). This check will include:
    - Head and chest circumference
    - Length and weight
    - General appearance (activity, tone, cry)
    - Skin
    - Head and neck
    - Eyes
    - Ear, nose and throat
    - Abdomen
    - Heart
    - Genitals
    - Reflexes
    - Spine and anus
    - Lungs
    - Hips

3 **Vitamin K** The Department of Health recommends that all newborns are given a vitamin K supplement at birth to avoid a rare but serious disorder called vitamin K deficiency bleeding. This disorder happens to about one in 10,000 full-term babies (some die of it). Vitamin K can be given by mouth (three doses) or injection (one injection). Some studies in the 1990s raised concerns about the link between injected vitamin K and childhood cancer but the current scientific consensus is that there is not enough evidence to support this, and that vitamin K is safe. You should be given information and the chance to discuss this with your midwife, before the birth.

Real birth tips: how the baby looks

Head shape *'I thought Sadie was deformed when I first saw her,'* says Kate, 40. *'Her head was such a weird shape.'* Your baby's head may indeed be a strange, alien, 'cone-shape' (like a purplish party hat) because the tiny bones have folded together slightly as she was born. This is normal. In a day or two it'll become more rounded. She will also be covered in a combination of vernix (white, lotion-like substance that covers a baby in the womb), amniotic fluid, possibly meconium (newborn's first poo) and blood. She will smell sweet, a bit sweaty and doughy.

Pigmentation Babies of colour can take a few days to develop their pigmentation. Jaye, a doula, says *'I had a first-time father who flipped-out at the birth, thinking that the baby was not his because of the baby's ashen colour. He began yelling "That's a white baby!" to his distraught Hispanic girlfriend. No one had bothered to let these parents know that their baby may not be brown upon birth, and it took us some time to calm them both down.'*

Mongolian marks These can look like awful bruises, but are pigmentation marks that usually fade as the child grows. *'Both of our boys were born with dark blue and grayish marks (closely resembling light bruising) on their bottoms. We were very sure to have the hospital and their GP record this to protect ourselves (from any accusations of child abuse).'* Michelle, mother of Joey (7) and Justin (4)

A WORD ABOUT MATERNAL BONDING | You may fall instantly in love and be flattened by awe and amazement. Then again, you may not. Many women say they were too exhausted and distanced by the birth itself to feel much at all about this strange being that they'd produced. This means nothing about the sort of mother you'll be. Julia says, *'I didn't bond with my first son Keaton until he was three weeks old. When I first saw him I handed him over to Buckley and threw up...'*

The best place for your baby, once she has been checked, is naked on your naked breast with warm blankets on top. Many childbirth experts say that privacy, dim lights, skin-to-skin contact and calmness are as crucial in this stage as they are during labour, so you can release a cocktail of hormones that will help you bond with your baby. Breastfeeding immediately, if your baby wants this, is certainly a good idea. It does many amazing hormonal things for both of you – and can help your womb to contract and expel the placenta.

BIRTH EMOTIONS

What women feel immediately after giving birth:

- thrilled it's over
- worried that the baby is OK
- surprised at the look, feel, smell, size (big or small) of the baby
- astounded that they have produced a real baby
- relieved they are not split in two
- worried how their partner is coping
- wanting to phone loved ones (yes, this soon!)
- panicking ('What do I do with this baby?!')

After the birth comes the afterbirth

While all this is going on, you will give birth to your placenta, something that seems, at the time, fairly insignificant, given the massive distraction you have just produced. Contractions will stop after birth, but soon (usually within 15–20 minutes) another set of (usually milder) contractions will start to force the placenta out of your womb. If you are bleeding unusually, the midwife may massage your abdomen to hurry this along. This can be painful, and distracting. Some women hand the baby to their partner so they can get on with it. Others find holding, breastfeeding and looking at their new baby takes their mind off it.

A few more pushes from you and the placenta comes out. It is softer and smaller and much squishier than a baby's head, but it can still be painful when it goes past your sore perineum. The midwife will check to make sure the placenta is intact and that none of it is still in your womb (this could cause an infection that would totally screw up your postnatal plans).

The placenta is a complete organ – often surprisingly large (it usually weighs about a pound) – created by you to protect and feed the baby you've just produced. It is the only organ in the human body designed to be disposed of after nine months, and has a surprising range of functions, including communicating with your baby to decide when it's time for labour to start. Most of us hardly give ours a glance, but the placenta gets reverential treatment in many other cultures. Apparently, in New Zealand, the Maori tradition is to decorate a pot or gourd before the baby is born for the 'whenua' (placenta) to be put in after birth. It is then buried in a special place. In Guatemala, some midwives believe that if the cord is cut before the placenta is out of the mother, the placenta will rise into the throat. In India some people bury or burn it as the 'other mother' or 'sibling' of the baby. In Papua New Guinea, if the placenta does not come out, the woman is taken to the sea to bathe while the midwife massages her abdomen. She then lies by a fire to help dry the blood of the birth. Once the placenta is out it is scooped up with a shovel and buried on the beach. Here, the hospital disposes of it (unless you want it for dinner, that is).

STITCHES | You may need to have some stitches to your perineum, vagina or labia. Your midwife will give you a local anaesthetic, by injection, before sewing up any tears that need to be sewn. How hard this is for you will depend on what your tear is like. I think I was actually phoning my mother-in-law when the doctor stitched me up after Sam's birth – the stitching was uncomfortable, but not painful, just a pulling and tugging sensation. After Ted's birth, the tear was more complex. I had to go to hospital and there was a long wait for the doctor to come and sew me up. It was extremely painful. Be prepared to use all your labour coping techniques again if you need to and **if you have any choice in the matter** get stitched up as soon as possible after the birth while you still have endorphins swimming around your system.

FINALLY... | The kind of birth described in this chapter may not happen to you. Yours may well be more complex and medical; far less 'natural'. Some of the above may happen to you, some may not. We have outlined birth this way to prepare you so you know what a 'normal' birth *can* be like: you don't want to be freaked out by normal events. If yours isn't like this **you have not failed and you're by no means alone**. The following chapters will give you strategies and options that will help you to be happy with your experience, whatever course it takes.

* *

FIND OUT MORE

If this is your second or third baby, this information is for you too: you may learn a thing or two you didn't know last time.

What to pack for the hospital

1 A t-shirt you won't mind getting messy
2 2 packs of maxi sanitary pads
3 5–10 pairs of disposable knickers (yes, really – alternatively, some cheap undies from Tesco or old horrid ones that you can throw away)
4 A big, soft robe
5 2 pairs socks
6 Slippers/flip flops for padding around the hospital ward/dealing with communal bathrooms

7   A couple of breastfeeding bras (they may get messy)
8   Moisturiser. Hospitals can get very dry
9   All your toiletries and don't skimp: toothbrush/paste, your favourite soap, shampoo, conditioner, lightly (or un-) scented shower gel, lotion, deodorant, comb/brush, lip balm, hair scrunchie/hair clip, mascara – the works. You'll deserve treating yourself (and you'll look gorgeous in the zillions of photos).
10 Snacks. Pack as if you will be mountain climbing: protein in nuts, natural (no sugar) sports drinks, energy bars and juices, for labour and after. Also don't rely on the hospital to have healthy food (or indeed any food) for you after the birth. Astoundingly, it's possible to have been in labour for days, finally deliver a baby, and find yourself with only a vending machine for sustenance.
11 Glasses/contact lenses. Glasses can be worn in labour, but not contacts
12 Your phone book
13 Two cameras. It's a heartbreaker when one conks out. Take a back-up disposable camera. Check batteries (take extras), film or photo card and that the flash works.
14 Camcorder, batteries and tapes
15 An outfit for going home in, and don't think you'll be your pre-pregnancy size. (Bring your favourite maternity outfit and expect to be in it for a while.)
16 Earplugs (can help in the ward if your partner has the baby and you want to sleep).
17 A tub of antibacterial wipes to wipe the loo (and anything else you might question) at the hospital and reduce your risk of hospital-borne infection.
18 This book.

For labour bring:
1   Lollipops to keep your mouth moist, knitting, books, magazines, crossword puzzles or other busy activity in case you have to be there for early labour, or have a very manageable labour (or a particularly restful epidural).
2   Change of clothes and toiletries for your partner
3   Snacks and drinks as above.
4   Beanbag/cushions/comfort blankets
5   Picture or something to focus on during contractions
6   Anything else you've planned to use in labour e.g. essential oils, massage oil, fan, cooling Evian spray for your face etc.

For your baby:
- At least 4 softest t-shirts or vests (preferably the kind that snaps up the front so you don't have to bother him by putting it over his head), socks and hat.
- At least 4 babygros (he may poo or wee on some)
- Jacket or outer clothes
- Newborn size nappies and wipes (hospitals will often stretch to one nappy for your baby but no more!)

- Blanket (hospitals have these, but you'll need one for journey home)
- CAR SEAT!! (the hospital will not let you leave without one).

Real birth tips:
- Never feel embarrassed to have a lot of luggage. Pack for a week away, expect to be gone maybe two nights. It's never a bad idea to be surrounded by things from home. Your own blanket can cover those awful hospital ones. Take all you might want – even if you use none of it. Better to prepare for a long haul, and then laugh about how much stuff you had.

- In hospital: find the kitchenette, work out where any available food and drink is, blankets and towels etc. Ask, and open every cabinet to see what's there.

- If you want and can afford a private room for after the birth, ask your hospital in advance what is available, the cost and how to sort it out. Most hospitals have fewer rooms than they need, so this may not be an option. But if you can get one, it's worth a lot, as wards can be noisy and exhausting.

- Tell your partner not to bring it all in when you first get to the hospital, in case you are sent home again!

- Pack nice things for yourself too, for after the birth – you'll deserve them.

Emergency delivery

Believe any pregnant woman when she says the baby is coming now! Take her seriously and get into action. Take a look: do you see a baby's head, are fluids trickling/gushing from her vagina? Is she panting? Even if the answer to these is no, if she says the baby is coming, start to do this:

- Stay calm (or fake it really well). Scaring her is going to make things worse.

- Call 999 if you have access to a phone. If you don't, round up neighbours; drivers in the car next to you; the farmer in the next field – you need to know that medical help is on the way.

- Give instructions to everyone. This will comfort the mother and remind you that you aren't alone. If you are alone, take a deep breath. **Women have been giving birth, just like this, for centuries.**

- Gather towels, blankets, clothing while keeping the mother calm and urging her to breathe through her contractions. Tell her not to push, and reassure her that she will be fine.

- Set up a comfortable place for her and a soft place for baby to land. Babies can come fast and are very slippery.

- Wash your hands if possible – but don't leave her all alone while you are doing this.

- Get her to lie on her side – this might slow the labour and will help you catch the baby. Help her to pant not push.

- When the head is out, the baby will turn toward one side and with the next contraction will most likely be pushed out. Keep your hands on the baby.

- Check to see if the umbilical cord is around the baby's neck. If it is, get her to pant (and not push) while you untangle it/lift it out of the way.

- Wipe the baby quickly and put him on his side or stomach on the mother's naked abdomen. She is the warmest place for him. Cover him with clothing, blanket or towel. Keep his face out of the blankets, but keep him warm. Only put him as high on her abdomen as the umbilical cord (still attached to the placenta inside her) allows.

- Wipe away mucous, blood or vernix (looks like body lotion) from the baby's nose and mouth and dry his hair. Rub him quickly on the head, back and chest. He's very unlikely to need extra help beyond this.

- Don't put the baby on his back. It is safest for baby to be on his stomach with his head lower than his body so that he can spit out any mucous and breathe.

Placenta

Don't give a thought to the cord – it's fine where it is and the blood flow stops minutes after birth. Never pull or tug on the cord. The placenta will come soon – within half an hour or so. Get the mother to squat to speed this process. Catch the very slippery placenta in a bowl, blanket, bag or piece of clothing. It's messy, and if you've never seen one you are probably now in shock: you will cope fine. Remind yourself that help is on the way. Set the placenta next to the baby (who is still connected to it). Get the baby to suckle on the mother's breast.

Should the placenta not come within half an hour, stimulate the mother's nipples (causing uterine contraction that will cause expulsion of placenta), get her in a squat or a stand. **Never tug on the cord.**

If it still doesn't come after another half hour, she needs medical help immediately.

What to do if the baby is not breathing
by paediatrician Renée McCulloch

'Many babies look blue or dusky purple at birth. This is normal. Once they start to breathe (or cry) they pink-up. However, sometimes they need some help or stimulation *to encourage them to breathe (or 'wake them up'). You can do this by wrapping the baby in a towel or blanket and gently rubbing her tummy or back, as if drying her. It is extremely important to keep the baby warm because a cold baby uses energy to try to keep itself warm, rather than to breathe.*

Very occasionally the baby might be shocked by the birth. The baby will seem floppy, blue and unresponsive. Often she will just need some gentle stimulation. It can take a good thirty seconds or so for a baby to breathe so don't panic.'

- Wrap the baby up in a warm towel, blanket or anything you have to hand (a pullover or even a t-shirt is better than nothing)
- Rub him briskly
- Call for help
- Lay the baby on his back on a flat surface (i.e. a towel on the floor). Keep his head in the natural position rather than tipping his chin upwards too far: this actually closes the wind pipe in babies (quite different from adults).
- Put your mouth over his nose and mouth. Don't blow hard! He has tiny lungs. Puff gently until you see his chest rise a little. If you can't see the chest rise, gently lift the chin with your thumb a small amount (we call this the 'sniffing position') and try again.
- Do this every three seconds until he breathes on his own or until help comes.

Further reading

Good places to start
Pregnancy, Childbirth and The Newborn, revised and updated: The Complete Guide by Penny Simkin, Janet Whatlley, and Ann Keppler (Meadowbrook Press, US, 2001)

National Childbirth Trust booklet: *Guide to Labour: A Step-by-Step Guide for New Parents* (2002) available from the NCT sales catalogue. www.nctsales.co.uk

Birth and Beyond: Pregnancy, Birth, Your Baby and Family – the Definitive Guide by Dr Yehudi Gordon (Vermilion, UK, 2002)

The Complete Book of Pregnancy and Childbirth by Sheila Kitzinger (Knopf, US, 2004)

Light reading for a first timer
The Rough Guide to Pregnancy and Birth by Kaz Cooke (Rough Guides, UK, 2001)

Interesting reading to explore natural birth further
Ina May's Guide to Childbirth by Ina May Gaskin (Random House, US, 2003)

Birthing from Within: An Extraordinary Guide to Childbirth Preparation by Pam England and Rob Horowitz (Partera Press, US, 1998)

Active Birth: The New Approach to Giving Birth Naturally by Janet Balaskas (Harvard Common Press, US, 1992)

The Gentle Birth Method: The Month-by-month Jeyarani Way Programme by Gowri Motha, Karen Swan Macleod (HarperCollins, UK, 2004)

Online

National Childbirth Trust www.nctpregnancyandbabycare.com. This has good solid information on pregnancy, birth and parenting, plus great resources for finding out more about special issues.

Baby world www.babyworld.co.uk includes birth stories and an ask-an-expert section.

Baby Centre Lots of basic information on birth stages, choices etc. www.babycentre.com

Homebirth Thorough, not bonkers or fanatical: plenty of birth stories and resources and worth browsing, even if you're not having a homebirth, to get a sense of what birth can be like. www.homebirth.org.uk

The Active Birth Centre Pro-natural birth, but worth a read through even if you think you're not 'natural birthy'. www.activebirthcentre.com

Birth videos You can buy DVDs and videos about birth that cover the subject from all angles. You might need to brace yourself to watch the graphic ones, but if you can bear it, do so: it can be genuinely useful to actually SEE women giving birth before you do it. This website contains a selection of good birth resources – you can choose the one that most appeals to you. www.worldofhealth.co.uk/acatalog/Pregnancy_and_Birth.html

Glossary

Braxton Hicks Contractions 'Practice' contractions – a tightening feeling (usually, but not always painless) around the tummy from as early as 20 weeks, getting progressively more noticeable during pregnancy.

Cardiotocograph Measurement of the fetal heart rate and contractions on a machine (electronic fetal monitor or EFM) that is able to provide a paper print out of the information it records.

Cervical ripening Process by which the cervix changes and becomes more susceptible to the effect of contractions. A 'ripe' cervix is more ready for birth.

Cervix the neck, or opening of your womb – the bit that dilates.

Dilation The opening of the cervix (neck of the womb) measured in centimetres. A fingertip dilation is 1 cm and 10 cm is full dilatation, as felt in a vaginal examination. Jenny Smith says, *'A helpful analogy is to think of the baby's head going through a polo neck jumper [your cervix]. It can't get through until the whole head has pushed through the top of the jumper.'*

Effacement Thinning of the cervix in preparation for birth. The thinner the cervix at the start of labour, the more easily it should dilate. First timers tend to efface before the cervix starts to dilate (i.e. before contractions begin). But second time around the cervix usually dilates and effaces at the same time. A vaginal exam will determine where the cervix is between 0 (meaning it has not yet begun to thin) and 100 per cent effacement (meaning it has thinned completely).

Induction of labour This is when you need help to get labour started because it is not starting by itself (see Chapter 5: Your options, page 155).

Macrosomia A large baby (over about 9lb).

Malposition When the baby is head-down, but not in the optimal position for birth.

Malpresentation When the baby's face, brow or shoulder or some other part of it is presenting first. Breech (when the baby is coming feet first) may be included in this category.

Meconium Your baby's first poo. This can' happen before the baby is born, and will be seen when the waters (amniotic fluid) break and come out brownish or green in colour. Sometimes this means the baby is 'in distress' and, if monitoring of the baby's heart rate confirms this, the baby may need to come out more quickly.

Perinatal Events surrounding labour and the first seven days of life.

Postnatal period Strictly, a period of not less than ten and not more than 28 days after the end of labour, during which time it is a statutory obligation for a midwife to attend you and your baby regularly.

Postpartum After the baby is born.

Presentation The position the baby is in, any time from the 3rd trimester onwards.

Station The progress of the baby's head down into the pelvis, as measured in relation to bony landmarks called the 'ischial spines' on either side of your mid-pelvis. Each 'station' is 1 cm. A baby that is just beginning to descend would be at -5 or -4 station. It would then progress during labour to 'engagement' which is 0 station. As the baby starts to come out of your vagina, it moves from 0 to +1 and so on. Crowning of the baby's head (i.e. when it is about to be delivered through your vagina) is +2. Plus or minus tells your midwife where the baby is in its descent.

Uterine involution The process of gradual shrinking of your womb, which starts when labour finishes.

Chapter Three:
Fear and pain

'I know about childbirth. My mum told me.
First, you go into labour and it really hurts
so you hurry up to the hospital. Then
there is some sort of huge emergency and
the baby could die at any minute. Then you
come home and everything is fine.'

ANNA, 15, NO CHILDREN

Fear

SIX USEFUL THINGS TO KNOW ABOUT YOUR BIRTH FEARS

1 Your midwives *want* you to talk about them
2 Virtually all pregnant women have them to some extent
3 Your fears can tell you a lot about how you should prepare for birth
4 Overcoming them can help you have a better birth
5 There are many things you can do that will help you overcome them
6 Your fears are reasonable: pregnant women are incredibly intrepid but giving birth is a big deal

Why is fear relevant?

Apart from the fact that it's turning you into an unreasonable nutcase at 2 a.m., there is a good solid argument for conquering any fears you have about this birth: doing so can really improve your experience.

There are some physiological reasons why fear can affect how your body works in labour. At its most basic, the argument goes like this: fear – particularly when you are in a stressful situation like childbirth – makes your body produce stress hormones (called **catecholamines**) which trigger your body's instinctive 'fight or flight' response. In this state, your muscles (including your womb) tense up. This, in turn, can inhibit labour, slow your contractions and heighten your sensitivity to pain. If, on the other hand, you are relaxed and relatively calm during labour, your body is likely to produce fewer catecholamines and more hormones called **endorphins**. Endorphins are as potent – if not more so – than morphine (you'll hear people claiming authoritatively that endorphins are *five hundred times* stronger than morphine. This kind of thing is clinically hard to prove, but you get the idea). Endorphins are often called the body's 'natural pain killers'. Another hormone you want lots of in labour is **oxytocin**, the so-called 'love hormone' which tells your womb to contract. (Your body produces oxytocin during orgasms and breastfeeding too.)

fear ···> *stress hormones* ···> *fight or flight* ···> *tension* ···> *labour inhibited*

Tip for understanding this:

'Imagine a rabbit in the field trying to decide if it's safe to give birth....Her labour starts off slow and tentative, because, if she hears a fox coming, she needs to be able to run away. Human beings are also capable of stopping early labour if we are anxious and nervous.' Writer and childbirth teacher, Janelle Durham

Recognising where your fears come from, decoding them and doing something about them can help you feel more relaxed when you finally go into labour. This will help you cope with pain, and may also help your labour to progress more smoothly.

THREE HANDY THINGS TO KNOW ABOUT ENDORPHINS

1 **Endorphins are mood elevators:** they not only make you feel less pain, they also make you feel happier about it.
2 **Endorphins hang around for a bit after the birth:** this helps with breastfeeding and recovery, and can give you a real high.
3 **Endorphins have amnesiac qualities:** this is why many women say they don't remember the pain of birth once it's done.

If this is not enough to convince you that giving birth is going to be fun you're not alone. Studies have found that nowadays we're more anxious about labour than ever before. Two psychological studies, 13 years apart, found that the proportion of women who reported feeling 'very worried' about the prospect of pain in labour increased substantially between the two dates. In 1987 9 per cent of first time mothers felt very worried about pain in childbirth. By 2000, this had risen to 26 per cent.[1]

Psychologists and birth experts have many explanations for this (we cover the main ones below). But it certainly looks like our increased fear of giving birth is starting to have an impact on how we do it: nearly twice as many of us are now asking for caesareans as we were ten years ago. Rather than being 'too posh to push' it could be that some of us are 'too scared to push'. (See Chapter 6: Surgical Birth). Of course, you can't put our entire changing experience of childbirth down to heightened fear, but there could well be a link between your fear of birth, and what happens on the day. *'We know from studies that fear can inhibit the progress of labour,'* says psychologist Professor Josephine Green of Leeds University. *'In our studies the more worried a woman was, the more likely it was that she would need an epidural.'* Epidurals are associated with more obstetric interventions (including caesareans) and, says Green, *'not having a "normal" delivery may also be associated with a worse psychological outcome.'* In other words, you may feel more upset by the birth afterwards, and, possibly, feel more worried about doing it next time too.

> **Where to go for help:**
> **The Active Birth Centre website** has information on creating a 'hormone-enhancing environment' for birth.
> www.activebirthcentre.com

How important it is to overcome your fear

In a nutshell, the available evidence suggests that **more fear is linked to more interventions which are linked to less satisfaction with the birth.** In other words, don't ignore your fears, however obvious they seem. *'It is vital to address your fears,'* agrees midwife Jenny Smith. *'Your midwife can help you work through* *your specific worries about the birth – whatever they are – or refer you to a counselor if you need it. '*

Many of us don't properly discuss our worries about giving birth with our midwives, either because we think they 'go without saying' or because we don't want to bother her or take up too much of her time. This is a mistake. *'Any good health professional in this situation will want to know how you feel,'* says Jenny Smith. *'We are service providers – the more you can communicate with us, the better the outcome will be. In the end, if you don't discuss your fears with us the only person who will really suffer is you.'* If you're still feeling shy, you'll be glad to know that studies reinforce the importance of getting help. One study[2] of women requesting caesareans out of fear showed that if they got psychological help with their anxiety during pregnancy more than half (62 per cent) withdrew their request and had normal vaginal deliveries.

In this chapter, we're going to give you some practical ways to get your head in the right place for this birth. We'll help you work out what your fears are, where they come from and what you are going to do about them.

Why are we scared?

First of all, there are degrees of fear. There is a medical name for extreme fear of childbirth: 'tokophobia'. This level of 'morbid' anxiety requires treatment from a psychologist who understands the condition. Tokophobia can be so extreme that some women, who long for children, actually stop themselves getting pregnant because they are so scared of what it would be like to give birth. We're assuming here that your fear levels are not all-out terror (you were, after all, brave enough to get pregnant). But if they are preoccupying you, discuss them with your midwife or doctor and ask for a referral to a counsellor who knows about fear in childbirth.

Tokophobic or not, there's an obviously alarming fact staring you in the face every time you try to bend down and paint your toenails: you're going to have to squeeze a baby out of your vagina. I remember looking down at my humungous belly as Izzie's due date loomed and feeling a surge of genuine panic. It looked *dauntingly* huge. I could not conceive of how I'd possibly get all that out of such a small opening. This may sound silly and obvious, but if such thoughts are crossing your mind then it's worth reminding yourself that much of your belly's enormity comes down to amniotic fluid, blood, a nice layer of fat (yes, sorry), and a large (but *squashy*) placenta. It's not *all* baby. It's also worth reminding yourself that, despite what your logical brain might be saying, your body is perfectly *designed* to do this.

Having said this, the thought of pushing out a seven or eight pounder is still enough to keep many of us up at night. Studies into anxiety and childbirth have found that the following things contribute to our fear:

- a negative mood
- negative stories told by others

- being given alarming information
- having negative past experiences of birth.

Birth has become scary, in part, because it's so 'other' to us nowadays. It feels genuinely alien to our largely controllable, pain-free lives. We associate birth with hospitals, risk, illness and crisis. Few of us have ever witnessed a birth in real life (i.e. not on TV). And all our preparation for birth seems to centre on 'reducing risk'. Medical advances, of course, have their advantages (the decline in infant and maternal mortality springs to mind). But there's no doubt that we are becoming more neurotic and distrustful about giving birth than ever before. This is somewhat ironic of course since childbirth, officially, has never been 'safer'. Part of the blame, here, has to lie on the shoulders of the wicked media.

The wicked media

'I HATE YOU! I HATE YOU!' screamed Salma Hayek during the birth scene in the movie 'Fools Rush In'.

'I CAN'T DO IT!' screamed Geena Davis during the birth scene in the movie 'Angie'.

'GIVE ME DRUGS OR I'LL KILL YOU!!!' screamed the character Chrissy during the birth scene in the movie 'Now and Then'.

'LORDY BE! MISS MELANIE'S GOING TO DIE, AH JUST KNOWS IT! HELP! HELP!' screamed Butterfly McQueen during the famous birth scene in the movie 'Gone with the Wind'.

'*Our media images of birth are not about women's fears of childbirth at all,*' says Rhonda Griffin, a psychotherapist specialising in birth trauma. '*They're almost always written from the male perspective and are in fact portraying men's fear of birth, not women's.*'

Towards the end of my last pregnancy I was watching ER. This is a rash thing for any pregnant woman to do but I thought I'd got away with it as there seemed to be no gruesome birth subplots. But then they chucked in a gratuitous little left-fielder: a perfectly healthy young woman is brought in, 36 weeks pregnant, complaining that she's having mild contractions (why she'd be there, and not at home or in a maternity unit is not explained). Her waters break while she's waiting in the examining room, after just a few Braxton Hicks-type contractions. In real life, the doctors would then check to see if she was dilating, and keep an eye on her to make sure her active labour started within 24 hours. On TV birth is different. A maelstrom of medical panic ensues: two doctors and two or three nurses sprint towards the cubicle, sweeping up equipment, pulling curtains round the bed. 'Don't PUSH!!' yells Dr Lewis, 'I need to examine her!! Abi, get me a fetal monitor!!'

No wonder we think of birth as a crisis.

So called 'reality' TV is almost worse. 'Every woman in labour hates her husband,' said a woman on a recent US talk show. This type of show makes grimly compelling viewing for a pregnant woman (especially one at home, a week or so away from the birth, feet up in front of *Trisha*). These programmes appear to be democratic and representative – they show 'real women' talking about 'real' life. But they're as skewed as the rest. Producers need viewing figures. They don't want dull 'the birth was surprisingly manageable' stories. Their bread and butter is pain and crisis; emotional ruction; husband-wife estrangement. Julia still has a vivid memory of a TV programme she watched seven years ago when pregnant for the first time. *'Oprah did a show on "Women Who Won't Give Birth Again" and I sat glued to it while women told horrific gruesome stories about things that had happened to them – unbelievable things. I couldn't switch off the TV but when it was over, I sobbed for an hour.'* If this is what telly provokes in a woman, a *doula*, who had seen many lovely healthy births in real life, what hope is there for the rest of us?

It's not just about having a bad dream that night. Research in sociology and media studies suggests that TV can affect our perceptions and even our behaviour. And when it comes to violence, bloodshed, trauma and crisis, birth in the media is up there with *Reservoir Dogs*. You might be able to distance yourself from this on a rational level. But you'd be unusual if the doubt did not creep in somewhere.

The simple truth is that most of the images of birth you absorb day after day from the media are **not realistic**. One 1995 study[3] analysed 92 births shown in one year of television. Out of these births, four babies and one mother died and five babies and four mothers experienced life-threatening complications. This morbidity and complications rate is ludicrously out of step with real life. Labour, in these shows, tended to be depicted as a rapid and unpredictable process, with little or no pain relief, that ends in an unexpected way, such as giving birth in a strange place without a medical professional in attendance, or without the intended birth partner. Getting from this perception to a genuine acceptance that birth is mostly safe and normal, isn't usually precipitously fast and is something you will cope with very well if you've prepared properly for it, can be quite a leap of faith.

So how **do** you get past these images? The obvious answer is turn off the TV, don't read the tabloid story about the dead baby, put down that book or magazine, walk out of the movie when she starts tearing her hair out. Of course, you'd have to be pretty obsessed, and dare I say it anal, to block out all negative images of childbirth from your life like this. But do try to recognise what's going on around you, and deal with it consciously.

SIX TIPS FOR MANAGING THE MEDIA

1 **Switch off the TV** if there's a nasty birth on it (get your partner to agree to do it for you if you're frozen in horror – he doesn't need to watch that sort of stuff either).
2 **If you can't switch off,** try and laugh about it.

3 **If you can't laugh,** remind yourself that TV executives need to make money for their Surrey mansions and that studies have shown that TV images of birth are hyped and warped.

4 **Stop reading** any magazine or newspaper article that has anything to do with births going horribly, tragically or freakishly wrong.

5 **If you can't stop, remind yourself** that it is incredibly rare for this to happen. This is why the story is in the paper in the first place. (I say this as a guilty journalist: I have written many articles about disastrous pregnancies and births and almost always sprinkle in 'this is very rare' caveats which most pregnant readers will of course ignore.)

6 **Be sceptical.** Remember that while screaming, shouting, bloodshed and knife-edge life-or-death scenarios make fabulous media fodder, they're not reality for most of us. Portraying a 'realistic' birth – 30 hours of slow, boring contractions and position changes, maybe gas and air or an epidural, followed by a lot of concentrated grunting would make unfeasibly dull telly.

On a brighter note, birth images in the media may be gradually changing. In the *Friends* episode where Rachel is in labour, she lingers for hours in the ward having contractions and watches in growing despair as other women come and go, having had their babies. Long first labours are certainly a reality for many of us. Rachel also – radically for a TV show – moves around, makes noise and keeps a sense of humour during labour (though unlike the rest of us, she continues to look fabulous while she's at it).

Other people's birth stories

It's not just the media that will affect your attitude to birth. Since the day you first lisped 'but mummy, how does the baby get OUT?' your own mother has probably been influencing your preconceptions. If not your mother, then it could be some other influential older woman in your life – an aunt or grandmother perhaps. I remember the wild-eyed look my own mother used to get when I asked her what giving birth was like for her, first time around. Her first experience of childbirth was a 48-hour labour, addled with sleeping drugs given to her by the hospital and ending in forceps (no epidurals in 1964). She thought my brother was dead for several hours after the birth and no one told her otherwise. This, 40 years later (and hardly surprisingly), can still bring a tear to her eye. When I was pregnant the first time she'd say breezy things to me like 'you'll be fine'. She really wanted to reassure me. She told me my sister's 'good' birth story (her second child) as many times as she told me about my brother's birth. She told me that my own birth had been long and 'difficult' but not horrendous. But my brother's birth – the horror story – was the one that stuck. This is not meant to be a critique of our mothers – what else can they do, after all, you did **ask** – but it's worth recognising that your mother (or aunt, or whoever) may be passing down some pretty hard-

'When I knew I was pregnant for the second time,' Julia remembers, 'the first thing I did – before I even told my family I was pregnant – was see a counsellor. We went through the births I'd seen as a doula, and separated them from my life. I had to remember that I'd not made the marriage, nutritional, emotional and hospital choices other women had. In fact, just talking about those births relieved me. Once I got over my initial feelings of shyness it took only two visits to release my fears.'

core memories. These stories will affect, in some way, your idea of birth. It can be immensely helpful, then, to recognise your preconceptions, understand where they come from and do something about them **before** you're in labour.

If you are squeaky clean on this one – if all your family stories are lovely positive ones – then this is fantastic news. These empowering stories are the 'normal' things you should cling to when you are hearing from friends, women in the street, online or in magazines, that childbirth is dangerous and awful. But remember that even the positive stories are not about *you*. No two births are the same, shared gene pool or not.

FOUR STEPS TO SANITY:
HOW TO HANDLE OTHER PEOPLES' BIRTH STORIES

1   Respect the story – she may be exaggerating, but it's not for you to judge.
2   Distance yourself from it. It's not your story – you've made different choices.
3   Work out how this story has affected your attitude to this birth: are you scared of something you weren't before?
4   Break down these fears: write a list. Are they realistic? What can you do to handle each one should it happen?

Family birth stories

If you're adopted, or your mother never said a word about birth to you, you'll have no familial birth stories to get hung up about. This can be an advantage – it is harder to make assumptions about your own genetic incompetence – but it can also be worrying. Betsy, who was adopted as an infant and is now the mother of two says: 'There was always a big nothingness about birth for me. Perhaps being adopted and not hearing many birth stories contributed to this blank feeling, but I possessed nothing less than sheer determination to meet my first biological connection [her daughter Selah] on my terms. I researched endlessly, for both births. I read and asked question after question. My anxiety, I think, was far greater than it would have been if I had had something genetic to go on.'

Coming to terms with your blank sheet – what fears or issues it raises for you – can be just as important as dealing with the horror stories.

More specific fears

If you go through the zillions of popular pregnancy books out there you'll find that hardly any discuss fear of childbirth properly. As Mary, a doula from California, puts it: *'What's scarier than fearing something and then feeling like you're the only one?'* **You are not the only one**. Doulas are often privy to women's deepest fears (it's their job, after all, to get this information out of a client and then do something to help her handle it) and any midwife will tell you that pregnant women are capable of worrying pathologically about any aspect of birth.

THE TOP FIVE FEARS

The doulas we interviewed for this book say their clients are most often afraid of:

1 **Not coping with the pain**
2 **Losing control**
3 **Having an emergency caesarean**
4 **Having an episiotomy or bad tear**
5 **Something being wrong with the baby**

Dealing with fear in general

Some health professionals may not be brilliant at dealing with your fears. It is worth preparing yourself for this, and finding alternatives if yours proves unhelpful. Julia experienced this in her first pregnancy.

'I once attended a childbirth class (not run by Kim, my midwife!) aimed at women who wanted a home birth. One night was set aside for what would happen if you have to go to the hospital. A woman in my class left during the film of a very clinical hospital birth. We heard sobs from the hall. Her fear of childbirth was huge. Our midwife/childbirth teacher went to the hall with her, calmed her, helped her to her car and returned to us – pale faces and freaking out now ourselves. She then said NOTHING *to us. Nothing about fear of labour. Nothing about why it was good/bad that this woman had broken down. Not even just a question about how we were all feeling about labour. We just never saw that woman again. If this midwife didn't know or didn't want to deal with our fears, how were we supposed to?'*

SIX GOOD WAYS TO COMBAT YOUR FEARS

1 **Talk to your midwife or doctor**. If they are not listening, talk to them about your frustration, or switch to a different one.
2 **Join a good childbirth class:** one that suits your frame of mind, whether it's an antenatal yoga class, the NCT or your hospital classes. You need to be able to talk to the teacher, and the other women in the group. The teacher needs to be someone who will listen to you, take your

fears and concerns seriously, and help you with them. She should be well-informed about birth options and birth in general.

3 **Learn relaxation and visualisation techniques** and take them seriously.

4 **Practise** these religiously while pregnant so that you can also use them without thinking when you need to be most calm: in labour.

5 **Try alternative therapies.** Even if you think you're a sceptic, you may be surprised how good things like acupuncture or reflexology are at calming you.

6 **Investigate having a female birth partner as well as the baby's dad at the birth:** a doula's job is to help minimise both your fear and your pain and an experienced woman friend or relative can really help with this too. See *Chapter 9: The Love of a Good Woman* for how.

Pain

SIX REASSURING THINGS ABOUT LABOUR PAIN

- **It is finite**: once your baby is born, it ends.
- **It is a productive, healthy pain.** It does not (necessarily) signal that something is wrong.
- **It usually comes and goes**: there are normally pain free bits between contractions.
- **If you are safe and relatively calm in labour,** your body will produce 'endorphins' and other hormones to manage the pain.
- **Pain relief in labour doesn't necessarily mean drugs**: it can mean tons of things before it means intervention or medication.
- **Drugs are an option:** modern obstetrics offer a range of pain-relieving drugs: if you know your options you can choose to use them if you need them.

Most of us are, to varying degrees, anxious about pain. But few of us know that labour pain can actually help labour to progress. *'The cervical nerves, pelvic floor muscles and vagina transmit a stretching signal with the pain. That then tells the pituitary to produce more oxytocin, which in turn kicks-up the labour's intensity, helping the cervix to dilate and giving that blessed urge to push,'* explains midwife Kim Kelly. Labour pain is not, then, as women were told until as late as the 1940s, merely a punishment for our natural sinfulness.

This may not stop the prospect of pain being scary. The most difficult thing about labour pain, for first timers, is probably that it's unknown. Nobody can tell you how you will experience pain because every one of us feels it differently. *'The pain of birth is like a huge wave,'* says Adrianne, 40, mother of three. *'It knocks you down while you're in it, but, like a wave, it passes. It's finite. Knowing this, while you are in labour, can make contractions do-able.'* This is certainly true of a 'normal' labour, but sometimes labour may not be 'do-able' at all. Your mindset, body, baby, surroundings – everything – will influence how the contractions feel to you. But most women would probably say that labour pain is like nothing they've ever encountered.

My own experience of unmedicated birth was that the pain was always manageable, though sometimes extreme. I'm not a masochist and in every day life I am utterly lily-livered about any physical discomfort. I would certainly have had an epidural if I'd needed one. But I never thought that I would die and I never panicked. Labour hurt but my entire body and soul was somehow focused on coping with it. It felt a bit like surrendering to something far bigger than me. (I used relaxation, breathing, movement and solitude, the room was dark and quiet, I felt safe and both times had fantastic professional and emotional support.) I was lucky enough to have no complications and in these conditions, my body got on with giving birth, and it felt triumphant.

Julia felt pain very differently in her unmedicated birth. This shows how unique and contradictory labour pain can be:

'My labour with Larson, my second baby, went perfectly. Except for one thing: I knew I was not going to live through the pain. At one point I was moved out of the tub so my progress could be checked. As I lay there on my own couch I had a very calm thought about my impending death. I thought about how my husband would raise our sons in this house, and how hard that would be with the memory of me in every room. I then saw my four-year-old's favorite train pulling over me, and, as it did, I dilated from 5 to 10 cm. Recently my mother-in-law remarked on how lucky I was to have such "pain free births". The pain of Larson's birth was exquisite.'

Labour pain doesn't really make sense. And this is, perversely, the point. When people say things like 'you wouldn't have a tooth pulled without pain relief' they're right. You'd have to be bonkers. But this statement has nothing to do with how your body might manage the pain of a straightforward, healthy labour – a pain it was designed to withstand. Now, of course, the reality is that your birth may not be simple. You may want, and need, drugs. You may panic. You may feel you can't cope. Things may become obstetrically complicated. You will need a mechanism to deal with this and that mechanism could well involve hefty doses of analgesia. If you're thinking you're going to breathe the baby out, and the baby happens to be in the wrong position, or your cervix happens not to be dilating, or you end up with some difficult medical interventions, or it just *hurts too much,* you may want drugs. We cover all this (there are always pros and cons to different kinds of medication) in Chapter 5: Your Options.

The crucial thing about pain in labour is that you should – as far as possible – be realistic about it. **Labour hurts**. *'If we downplay labour pain with the idea of protecting those we love from distress, we're actually sending expectant mothers into* a realm that they have no means to define, accept, or use to their advantage,' writes Gayle Peterson in *An Easier Childbirth*.[4] For most of us, accepting we might experience pain is a huge challenge. But you will be more likely to cope with pain in labour if you're expecting labour to be painful.

Most of us are not used to pain in our lives. We think of pain as 'bad', 'scary' or 'dangerous'. We hear women's stories of childbirth 'agony' and can't help but conclude that birth (without an instant epidural) must be an appalling ordeal. When I was trying to work out what I was most scared of before my second birth, I was surprised to find that it wasn't the thought of another caesarean that worried me most, or even the thought of my caesarean scar rupturing during the birth (which I knew was incredibly unlikely); it was the notion that I would have to pass through some 'dark continent' of agony in order to produce my baby. I just didn't know how I would survive this unknown, horrendous place. I'd only made it to 3 or 4cm with my first labour and that had been very painful indeed. The notion of what **real labour pain** could possibly mean filled me with dread. I eventually liberated myself from this by realising that if I wasn't coping I'd just have drugs and accept any side-effects as part of this informed decision. Labour pain, then, is something about which you have to keep a certain perspective: you're living in the 21st century and you don't need to martyr yourself in the name of any childbirth goal.

'First time around I'd got myself into such a positive mind frame about birth,' says Beverley, 37, mother of three, 'that I genuinely thought it was hardly going to hurt if I just did my yoga positions and stayed focused. I was horrified by the reality. I ended up with an epidural at 5cm, and a forceps birth. The second time I was much more prepared for how hard it might be. I'd done much more research about how to handle contractions, and I had a very supportive and helpful midwife. This made me far more able to handle the pain. I could cope with it mentally in a way I couldn't the first time.'

How fear affects pain

Many women, particularly first time around, find that labour slows or stops or becomes more painful when they get to hospital. The unfamiliar surroundings and anxiety about what's ahead (even the noises of other women giving birth, which can sound scary to the untrained ear) can all trigger tension. This tension can in turn produce more of those adrenalin type hormones, which can inhibit labour and may stop you coping with the pain so well. In short: now is the time to get on top of your fears.

FOUR MORE THINGS TO REMEMBER ABOUT LABOUR PAIN

1 **Most labours start slowly:** most women are not thrown into instant, unmanageable, constant pain.

2 **Many labours start with low level, intermittent contractions:** this gives you valuable time to practise your pain-coping techniques and cope with the realisation that the birth is beginning.

3 **Most contractions last no more than a minute.**

4 **Many labours continue with the 'contraction – break – contraction' pattern all the way to transition** (See Chapter 2: Birthing for Beginners, page 53), then you get a 'break' with fewer contractions before you push.

Some ways women describe labour pain

As you can see from these responses, we all feel it differently:

'My contractions were an intense clenching feeling round my middle, overwhelming while they were happening, but not what I would describe as painful.' Tina, 38, mother of Michael (1)

'It felt like an acute period pain, a gripping feeling. When my labour was at its peak the gripping felt overwhelming but most of the time it was manageable. The pain when pushing was completely different. Far less onerous. I felt I was controlling it, pushing the baby into the right position to crown. With my first baby, the midwife told me to keep going – that I would feel like I was splitting apart. Funnily enough, this helped – I wasn't scared by the feeling because I knew it was OK.' Sarah, 35, mother of Margaret (18 months) and Thomas (6 weeks)

'I found the pain of early labour the toughest to handle. My labour started very slowly – I had painful, regular contractions for three days with no dilation. On day four I was going out of my mind with boredom, sleeplessness and the relentlessness of the pain. When labour got going I found it easier rather than harder: the pain became intense but I knew it was going somewhere at last.' Lilian, 38, mother of Jacob (4)

'Each contraction felt like nothing I had ever known, but the feeling of coming through each one was exhilarating. I kept visualising a mountain – getting to the peak and down the other side.' Susan, 34, mother of Lorelei (3)

'I remember wanting to curl my toes and thinking "this is what 'toe curling' means". It was an unbearable ache – not a sharp pain, though a short lived one – like someone squeezing your insides, like a really intense period pain. Pushing was a really positive pain, quite productive and when the head crowned it was an intense burning pain, but one that seemed more bearable than the contractions. Despite this, it's incredibly fulfilling – it's the best feeling in the world when the baby is born.' Lucy, 35, mother of Harry (2) and Emma (1)

'It was a gripping feeling round the middle – intense and engrossing, like a highly magnified period cramp with backache – and, with my second baby, pains running down the front of my legs. There was something tingly about this pain, like my nerves were on end. When it came to pushing I thought it wasn't supposed to hurt any more

and was surprised how much it did: the pain was the same kind, but lower, more grinding, and more controlled. I was also surprised that after the baby was out, the contractions continued to get the placenta out: somehow I hadn't anticipated that. They were weaker, but still painful.' Freda, 35, mother of Annaliese (2) and Joshua (3 weeks)

'My pushing stage was extreme; totally instinctive – it felt like my body was literally vomiting out the baby – I had to just give in to it. On one level I was steamrollered by the pain, but on another I was totally rational – feeling really excited that I was going to meet my baby any minute.' Polly, 30, mother of Finn (4 months)

'My first labour was uneventful – gas and air helped. The contractions were squeezing, tight like you can't breathe, but OK. My second was a back labour; it was agony – constant back pain, shooting pains down my legs, no let up… I had an epidural as soon as I could.' Margot, 29, mother of Arnauld (3) and Amelie (5 months)

'Though it was the most extreme pain of my life, I can't say it felt 'bad' exactly, or even really out of control. It's pain for a reason. You know it's OK and you get through it somehow – however you can – and the result is so worth it.' Clara, 30, mother of Rosie (1)

Julia's pain code tip:

Since pain is so subjective in labour, and women are often in a state where they say and do odd things, Julia uses a special 'code' with her clients when it comes to communicating about pain in labour (specifically, the need for pain relief).

'This tactic can be incredibly useful if you are keen to avoid unnecessary interventions, but want to know that if you're not coping, drugs will be forthcoming. My clients pick a word that would not regularly be heard in a delivery room – one client used the word "Pickle". During labour women sometimes ask for medication or an epidural. But these can become general words – words that mean she's asking for help of some kind – not necessarily medication. Not until she uses her code word do we really know she is coming close to her limits. This agreement empowers her to know that:

1   No one is going to withhold medication from her or make her suffer.
2   Nor is anyone going to suggest medication to her when that's not what she is really asking for.
3   We are really listening to her.
4   Medication is an option she has up her sleeve that gives her the strength to face the pain.
5   She knows that when she says the code word, we go into action.

If she says the other words – the words women so often say in labour – then we still listen and talk to her but we take those words to mean she needs general help and comfort measures, not hard core medication!'

A WORD ABOUT PAST SEXUAL ABUSE | For some women past experience of sexual abuse is inseparable from the fear of losing control. Julia has heard countless stories of sexual abuse from the women she has worked with. If this has happened to you, it is worth knowing that your experience could affect – profoundly – how you experience childbirth. As Julia says: '*The women I've worked with often continue to carry feelings of shame, guilt and embarrassment without telling their midwife. Childbirth roars through us with a powerful energy. It is really important to choose caregivers you trust and to tell these people what has happened to you. If you don't you could be setting yourself up for some powerful images to be revisited when you are giving birth.*'

'*We really, really need to know,*' says midwife Jenny Smith, '*about issues like past sexual abuse. They can deeply affect how a woman gives birth. And unless we know, we cannot take the steps necessary to make the experience of childbirth as untraumatic as possible for you.*'

Julia had one client who is a great example of how positive it can be to talk about your past:

'*A week or so before the birth, Patty told me she was raped aged 15 and hadn't mentioned it to the midwife. We talked it over calmly, and eventually she decided to phone her midwife. We then focused on the pain code (mentioned above) and I assured her that no one in her labour room would be expecting this revelation to cause any problems at all – but now that we knew, we would be prepared if it did. She had a ten-hour straightforward birth, with a long pushing stage that the midwife handled very sensitively. She told me later that the pushing stage was the single biggest surprise of her life: we talk about it as being so painful, but for her, it was her chance to reclaim her body, revisit its power and heal herself in a very poignant way. Patty did two things very right: she had counselling before she became pregnant. And she told those that would be caring for her in labour. When the time came, she felt safe and protected and so she was able to separate the experience of giving birth from her past rape. I have worked with young girls who did not have the advantages of counselling and time that Patty did. (These are young girls who have been raped, and are pregnant as a result.) These are the gut wrenching births – they have no time for separation from rape to birth. Patty used her labour as a surprising reclamation of her body. But a woman whose rape was recent, no one should expect her to be empowered or healed so soon. She needs to cope, to be reassured and to be heard. If you have been abused tell your midwife as early in pregnancy as you can.*'

Where to go for help:

Rape Crisis A non-profit organisation that has groups across the UK and Ireland offering support and information. This website has local helpline numbers, but you can look in your local phone book if you can't get online. www.rapecrisis.org.uk

The Rape and Sexual Abuse Support Centre Support and information for women and girls who have been raped or sexually abused, however long ago. Call their local rate helpline 0845 1221 331 (Mondays to Fridays 12 p.m.–2.30 p.m., 7 p.m.–9.30 p.m., weekends and bank holidays 2.30 p.m.–5 p.m.).

NAPAC (The National Association for People Abused in Childhood) provides support no matter how long ago the abuse took place, helping people to take control of their own recovery. Call their free helpline 0800 085 3330 (Mondays to Fridays 9 a.m.–1 p.m.). Also check out their website at www.napac.org.uk.

Further reading:

When Survivors Give Birth: understanding and healing the effects of early sexual abuse on childbearing women by Penny Simkin and Phyllis Klaus (Classic Day Publishing, US, 2004)

Losing control

'The worst thing for me first time was the sense that I had no control whatsoever over my body, or what was being done to it,' says Francoise, 30, mother of Maude (3) and Pierre (1). 'They nominally asked me before they did things, but I had no idea how to make these choices–I was scared, immobilised by the epidural, totally overcome. I felt really violated afterwards.'

Psychological studies have found that a major factor in how we cope with birth is not so much what happens to us, but whether or not we feel consulted and 'in control' of what happens to us. It's not the actual intervention that's a problem. It's how you feel about it. Feeling that things are being done 'to' you, that you don't understand why, and that you are not being respected or consulted, can lead to what psychologists call 'negative psychological outcomes'. These can range from just feeling upset by the birth, to feeling downright traumatised by it.

THINGS YOU CAN DO TO MAXIMISE YOUR FEELINGS OF CONTROL

- **Accept that you cannot hope to have 100 per cent control** over what happens during this birth (though you can influence many aspects of it). (We talk about this in detail in Chapter 7: Expect the Unexpected.)
- Remember that you can **influence your reactions** to what happens, and that this can make a vast difference to your feeling of control.
- Really **inform yourself** about birth so you understand the issues.
- Write an **informed birth plan** (see Chapter 7) so things will not be done 'to' you without your consent.
- Make sure your **birth partner** is fully aware of his/her role in supporting you.

- Consider **hiring a doula** or having some other female birth partner as well as your baby's dad: a big part of her job will be to keep you feeling informed and respected.

Emergency caesarean and other interventions

This is a complicated issue, but not one to fear. If this is something that scares you, don't dismiss it. There is a lot you can do to tackle this worry and to maximise your chances of avoiding an unnecessary caesarean. (We discuss this fully in Chapter 6: Surgical Birth. We also discuss coping with interventions in Chapter 5: Your Options, page 165.)

Fear of episiotomy or tearing

An episiotomy is a surgical cut to your perineum that allows the baby to be delivered quickly. It used to be virtually routine but is far less common nowadays because the thinking is that a tear generally heals better than a cut. Episiotomy is most commonly used when forceps are necessary, or when the baby is showing signs of distress and needs to come out very quickly. In this situation, which is relatively uncommon, you will just want the baby out safely. Again, there are ways to cope during this intervention (see Chapter Five, page 165), and many ways to soothe your perineum when it is healing (see Chapter 10: Frozen Peas and Pyjamas).

WAYS TO AVOID EPISIOTOMY | Put on your birth plan, clearly, that you do not want an episiotomy unless it is a medical necessity (this way, even if one is necessary you will be consulted, and will fully understand the reason). Stay upright and move as much as you can during labour to use gravity to help your baby descend and to maximise the efficiency of your contractions.

TEARING | Many women have minor tears to the perineum when they push the baby out. This sounds awful in advance, but usually the tear happens and then the baby is out, and you're utterly distracted and elated. Tears like these heal quickly and are rarely a problem. More complicated tears do happen. These can be harder to handle but, again, there are things you can do to minimise the chances of this happening to you, and tons of things you can do to cope afterwards.

THINGS YOU CAN DO TO AVOID TEARING

- **Perineal massage:** discuss with your midwife how to massage your perineum in the six to eight weeks before the birth. Studies have found that this can help the vagina and perineum stretch more easily, and tear less, when you are giving birth.[5]
- **Rethink your desire for a fast pushing stage.** In fact, you are more likely to tear in a fast delivery. Longer pushing stages can lead to gentle births.

- **Consider your position while pushing.** You want to use gravity, but you don't want the baby to fly out. Consult your midwife for the best positions to help you avoid episiotomy or tearing (for example, giving birth on all fours).

- **Consider a water birth.** Proven to be gentle on the perineum but do investigate the risks and benefits, see Your Options, page 175.

- **Talk to your midwife** who will explain the ways she can reduce the risk of tears during the birth. A midwife's techniques can include: massaging your perineum during the birth to help ease your baby out; using cold or warm compresses and slight counter pressure to keep the baby from coming too fast; using oil to lubricate and gently stretch your perineum when you are pushing.

Fear that something will be wrong with the baby

This is something virtually all of us worry about at some point during pregnancy, and often during the birth too. It can be a concern even if you have absolutely no reason to suspect anything may be wrong. My first words, on giving birth to Sam, were, *'Has he got Down's?'* I just couldn't believe that the birth had gone so well: something had to be wrong. If you already have had a baby with a birth defect, have been through the trauma of a stillbirth, or have had a baby that has had to go to intensive care, this fear becomes very real, and very pressing.

THINGS YOU CAN DO

- **Talk to your midwife and obstetrician** about your specific fears. Don't be fobbed off by 'don't worry, it won't happen again'. You need more facts than this if you're to stop worrying.

- **If this is not your first baby** understand what factors are different this time and why.

- **Make sure that you are genuinely happy with the choices** you have made for the birth, and with the care you are getting.

- **Investigate other care options** if not.

- **Educate yourself** on anything you can do now to prevent the specific problems you encountered last time. Talk to your midwife/obstetrician about the latest studies and how you can work with them to reduce your risk.

- **Get as much information as you can.** Many birth defects can be detected with antenatal screening tests (many can also be ruled out antenatally, see Chapter One, page 47). But remember that screening can be inaccurate.

- **If you know your baby is at risk of being born with a specific birth defect**, arm yourself with information now. There are support organisations out there for almost every condition you could think of. Contact the one relevant to you, and get specific advice from them about your baby's condition. Then join a support group of parents who have been where you are now. If your hospital does not have information on support groups for your baby's condition (it should) hit the internet.

- **If your screening tests have ruled out most defects**, try and let it go and be grateful. If you can't, and it's obsessing you, get help from a counsellor.

> **Where to go for help:**
> **Birth Defects Foundation**, UK BDF Newlife, BDF Centre, Hemlock Business Park, Hemlock Way, Cannock, Staffordshire WS11 7GF 01543 468888
> www.bdfcharity.co.uk

Some 'mind-body' ways to manage fear and pain

If you're an 'alternative medicine' sceptic, don't skip this section. Remember the documented physiological links between fear, tension and pain. Midwife Jenny Smith encourages her patients to explore all kinds of alternative techniques: '*Many women I work with find alternative therapies, like visualisation, yoga, aromatherapy or hypnobirthing incredibly calming and helpful, both when pregnant and during childbirth.*' Sue Macdonald of the Royal College of Midwives agrees: '*In my experience as a midwife, women who are relaxed during labour do not experience pain in the same way as women who are tense. Techniques like self-hypnosis, relaxation and yoga can be very useful indeed in managing the pain of childbirth.*'

Julia is a trained hypnotherapist, and many of her clients (including me, your average sceptic) have found the techniques she teaches really useful for dealing with both fear and pain. See Find Out More on page 108 for simple self-hypnosis/relaxation methods.

EIGHT ALTERNATIVE THERAPIES THAT MANY WOMEN FIND USEFUL

For the best recommendations of experts working with a pregnant body, start with your midwife. (We have details of how to find practitioners in Chapter 5: Your Options, page 180.)

1 **Acupuncture** There are few clinical trials to 'prove' anything, but many women swear by acupuncture for both pregnancy and labour. Choose a registered, recommended acupuncturist who specialises in working with pregnant women. In some parts of the country you may find an 'acupuncture for childbirth' group. Ask your midwife for a recommendation.

2 **Affirmations** Studies have found that a 'negative attitude' to birth can influence how women feel during the birth (including how we experience pain). If you feel doomed to have a disastrous time of it this may influence how you cope on the day. When I hired Julia, one seemingly mad thing she made me do was stick up little cards around my house saying things like: *'Childbirth is a normal, healthy event'*. I found this a bit embarrassing, but the 'affirmations' gradually started to sink in and after a few months I realised I was actually starting to **believe** that I could have a normal birth which would not be a medical extravaganza. You can also have specific sessions with therapists trained in childbirth issues, during which you hear positive affirmations about the birth. You can listen to positive affirmation birth tapes. Or you can just put up little embarrassing notes on your mirror like I did. (See Find Out More for affirmation techniques, page 108.)

3 **Antenatal yoga** This will teach you breathing and relaxation techniques. It will also, hopefully, give you a sense of what an 'active birth' might be like, and should give you confidence in your body's ability to give birth. As with all of these approaches, it's important to be realistic: yoga can help you whatever kind of birth you have, but no amount of yoga can **guarantee** you an earth-mother experience of childbirth.

4 **Aromatherapy** In some hospitals midwives are actually trained in aromatherapy techniques so this is not as ineffectual as you might think for pain relief and relaxation in labour. Essential oils should be diluted in a light massage oil (almond oil is good as a base). Good oils for labour include: lemon for anti-nausea, lavender for relaxation and peppermint or eucalyptus for energy. Talk to a trained aromatherapist for more ideas.

5 **Homeopathy** Studies are not conclusive on the use of homeopathy in pregnancy and birth but many women (midwives included) believe it can work well for quelling fears or tension as well as inducing labour, keeping labour progressing or soothing pain. See a registered homeopath and check that your midwife is OK about any specific homeopathic remedies you want to take.

6 **Hypnotherapy** The word, for most of us, conjures up zombie-like figures under a hypnotist's control. In fact it's mainly about deep relaxation techniques which can be immensely useful for managing fear, tension and ultimately pain during childbirth. There's a distinction to be made between general hypnotherapy techniques (for instance, deep relaxation methods, positive affirmations and visualisations) and a specific birthing philosophy known as HypnoBirthing®, (see Chapter 5:

Your Options, page 179). Most midwives will tell you that self-hypnosis and relaxation techniques are well worth learning – and practising – in advance. Some hypnotherapists specialise in pregnancy, labour and birth.

7 **Massage** This has obvious relaxation and de-stressing benefits for before, during and after labour, and can be brilliant for pain relief in labour. Find a practitioner experienced in pregnancy massage as someone who does not understand the pregnant body may actually do harm.

8 **Visualisation** This is often part of hypnosis courses and can also be a good relaxation tool (again, try not to balk at the word hypnosis: nobody will make you put your pants on your head in public). Some techniques you can learn using visualisation involve 'dissociating' yourself from your body (i.e. the pain) by imagining going to a safe, lovely, relaxing place in your head. Others involve you picturing your baby's head descending through your pelvis, while you are actually in labour. Again, the biological fear-tension-pain explanation makes perfect sense here. (See below for Julia's *3 Steps* method.)

Three steps to understanding your birth fears
(N.B. *Save these results for writing your birth plan*)

STEP 1: IDENTIFY YOUR FEARS | Make some quiet time for this, get a pen and paper and switch off the phone. It might help to set a timer – then you'll know there's a beginning and end. If this is not your first birth and your last birth was traumatic you might find this exercise too upsetting. If you get distressed, stop. Go back and talk to your midwife about the fears you have left over from that birth.

- **Draw a picture of birth, the way you imagine it** – whatever comes into your head.
- **Is what you've drawn surprising**? If so, why? Write down your answers.
- **What one word** describes your feelings about birth?
- **What are your greatest fears** for this upcoming birth? List these slowly and think about them carefully.

STEP 2: TALK ABOUT IT | Now you need to get comfort and answers. Hopefully this book will arm you with information. But talk to your midwife (and doula if you have one) now, taking your list of fears to your next appointment. Also, talk to your partner about his idea of birth (he can even do this exercise himself).

STEP 3: MOVE ON | Easier said than done but by now you should understand your feelings more. The next thing to do is get practical and start making good choices so that this will be a positive birth. Ask yourself:

- **Do I know ways to prevent my labour fears from happening**? (see Chapter 5: Your Options)
- **Do I know how to cope should they happen despite all my efforts**? (see Chapter 7: Expect the Unexpected)
- **Do I feel comfortable with my midwife's answers** and with her attention to my fears? If not, go back and talk it through again. If you still don't find that she's sympathetic or helpful, or worse still you feel that she's not *listening*, see Chapter 5: Your Options and Chapter 9: The Love of a Good Woman for ways to get the support you need.
- **Where else can I get support or help?** Your childbirth teacher, a doula, specific support groups, counselling – do whatever works for you.

· ·

FIND OUT MORE

Three steps to self-hypnosis (or, how to relax and think positive thoughts about birth)

Step 1 – Start some affirmations

The idea here is that you 're-programme' your own mentality about birth by saying positive things to yourself over and over again, when you are in a 'suggestible' (i.e. relaxed, safe, quiet) state. Studies have shown that a woman's attitude – positive or negative – to birth can be an important factor in how she experiences it. So this really is worth a go. You will feel silly at first, but persist. Your partner, of course, may also laugh at you when he finds you doing this. Try explaining the rationale but if he's still going to chortle away distractingly, just do these affirmations when he's not around.

Start tonight and continue for the next seven days.

1 **Repeat an affirmation** – one that you have decided on for yourself – ten times when you go to bed, just before you are ready to fall asleep. Your affirmation should be positive, simple and believable. Always phrase it in the present tense. For instance:

'I know my body is strong enough to give birth'
'My body knows how to give birth and I will let it'
'Childbirth is a normal, healthy event'

While you are saying it to yourself, imagine – in any way you can – feeling strong, safe and powerful in labour (or whatever matches your suggestion).

2   **Keep count.** Every time you say your affirmation, press down with each finger of your right hand. Then continue with each finger of your left hand until you've completed the affirmation ten times. This is to stop you falling asleep before you're done.

3   **Do it every night.** This may feel silly at first. But do this exercise **every night** without falling asleep until you've completed the repetitions.

The idea is that you establish a habit pattern and 'programme' yourself to think more positively. Gradually, you'll find yourself reacting more positively to your affirmation.

Step 2 - Learn how to relax

After you've practised your affirmations for seven days, you then start learning how to relax. Continue with your affirmations every night before bed, too. But add this:

Twice a day – before breakfast or lunch, say, then once after dinner – you practise relaxing yourself and staying in that relaxed state for two to three minutes, then waking yourself up.

Here's how:
- Sit in a comfortable chair with your back supported
- Focus your attention on a spot opposite you, slightly above eye level
- Take three deep breaths – slowly.
- Hold the third breath in for three full seconds as you count backwards: 3...2...1...
- Close your eyes, exhale and RELAX your body (try quickly scanning all your body parts starting from the top of your head, your face, your neck etc. to make sure the muscles in each are relaxed and limp). Allow yourself to go into a deep rest.
- Stay in this state for about two to three minutes by counting down slowly from 25 to one. It will help if you allow yourself to visualise or imagine each number being written on a blackboard or shown on a computer as you count backward.
- To wake up, count FORWARD from one to three. You should wake up refreshed, alert and energetic.

Step 3 - Relax and read your affirmations

Once you've mastered Step 2 (try doing it for seven days) and are good at getting yourself quickly relaxed, you can move onto this step. Once you start this step, you no longer have to do Step 2.

For this step you need a small card that you can carry with you. Write your affirmation on this card (or go to www.bloomingbirth.net for affirmation cards ready for you to print and use).

- Sit down and choose a spot opposite you, slightly above eye level to focus on. Hold the card in front of the spot and read the affirmation to yourself three times. Allow yourself to visualise actually doing what is written on the card (yes, really see yourself pushing the baby out, or whatever).

- When you've done this, drop the card and take a couple of deep breaths, then a third breath – hold it , close your eyes and count backward from three to one. Exhale, and go deep into your relaxed state (you should, by now, be good at doing this as you've practised it in Step 2).

- At this point, instead of counting backward from 25 to one, like you did before, just sit there and let the affirmation repeat over and over in your sub-conscious mind. At the same time, visualise doing it. You'll find that at times the words start to break up and become fragmented. That's perfectly OK.

- In a few minutes you'll have a feeling it's time to stop and wake up. This rough time limit was set when you established it as a habit in Step 2. At this point you just count forward: 1...2...3... open your eyes and get on with your day, hopefully feeling refreshed and relaxed and terribly confident about this birth.

Affirmation tip:
It can take a couple of weeks, or more, for you to start feeling the affirmations are believable, or having any affect on your mentality.

Relax! Damn you

Two easy relaxation methods
Practise these repeatedly during pregnancy, make them second nature and use them when you're in labour: both between contractions **and** during them – whenever you need a way to let tension go.

BODY SCAN | You can do this alone, but it's easiest to get your partner to read these instructions to you while you do it.

1   **Sit or lie down,** using pillows to get really comfortable.

2   **Be aware of your breathing.** Close your eyes and sink into your pillows, imagining they are sand on a beach or clouds supporting you.

3   **Become aware of the top of your head.** Your partner can put his hands there while gently asking you to release tension in your head (don't question 'how?'-just think it). If you are alone, imagine a light, a colour or some kind of energy moving into your head, gently untying the knots and tensions. Do this for as long as you like (a minute or two is usually enough).

4 **When you are ready, breathe out,** release all the tension that your head was holding. If your partner has his hands firmly on your head, he should now take them off and move on to your neck. Think about releasing the tension there. If any other thoughts come to your head while you're doing this, don't worry that you're doing this all wrong – just tell yourself you'll think about them later and go back to imagining the relaxing colour/energy/light moving through that part of your body.

5 **Carry on 'scanning'** through the different parts of your body slowly, re-programming each tense part and not moving on until you feel some release. Eventually, imagine this de-stressing light or energy moving out through the soles of your feet.

N.B. Pay special attention and time to your shoulders, heart, back, and if you previously had a caesarean give extra time to visualise your scar 'healing'. Of course your scar has healed, but really try and 'feel' or 'believe' that it has indeed healed. Don't neglect your poor perineum and vagina – you wouldn't think it, but it's surprising how tense they can be!

Relaxation tip:
Many pregnant women fall asleep during this process, so don't worry if you nod off. At least it shows you are relaxed.

MEDITATIVE BREATHING | This is used in transcendental meditation but you don't have to be a spiritual guru to benefit. Many antenatal yoga teachers use similar methods to enhance relaxation through controlled breathing.

1 **Choose any calming, comforting word** you like to repeat (Om, Allah, Baby etc.).

2 **Get in a comfortable position** e.g. sitting on cushions, or lying on your side supported by pillows.

3 **Close your eyes and repeat the word** over and over again as you breathe. If it helps, think of breathing the word in, then breathing it out. If any other thoughts come into your head, just move them to one side for later.

Variation: using a simple affirmation and image Do the same meditative breathing exercise using an affirmation and visualising yourself actually doing it (e.g. feeling really powerful while giving birth/having a calm, safe birth etc.). You can also do this exercise while looking at a photo or picture that you love (anything will do). This is a good idea, because you can then take that picture with you to the labour room and focus on it while you are actually in labour: it can be a kind of comforting 'trigger' for your relaxed state.

Further reading

Coping with Labour Pain: A Comprehensive Guide to the Best Ways to Alleviate It by Nicky Wesson (Vermilion, UK, 1999)

Mind over Labor: A Breakthrough Guide to Giving Birth by Carl Jones (Penguin, US, 1988) (includes meditation techniques)

An Easier Childbirth: A Mother's Guide for Birthing Normally by Gayle Peterson (Shadow and Light, US, 1993). Helpful for getting past previous childbirth experiences.

Having a Baby: Mothers Tell Their Stories (A Celebration of the Joys of Childbirth) by Patricia Bernstein (Simon and Schuster Pocket Books, US, 1993)

Childbirth without Fear by Grantly Dick-Read, foreword by Michael Odent (Pinter & Martin, UK, 2004). This classic contains much that is still relevant today.

Resources

British Association for Counselling and Psychotherapy has a 'find a therapist' function on its website www.bacp.co.uk. BACP House, 35–37 Albert Street, Rugby, Warwickshire CV21 2SG 0870 443 5252

Chapter Four:
Second time around

'After my first birth, I vowed I'd never do it
again. At the time, the doctor, midwives and
even my mother said it would be a doddle
next time. Well, next time is now imminent,
and I'm wondering: what if they're wrong
and it's a nightmare again?'

JENNIFER, 33, MOTHER OF HARRY (2) AND EXPECTING
HER SECOND BABY IN TWO WEEKS

TEN POSITIVE FACTS ABOUT SECOND (VAGINAL) BIRTHS

1 You are less likely to need an episiotomy
2 You are less likely to need forceps
3 You are less likely to need ventouse (helping the baby out with a suction cap)
4 You are less likely to have a caesarean (if you did not have one before)
5 Your induction is likely to involve less intervention and to work faster
6 Your cervix is likely to dilate more quickly
7 Your pushing stage is likely to be shorter
8 You are likely to tear less (or not at all)
9 Your age will not necessarily have any impact on how you give birth
10 You are more likely to cope better with the pain (both mentally and physically)

The importance of owning up

Like most women who had a complicated first birth, my biggest fear when facing it all for the second time was a repeat performance of the first. This may sound dramatic since the result of that first birth was Izzie, my beautiful, healthy baby girl and my main goal was, of course, to produce another unscathed infant. But I couldn't help feeling there must be a better way of achieving this – a less emotionally traumatic way that involved fewer scalpels and drugs. The problem was I had no idea what this 'way' could be.

My confidence in my ability to give birth was in tatters. Izzie's birth taught me that my body was an unreliable alien. It did unexpected, threatening, unreasonable things during childbirth. Things that hurt. Things, most importantly, that threatened to hurt the baby it had so brilliantly created during the previous nine months. Childbirth seemed perilous and unpredictable. And I was clearly no good at it.

This is not a good starting point when you know you want another baby. But for many of us these feelings are the reality of birth second time around (or at least, the run up to it). If you are generally a confident individual, used to taking control of your life; if you like plans, objectives and schedules, this feeling can be alarming and unfamiliar, if not downright scary. You may be haunted by the things you think 'went wrong' in your first birth: the epidural that did not work, the emergency caesarean, the unexpected ventouse, the difficult forceps delivery or the early labour that lasted for days. You may be worried that you will have to be induced again. Or that this baby, like the last, will shoot out too fast.

Most women, first time around, are inadequately prepared for the reality of birth and some are left quite shaken by it. Many psychologists now believe that this is a hugely underreported problem. Indeed, according to Dr Stephen Joseph, a psychologist who has researched the psychological effects of childbirth, *'About two to three per cent of women may have clinically significant problems of post traumatic stress after childbirth.'* Symptoms of post traumatic stress disorder (PTSD) after a difficult experience of childbirth include sexual avoidance, birth flashbacks, fear of childbirth and parenting problems. All of this sounds extreme, but the bottom line is that if your first birth was not a joy-filled epiphany, your feelings about this one will be very real.

And you are probably minimising them – to yourself, to your friends, to your midwife, to your family. This is the socially acceptable way to face a second birth. You are supposed to say, 'Oh, I'll be fine this time', despite your silent catalogue of personal evidence to the contrary. There are many reasons for the stiff upper lip approach to second births, each as deluded (and understandable) as the last. In Britain today we are allowed to whine about fame-hungry celebrities, our spin-crazy Government or the shocking lack of talent on the Turner Prize shortlist. But we aren't allowed to complain about things like personal pain, fear or discomfort, particularly not when they are connected to something as obvious as childbirth. We are supposed to be brave, selfless and stoic. We are supposed to face childbirth – and I use this cliché wisely – like a man.

And we all know how in touch men can be with their emotions. Childbirth is the most raw, extreme physical event you will probably ever encounter. It is also one of the most emotional ones (your body, your baby, life, death, agony, ecstasy: birth has it all). Yet you're supposed to knuckle down and get on with it, apparently feeling nothing beyond sweet maternal joy at the safe 'delivery' of another treasured progeny. It's not surprising, then, that many of us fail to discuss how we really feel about the prospect of re-entering the delivery room.

Your friends will tell you not to worry about this birth. And this birth may indeed be better than your last – the facts about second births are certainly in your favour – but there are no guarantees. You can, however, radically alter the way you cope this time. You will cope significantly better with whatever this birth has in store for you if you are first prepared to admit to your feelings and resolve them rather than sweeping them under your Formes maternity dress in the hope that they'll disappear. (We talk about how to handle fear and other powerful emotions in Chapter Three: Fear and Pain).

For many of us, just admitting that we feel crappy about our first birth is a big hurdle. If you are accustomed to success, if your career is stellar, you cook like Nigella and your friends all admire your social panache, you may find it hard to admit that something in your life did not reach a similar level of personal excellence. *'One important step for many women,'* says obstetrician Lucy Chappell *'is to realise that birth is not an exam – you don't pass or fail it.'* Even if you're not a perfectionist, admitting that your first birth floored you, you feel it all went wrong and you are scared it will happen again makes you vulnerable. But your midwife cannot help you resolve your fears or deal with specific issues if you are not prepared to mention them. *'Many women put a huge wall up between their past experience of birth and the next one,'* says midwife Jenny Smith. *'This is not helpful for us. Midwives often don't know the woman's worries; we find out too late to be able to resolve them. It is crucial to tell your midwife what you are really concerned about so that she can actually do something to help you as an individual.* **We need to know!'**

If you want to go into this birth with a deep-seated confidence that it will be better this time, perhaps the best place to start is by understanding the facts. Don't bother trawling through your old childbirth books in search of second birth facts. You might find the odd snippet, but you are more likely to emerge cross - they told you all that first time, and look what happened - than reassured. In the following pages you will find data and explanations that should answer any general questions you have about second births. If you have any specific medical condition, you should then do some follow-on research (start by asking your obstetrician about it).

Pregnant again

In her book about having a second child, Rebecca Abrams writes, *'As far as sympathy and support goes, whatever your age, you should steel yourself for something altogether less exalted this time round. The fact is, no one but you cares how often or for how long the baby kicked you in the night ....'*[1]

Pregnancy can certainly feel quite different second time around. The most obvious difference, of course, is that this time you're not on the sofa watching Fern and Philip all day with a tub of Haagen Dazs on your lap. No, this time you're wrestling with the complex emotional and physical demands of the child who is outside your body; the one who's wanting you to read stories, get up in the night, jump up and down on the trampoline, carry her to the swings and generally behave just like you always have - in fact, more so, because somehow, perhaps unconsciously (and virtually every pregnant mother reports this experience) she is feeling threatened by her growing sibling. 'Clingy Older Child' should, in my view, be a recognised side effect of the later stages of subsequent pregnancies.

Beyond this (and, possibly, your increasing terror at the prospect of dealing with two - or more - kids) you may encounter some physical differences between this pregnancy and the last:

SIX DIFFERENCES WITH SECOND PREGNANCIES

1 **Your belly will probably get bigger, quicker** (I was in my maternity jeans at eight weeks with Sam's pregnancy, and practically at conception with Ted, my third). This is not because you're gestating the next Giant Haystacks. It's because the muscles that run vertically from your breast to your pubic bone have stretched once, so will stretch more easily again.

2 **You'll almost certainly feel more tired** (unless you have a team of nannies, maids and housekeepers).

3 **You may be more, or less, sick.** Experts are divided as to whether morning sickness is more common second time around but it's certainly common to be *really* sick with one pregnancy, and fine with another (neither is a sign that anything is wrong).

4 **You may also have more minor side effects,** like heartburn, backache, anaemia, varicose veins and piles. The basic rule is if you got them before, you'll probably get them again, maybe worse, this time.

5 **You may be more incontinent** this time during the pregnancy (though not afterwards).

6 **You *can* get new stretchmarks** beside the old ones, usually in the last stages. I still – several months after Ted's birth – have a red and white striped belly to prove this.

Second pregnancy tips:

The books all tell you to 'rest when your first child rests'. Of course you won't. You'll be frantically stuffing laundry into the washing machine, mopping the floor, catching up on your emails, phoning your bank and generally doing all the stuff you can't do with a toddler on your heels. However, you are growing a baby and you **need extra sleep.** Go to bed an hour early (you'll feel like you don't have a life, but it's temporary). And arrange with your partner that he gets up for your other child during the night, not you (get earplugs and DON'T fall into the trap at 3 a.m. of thinking 'I'll just go to her – it'll be quicker').

When to break the news to your first child

There's no good time. When you do this will depend on your child's age, personality and disposition. Waiting until you're at least 12 weeks is an obvious tip, since you don't want to have to explain should anything go wrong with the pregnancy. Another nice tip is to phrase your announcement carefully. Something mildly duplicitous like: 'Inside my tummy is a little baby that really wants to meet you: you are going to be a big brother/sister!' is perhaps more tactful than 'I'm going to have another baby, darling'.

Your advancing age

The fact that you're older this time may slightly raise your risk of miscarriage. You are also more likely to have a baby with chromosomal abnormalities such as Down's syndrome as you get older (though remember it's a curve, not a sudden leap at 35 into a 'danger' zone). In your 20s you have a one in several thousand chance of your baby having a chromosomal abnormality. By the time you are 45, the chance is about one in 30. You may, then, be more likely to face a choice about whether to have 'diagnostic' tests during this pregnancy (see Chapter 1: Pregnancy for Busy Women, page 47).

Older mother tip:
Ask your midwife about screening tests as soon as you are pregnant so you don't miss any you may want. A nuchal scan plus blood test is a good way to screen for chromosomal abnormalities but it has to be done when you are 11 to 12 weeks pregnant. Not all hospitals offer this as part of your antenatal care although some will do it privately. It can also be done at private clinics if your local hospital does not offer it at all. For example, **The Fetal Medicine Centre**, 137 Harley Street, London W1G 6BG 020 7486 0476 Fax: 020 7486 0294 Email: enquiries@fetalmedicine.com.

Second births: the facts

FIVE THINGS WOMEN SAY ABOUT SECOND BIRTHS

1 It was quicker from start to finish
2 I dealt with the pain better
3 I had far fewer interventions
4 I knew what I wanted and was more confident in asking for it
5 I recovered more quickly

Your future is rosy: second births, in general, are simpler, faster and less traumatic than first ones. Research evidence backs this up. One survey[2], *Listening to Mothers*, based on interviews with 1,583 American women, found that those who had one or more baby already were far more positive about labour than first time mothers. They were less likely than first timers to have an epidural in labour, and less likely to report negative feelings about labour and postpartum. You might actually deal with pain differently second time around. One study[3] showed that women who have undergone at least one vaginal birth are actually more tolerant of pain than women who have never given birth before. Psychologist Professor Josephine Green, who has studied women's feelings of control during labour, says the psychological differences between first and second labours are marked: *'Our studies have shown that on average women having their second, or subsequent babies, feel more in control during labour than women having their first babies.'*[4] In short, as obstetrician Lucy Chappell puts it, *'First and second time mothers are a completely different ball-game.'*

Speed
'Second births, in my experience are usually – though not always – quicker, and less complicated than first ones,' says midwife Jenny Smith. Occasionally a second baby might be significantly bigger than a first, or might lie in a difficult position for birth, which can make labour slower. But this is uncommon. There is, however, no single, definitive clinical study that proves that second births are 'easier' than

first ones. This is probably because it is virtually impossible to pin down what 'easier' actually means when it comes to childbirth. Now, most second time mothers could come up with a suggestion or two on this one. 'Quicker' would be one – especially for those of us who took what seemed like a millennium to dilate to 10 cm (or never got there at all) the first time. If quicker means easier to you, here are some reassuring facts:

- In an average first birth, doctors would expect about 1 cm an hour cervical dilation.
- For a second birth, they would expect your cervix to dilate at about 2 cm an hour.
- If you have pushed a baby out of your vagina once before then your pushing stage is also highly likely to be quicker this time.
- Second time mothers rarely need a drip to speed up labour.

Midwife Kim Kelly explains why this is: *'If a baby has moved down the vagina once already, the vaginal tissues have stretched once already and will stretch more quickly this time. This helps a second labour to go more quickly.'* Think of what you do before you blow up a balloon: you stretch the neck of it a few times so the air goes through more easily. Your baby, sadly, will not pass through your 'birth canal' like a puff of air. But it is likely to require a little less pushing this time. *'The midwife actually told me not to cough,'* says Jan, 35, mother of Annabel (4) and Eliza (3 months). *'I had an epidural and had been asleep so I didn't know how far along I was. The midwife wasn't ready, she saw Eliza's head and didn't want her just to fly out.'* Eliza did fly out, after just two pushes, all 9lb 5oz of her. In fact, as Kim Kelly puts it, *'The big issue with second time mums is helping slow the urge to push so they don't tear unnecessarily due to a too fast labour.'*

To those of us who pushed for hours first time, stories like this seem inconceivable. But your body retains a kind of 'memory' of that first birth. Your cervix has dilated before, and so tends to dilate quicker this time. And if you have not been battling your way through days (and nights) of contractions you will be able to muster far greater resources to push your baby out this time. This – along with your more flexible friend, your vagina – is why women like Jan describe the ease of pushing with number two. They are not lying.

Of course, if like me you had a caesarean first time, the elastic vagina theory does not count. Your vagina has NOT stretched like this before. You are a novice pusher and your pushing stage is likely to be longer than most second births. We discuss vaginal birth after caesarean (VBAC) in Chapter Six: Surgical Birth. But it is probably worth mentioning here that many women who have a VBAC do not feel 'cheated' at having to push like a beginner. Many say afterwards that the pushing stage felt like a triumph. *'I was so delighted to be pushing at all,'* says Kate, 31, mother of Charlie, 7, and Leon, 1, *'I've never felt more determined to do anything in my life. The midwife asked me, after a couple of hours of pushing, if I wanted a ventouse and I actually laughed. There was no way anyone was coming near me at that stage.'* This is the kind of perspective you only get as a second timer, driven by a possibly negative past experience. Kate pushed her second son out half an hour later. *'I did not care a hoot that I tore,'* she says, *'Which amazes me now, when I think about it.'*

Rapid labour

An 'easier' birth is not necessarily a fast one though. You'd think that not having to spend hours yowling in a tub of lukewarm water would be a blessing, but if you woke up first time around at 2 a.m. with agonisingly strong contractions, and an hour later had a baby in your arms, the prospect of another rapid birth may in fact be far from comforting.

'My first birth took three hours from start to finish,' says Tracy, 35, mother to John-Paul (5), Remy (3) and Joe (1). *'I was hugely shocked at the level of pain that the human body can tolerate. I wanted gas and air but they refused, saying it would slow labour down and because he was distressed they had to get him out quickly so they gave me an episiotomy. I think fast labours are supposed to be more painful as you don't have time to release any of these so called natural painkillers, endorphins, and you don't get time to have drugs.'*

Facing her second birth Tracy was 'dreading the pain'. Remy was born in two hours, after three minutes of pushing, and she tore badly. *'I think everyone was taken by surprise both times at the speed of it,'* she says. *'I did not do anything to prepare for it being fast, and nobody gave me any tips on how to slow things down.'* Third time around she was more prepared, mentally:

'Joe was born less than an hour after the first contraction. He came out 20 minutes after I arrived at the hospital. I had written on some paper that I handed to them on my arrival that I wanted gas and air and that if they could, to slow it down to avoid a bad tear... When I felt Joe coming out the midwife told me to pant but I shouted "I DON'T CARE ABOUT THE STITCHES!!" as I knew the pain would be over once he was out. Yes, I tore again but it was worth it this time for the quick delivery!'

Known as 'precipitous delivery' or, by some, 'taxicab birth', such experiences can take their toll, both emotionally and physically. Some women, after experiences like Tracy's, say they missed the 'satisfaction' of pushing. Others say they found it hard to bond with the baby as they were in shock. If you had a short first labour you do need to prepare yourself for number two to zoom into the world with scant warning. There are, however, things you can do to make this fast labour safer and more manageable than your last.

SIX WAYS TO MANAGE RAPID LABOUR

1   Talk to your midwife about positions in labour which can work against gravity (e.g. lying on your side).

2   Talk to your midwife about breathing techniques – using gas and air – that fight or slow the pushing urge.

3   Tell the labour ward when you phone that your first birth was very fast, so that they can prepare for you.

4   Write in your birth plan (make it succinct) what your concerns are and anything you want the midwives to do.

5   Make solid arrangements well in advance: pack your bag early and get someone on standby to care for your first child.

6   There is a possible link between postpartum haemorrhage and rapid second stages so make sure your midwife/doctors are aware in advance that this baby could whiz out.

Fast birth tip:
'Second time around I carried the hospital number with me at all times,' says Judy, 28, mother of Jack (3) and Zoe (1), both born in under two hours. *'My bag was packed way in advance, my husband and mother both carried mobiles in the last two weeks and I made my husband read the emergency delivery chapter in our birth book again.'* Judy made it to the hospital just in time to push Zoe out.

Medical intervention and second births

Medical intervention is now the norm for women giving birth. NHS figures show that fewer than half of us (47 per cent) can expect to have a 'normal' labour and delivery (the rest will have some kind of medical intervention)[5]. 'Instrumental birth' – that is, when the baby is helped out using forceps (tong-like implements) or ventouse (a suction cap) – can be hard to handle. Episiotomies (a cut to the perineum: the skin between your vagina and anus) can be upsetting and a caesarean may leave emotional as well as physical scars. As anyone who has had a pair of forceps up their vagina will tell you, instrumental birth is not to be sniffed at. This is why many women are quite reasonably scared that they will encounter the same thing second time around. There are ways to cope with medical intervention in birth: we cover this in Chapter 5: Your Options, page 164 and in Chapter 7: Expect the Unexpected, page 228.

The good news is that first births are more likely to be 'instrumental' than subsequent ones. One explanation for this is that nearly half of all instrumental deliveries happen because of a prolonged second (i.e. pushing) stage. This is usually because the baby is not in an ideal position for birth. Second time round, our bodies are simply better at getting the baby into the correct position, our wombs are more efficient at contracting, and our vaginas are stretchier.

YOUR CHANCES OF INSTRUMENTAL BIRTH SECOND TIME AROUND[6]

- With your first baby you had about a 21 per cent chance of an instrumental delivery.

- With your second or subsequent you only have about a 7 per cent chance of instrumental delivery, as long as you aren't having a multiple birth. Twins, or any multiples, tend to involve higher rates of intervention.

- You are, then, three times less likely to face forceps or ventouse with your second (or subsequent) baby than you were with your first.

A WORD ABOUT EPISIOTOMY... | If you had one last time, you may be worried that this will have to happen again. As childbirth educator Sheila Kitzinger wrote: *'A woman who has had an episiotomy, especially if her permission was not asked beforehand, may also feel violated. That is a word many women use when talking about their reaction to episiotomy.'*[7] Kellee, who now has six children, still remembers vividly the pain of the episiotomy she was given with her first baby. After a rapid labour, *'he [her obstetrician] cut me without my permission....My recovery took longer and my stitches hurt immensely for weeks'*. Not all episiotomies are traumatic, of course; indeed, many exhausted women say theirs was their salvation, and many a pelvic floor has been relieved by a swift episiotomy after a very long pushing stage. But even if 'violation' is not a word you would use about yours, you may not relish the prospect of facing another one. The obstetric trend is, you'll be glad to hear, hugely in your favour.

QUICK FACTS: EPISIOTOMY[8]

- In the early 1990s more than 20 per cent of mothers had an episiotomy
- By 2002–3 this had dropped to 13 per cent
- 19 per cent of women have an episiotomy the first time
- With subsequent babies, only 7 per cent do

Again, this is partly because there are fewer instrumental births second time around (about 80 per cent of forceps deliveries and 60 per cent of ventouse deliveries involve episiotomy). It is also partly because your vagina and perineum stretch more readily in a second vaginal birth. *'Even if you have a scar from a previous tear or an episiotomy,'* explains midwife Kim Kelley, *'there will more than likely be enough stretch to let the baby out [without another episiotomy].'*

There is one caveat here: if you have an instrumental delivery second time around, your chances of episiotomy do rise again, regardless of whether this is your first or second baby.[9] But if you go into this birth calm, confident and with an armory of brilliant labouring techniques, the chance of either happening will be slim. And, if they do happen, your ability to cope with them will be superlative. (Read more about how to make informed choices about your perineum in Chapter 5: Your Options.)

INDUCTION OF LABOUR | There is, of course, a chance that your baby will need to be induced. Nowadays about one in five babies are. According to obstetrician

Yehudi Gordon, in second and subsequent pregnancies, you are less likely to give birth more than ten days past your due date[10] but there are few hard facts available on this one. *'We have surprisingly little data about length of pregnancy first and second time around but it seems that induction is more common with first pregnancies,'* says obstetrician Lucy Chappell. Even if you are induced again, you should know that second inductions usually involve fewer interventions than first ones. *'Your body is usually more efficient second time, even if you are induced,'* says midwife Jenny Smith, *'so second inductions are likely to be far easier – often just rupturing the membranes [breaking your waters] can trigger the labour and no more intervention is needed.'*

EPIDURALS | Because you are less likely to have an instrumental delivery this time, you are also less likely to need an epidural. Only 12 per cent of women whose labour begins unaided, and who do not need an instrumental delivery, opt for an epidural in first or subsequent births.[11]

CAESAREANS | If you had a caesarean last time, your chances of having another one *are* statistically high (about 67 per cent of women who had a previous caesarean have another one second time around)[12]. However, this is not because vaginal birth after caesarean (VBAC) is dangerous or doomed to failure.
It is because many women simply opt for a repeat caesarean. This may be partly because most of us are not given the support (medical and emotional) we need to give VBAC a good try. In fact, up to 80 per cent of women who have had one caesarean will have a vaginal birth if allowed to labour second time around. (See Chapter Six: Surgical Birth for tips on VBAC.)

If you did not have a caesarean last time, then the chances of you having one with this birth are very small indeed. However, it does happen: *'It never occurred to me that I would have a caesarean with my second baby,'* says Anna, 34, mother of Maisie (4) and Mattie (1). *'The labour was fast, but Mattie just got stuck. The doctors were worried about his heart rate, everyone was panicking, and before I knew it, I was in surgery. I was in total shock afterwards. And still am.'* Skipping Chapter Six: Surgical Birth could, then, be a mistake, no matter how unlikely you think a caesarean is in your case.

Your age and this birth

If you're somewhere approaching (or beyond) forty years old, you may have just read all these nice, positive statistics about second births thinking 'but this does not apply to me because I'm older this time'. Your doubts are understandable. If you are in your late thirties or beyond, your doctor may well have already mentioned potential 'complications' associated with your 'advanced maternal age'. It can feel particularly galling if you are having your second baby and your doctor tells you that this birth will be harder than the last simply because you are now officially, obstetrically, old.

If your first delivery was difficult, this 'fear factor' will probably escalate. Many doctors will look at your medical notes, see that previous prolonged first labour, that emergency caesarean, or the postpartum haemorrhage (all things that can happen to anyone regardless of age) and start twitching. Before long, the C-word will be bandied around, and you'll be feeling totally incompetent. There is, in fact, no conclusive medical evidence that your age in itself is a 'complicating factor' in your second birth or will necessitate a caesarean.

The fact that you are an older mother is not exactly going to make you stand out in the playground these days. If you started having children late you'll be – like Madonna or Cherie Blair – practically pensionable by the time you get round to completing your family.[13] And there's no denying it, childbirth, like looking good in a miniskirt, may well come easier if you are twenty-one. But if you are over thirty-five, in reasonable physical condition, and are suffering from no obvious pregnancy complications – even if your birthing track record is dicey – there is no reason why your second birth should be any more complex than any one else's.

You will read or hear that 'the older you are, the less supple your body becomes'. This is a bit misleading. Many of us – especially in this age of yoga and Pilates – are actually in better shape now than we were a few years ago. We probably know more about nutrition and health than we did then – and care more. Our minds may not be quite as helpful. As one Seattle midwife puts it: *'The basic fact is that the older you are, the less supple your mind becomes. With their first baby, most women are a clean slate: open to new experiences and seeing childbirth as an exciting venture. Fear can step in as we age.'*

Julia has seen this repeatedly with older clients who are having their second babies.

'Often, as we get older, we get more successful in other areas of life. We become used to controlling things, bossing people around, having things just the way we want them to be. Many of my older clients have achieved things in life through being organised, focused and unbending in their priorities. One such woman, Miranda, who was forty-two and had her first baby by caesarean, ran a string of brokerages and was a highly successful business woman. She would only speak to me with a huge filofax on her lap. She wanted a vaginal birth but was so trapped in her head – so orderly and organised – that I worried she would not be able to let go enough to trust her body to give birth. As the pregnancy progressed, I noticed that Miranda approached the birth like a business project. She researched and planned doggedly, reading everything she could get her hands on. I knew I'd been hired to help Miranda make a "success" out of this birth at all costs.

'But the sense that Miranda was thinking too much made me uneasy. I'd seen other women, in similar mindsets, fall apart during labour when their "plan" was derailed. So I suggested Miranda see a hypnotherapist. This worked fantastically. She was able to be logical with me (we talked through her fears and options in an orderly way). But she let herself go with the loopy hypnotherapist (they meditated those fears away). In the end she had a no-fuss vaginal birth. I believe that a large part of this

success was her discovery that she could go with the flow, lose herself in the birth and relinquish some control.'

If you find yourself strategising this birth like it's a new business venture don't stop entirely (you are, after all, probably in your comfort zone). But do make yourself pause from time to time and ask yourself how you are actually *feeling about all this*. Preparation for birth has to involve more than meticulous planning.

FOUR THINGS YOU SHOULD KNOW ABOUT AGE AND LABOUR SECOND TIME AROUND

1   If you had a vaginal birth first time, your age will not prevent your vaginal tissues from stretching more easily this time.
2   Your age will not necessarily prevent your cervix from dilating more quickly with your second birth.
3   Whether or not you have less stamina this time will depend on you: if you are in good physical shape you should not find yourself any more exhausted than you were last time.
4   Your overall physical health and level of fitness are more important to your stamina than your age (a ninety-year-old recently ran the London marathon, after all).

The rates of caesarean section do rise – statistically – as you get older. No one has established any definitive physiological reasons for this. Many of the caesareans in women over the age of thirty-five are elective repeat caesareans.[14] One recent study into maternal age and caesareans found that 'physician and maternal preference' was the most likely explanation for the higher section rates among older women. In other words, you are more likely to *opt* for a caesarean if you are older, especially if you had one before.

The statistics (above) on second births apply to second time mothers **of all ages**. Your age in itself is not a reason to believe that this birth will be complicated. You may, however, have to contend with doctors who are more 'hands on' than they would be with a younger woman.[15]

A WORD ABOUT FEAR, PAIN AND SECOND BIRTHS | Many of us, when facing childbirth for the second time, latch on to a throwaway comment made by a doctor or midwife about our last birth. This becomes the 'reason' for any problems we experienced and it looms when we think about doing it all again. But second births can confound such expectations. *'I was convinced I had a tiny pelvis,'* says Sarah, 33, mother of Jack (5) and Ella (1). *'Jack was born by caesarean after two hours of pushing and a 48 hour labour. I remember the consultant saying something like "there just isn't enough room for him". That's as much explanation as I got. But because I then believed my pelvis was too small, I planned to have a caesarean with Ella. The consultant said it would be safer that way. In the end I went* *into labour three weeks early. Ella was born after a seven-hour labour, an hour of which was pushing.'*

It is, in fact, relatively common for second babies to be VBAC (vaginal birth after caesarean) when they are even larger than the first one – despite the woman being told first time that her pelvis was too small to accommodate the baby. When you're expecting your second baby you may hear positive stories like Sarah's. But if you have convinced yourself that you are somehow 'abnormal' these will mean nothing to you. You *know* it won't happen that way for you: yours is, after all, the genuinely too-small pelvis or the unstretchy vagina or the too-high cervix; yours is the enormous baby, or the baby that will never get into the right position. The positive birth stories roll off your back but the gory ones stick fast. If you want a more manageable second birth then letting go of what happened last time – unpicking your own story, separating fact from fantasy and thereby defusing your fears – is really important.

HOW TO HANDLE YOUR FEARS

- **Talk to your midwife about your last birth** and how you feel about it.

- **Get hold of your notes**, and go through them with her, or with your obstetrician. Get them to explain exactly what the terms mean and what happened, especially if you had medical intervention. Sometimes, if you did not understand what happened last time, you may feel violated by something that turns out to have been a wholly necessary procedure.

- **If you have a doula or another woman to support you, talk to her in detail** about that birth.

- **Try and understand how that birth has affected your perception of childbirth generally.** See Chapter 3: Fear and Pain, page 107.

- **If you still feel traumatised, worried or upset by your first birth,** get help: see a counsellor, talk to your midwife and childbirth class teacher or try calling **Birth Crisis** which offers support to women who have had traumatic or difficult birth experiences. Helplines: 01865 300 266 or 01380 720746 or 020 7485 4725 or 01454 299449

- **Finally, if you find you can't stop talking about that birth,** consider whether some counselling might help. You don't have to become Woody Allen: even a one-off session (particularly with someone who specialises in birth fears) can really lay things to rest.

Getting your birth records tip:

Don't be surprised if what you see, when you get the records from your last birth, is very different from your impressions of what happened. See your birth records as another opinion; even though the forms look official (and are) they are not the only story here. Some of what happened might, in fact, leave room for debate: 'need for episiotomy' might mean you had a doctor who preferred delivering by that method, while a different one would not have decided it was needed. To apply for a copy of your maternity records write to the Data Controller, Medical Records Department, at the hospital where you had your baby. There may be a small charge.

A few other common fears for second timers

MEDICAL CONDITIONS RECURRING | In general, if you had a medical condition last time, talk to your doctor about it as soon as you know you are pregnant. Also, you might find it helpful to do as much research as possible, online or in a library, about your condition so you fully understand it. This way, if there is something you can do to prevent, or manage it, you can take action in good time.

- If you had **pregnancy induced hypertension** (PIH) you could well get it again (there are many factors that influence your likelihood). Talk to your doctor as soon as you know you are pregnant.

- If you had **pre-eclampsia** last time, there is a 10–15 per cent risk of recurrence; the earlier you delivered your baby last time, the higher your chance is of getting it again. It's usual to develop it four to six weeks later in your second pregnancy than you did in your first. Ninety per cent of women get it later and less severely in a subsequent pregnancy. (N.B. If you didn't get pre-eclampsia last time, you're even less at risk this time.)

- If you had a **premature baby** last time, you are more at risk of having a second (or third). If your last baby was a spontaneous pre-term delivery you're about three to five times more likely to have one this time too. Ask to be referred to the doctor at your hospital who specialises in prematurity. Sometimes there are ways to minimise the risk of your baby being born prematurely again.

BIG BABIES | If your last baby was big, it is likely that this one will be big, too. Often – though not always – second babies are actually slightly bigger (on average this baby will be about 150g bigger than the last). This can sound horrifying if you had a hard time giving birth to your last baby. However, all the cheery statistics about second births still apply to you: your vaginal tissues, your muscles and ligaments have opened once before for a big baby, and your womb is now a pro at positioning a baby, and contracting to get it out. All of this – and the fact that you are reading this book (so will know far more about preparation and good positions for labour) – makes it highly likely that you will cope superlatively with giving birth to a big, healthy baby.

Big baby tip:
Often your baby is big simply because your body likes to grow them that way. However, there may have been a cause. Talk to your midwife as soon as you are pregnant about gestational diabetes so you can rule it out as a cause, or manage it well this time if it is one. Beyond this, you might want to watch what you are eating. In *Birth and Beyond*, Dr Yehudi Gordon writes:[16] *'If your first baby was very large, avoiding fast-burning sugary drinks and foods during this pregnancy may help to reduce your baby's weight.'*

BREECH BABIES | If your baby was breech first time around, you may be wondering if its sibling plans to arrive the same way. Most breech pregnancies are unexplained. This means doctors can't tell you, for definite, whether it will happen again. If you've had one breech baby you are more likely to have another one than you are if your first baby was head down ('cephalic'). However, the majority of women who have a first breech baby, then have a second (or subsequent) cephalic one.

SOMETHING WRONG WITH THE BABY | The pessimists among us (and we are legion) often believe that our luck may 'run out' this time. We've managed to have one healthy baby, or more (even if the process was tough), so we're somehow 'due' for a disaster. *'It is normal for women to feel anxious, with their second or third babies, that something will be wrong,'* says obstetrician Lucy Chappell. *'But the huge majority will go on to have another healthy child.'*

POSTPARTUM HAEMORRHAGE | Jan, who haemorrhaged badly after the birth of her first baby, says the recovery was the thing she dreaded when she thought about whether she would haemorrhage again. *'I was severely anaemic. For the first week or so, whenever I breast-fed at night, James had to pick up the baby and move her from one breast to the other for me. I distinctly remember kneeling in front of the long mirror in our bedroom (I couldn't sit or stand) wondering how long it would be before I had the energy, or inclination, to hold a hairdryer at head-height.'*

About 7 per cent of women suffer postpartum haemorrhage (PPH)[17]. If you had it last time, you are statistically more likely to have it again. But there are many kinds of haemorrhage and it is important to get your medical notes, and fully understand what happened to you first time around. Why you had the first haemorrhage will be an important factor when it comes to weighing up any risk of it happening again.

A big part of the impact of PPH is psychological; it can leave you in a poor state to care for a new baby, and physical recovery can take a long time. *'My basic advice,'* says obstetrician Lucy Chappell, *'is to be proactive this time. Sometimes small medical intervention at the birth can make a huge difference to the kind of postpartum you have.'* Bombard your midwife or doctor with specific questions and get specific answers. What caused it first time? Could this cause it again?

What can you do to minimise the chances of this happening? Though it can be scary – not least for your partner – a postpartum haemorrhage is rarely life threatening if you have the right medical care and facilities. Some studies have suggested a link between epidurals and postpartum haemorrhage. Again, discuss this link with your doctor who will be able to give you the most up-to-date information and talk to you about a managed third stage (an injection to speed up the delivery of the placenta). Finally, ask what you can do to ensure you're not anaemic going into this birth (discuss with your midwife whether you need iron supplements).

POSTNATAL DEPRESSION (PND) | If you had postnatal depression last time, depending on the severity it may happen again. If you were admitted to hospital last time, for instance, you have a one in two to one in three chance of the depression recurring with this baby. But don't wait until it does: the system for helping women with PND in this country is, in places, inadequate, and if you wait until you are depressed, you may have lost some of the insight – and drive – necessary to find the help you need. You should not feel stigmatised by this: you simply need help, as you would if tackling any other pregnancy condition. Prophylactic care may be available: you might, for instance, be given anti-depressants to take after you have the baby. Talk to your midwife or doctor and ask for a referral to the psychiatrist. Also, prepare your partner, family and friends for the possibility that it will recur – they need to be aware of the signs so they can help you as early as possible this time.

Tip: Prepare yourself for something new

When I had Sam, I thought I would not need much help postpartum. I'd done breastfeeding, sleeplessness, burps and yellow poo before. I knew what I was doing. The first six months of Sam's life were largely hellish for me. I did NOT know what I was doing: I had a two-year-old and a newborn and, as one friend put it, 'One plus one does not equal two'. The same goes for birth. Second time around it's a different beast and you need to prepare for it, to handle your unique fears and issues if you want to be sure it will be better than the last one.

BIRTH SURPRISES THE SECOND TIME AROUND

The birth:
- The onset of labour may not be as clear cut with a second baby.
- You are more likely to feel Braxton-Hicks contractions (possibly more strongly) before you actually go into labour.
- Contractions may be faster and more intense when you do go into labour.
- This time you may want totally different forms of comfort/pain relief.

After the birth:

- Afterpains – in the hours and days after the birth – tend to be much stronger after each birth you have. Brace yourself for this, and stock up on paracetamol.
- Your vaginal tissues and pelvic floor muscles will recover just as well from this birth if you do your pelvic floor exercises (see page 30), and if you do them, you should not be more incontinent this time.
- You need to take postpartum seriously and prepare for it as much as you did last time, if not more (see Chapter 10: Frozen Peas and Pyjamas).

The onset of labour

As Scarlett O'Hara puts it in *Gone With The Wind*, *'Death and taxes and childbirth! There's never any convenient time for any of them!'* Many women find, if they have a vaginal exam near their due date, that they have actually been dilating for a few days in the run up to the birth without even knowing it. This can flabbergast you if it took you hours – if not days – of contractions to get past 'pre-labour' last time. But when labour does kick in, the contractions may feel less manageable than they were at the beginning of your first labour. *'I was bent double over my Safeway trolley, with Toby yelling at the top of his lungs,'* says Cassie, 31, mother of Toby (3) and Jessie (6 months). *'With Toby I'd been having contractions for 24 hours but the midwives sent me home three times saying I was not in labour. With Jessica, I thought things might be happening, but I remembered how depressing it was to be sent home so many times. So I tried to keep busy and took Toby to the supermarket of all places. The contractions were so strong, I had to call my husband to come and get us and take me to the hospital.'* This happens in second labours that are quicker. But do remember that not all second labours zoom by. Your second labour *could* be just as long as your first – and maybe even longer.

LABOUR AND YOUR FIRST CHILD | You may, then, find yourself baying on hands and knees with your three-year-old howling next to you. Some women want to have their first child at the birth of their second. But most of us categorically do not. We do, however, often end up with a little spectator – at least initially. If you have not prepared your first child for this, the sight of mummy bellowing like an angry bull is not going to be a reassuring one.

We are still incredibly prudish when it comes to discussing childbirth with our children. We may not explicitly mention storks these days, but we do say things like 'the baby will just pop out!' or '...mummy will say ouch and out he'll come!' Clearly, you do not want to terrorise your child with images of blood, sweat and tears. But since she may inadvertently witness your early labour she does need to be sensibly and honestly prepared for what it might look and sound like. How plainly you speak about this will depend on your child's age and temperament. Two- or three-year-olds do get scared easily and at this age they have not fully separated from you – effectively they still think on some level that they're still a part of you. When they see you in pain they can get pretty distressed. A panicky child clinging to your leg shouting 'no! mummy no!' is not a helpful labour companion.

Many of us go into hospital too early with our first babies. We get sent home or, even more demoralising, traipse for hours through depressing hospital corridors trying to 'get things going'. We vow, second time, to stay at home as long as possible. This, for most of us, is an excellent plan. As long as we have sorted our first child out. This means more than putting your babysitter on stand by. You have to actually talk to your first child – even if he is only two – about what is going to happen. He knows you are having a baby, but does he know it will not just plop out into your lap smiling and wanting to play? You'll be going away – maybe for a few days. You'll be tired when you get home. Does he know this?

'When I went into labour with my second baby, it was not as I had planned,' says Diane, now a mother of four. *'I was home sewing Alana's Halloween costume when I felt my first – surprisingly intense – contraction. It never crossed my mind to tell my four-year-old about labour. I think she said "Mummy, are you cross?" I shoved in a Snow White video. I think this reassured her a bit, but the half an hour before my husband got back was not the most comfortable of my life. If I had to do it again, I would have found a better way to have warned her.'*

And, if you find it hard to accept the notion of 'productive pain' and 'endorphins' think what these things will mean to a two-year-old.

TIPS FOR TALKING TO YOUR FIRST CHILD ABOUT LABOUR

- **Show her what you will sound like** when labour starts. Bellow with her for a bit – most kids find this hilarious – breathe deeply and loudly. Do these 'labour alarms' regularly in the last month of pregnancy. The noises you make when in labour are going to shock her if she's not heard them before. And if you're suppressing them when you're in pain, the pain is going to be a lot harder to handle.

- **Show her what you will look like** in labour: bend double, lie on the floor, go on hands and knees, grimace madly – whatever you think you're likely to be doing. You can look extremely odd during a contraction. If she's seen it before she won't be scared.

- **Normalise the parts of your labour that your child might witness,** using language she can understand. You know your own child, and can do it your way, but be honest (without being scary).

- Regardless of your child's age, listen to her concerns.

Most children's books about impending siblinghood involve cartoon animals and never deal with labour or birth at all. The aardvark goes to the aardvark hospital and comes home with a fully dressed baby aardvark in an aardvark pram. While this might be a nice way to start conversations about what it will be like to have a baby around, they are useless in preparing your child for your labour. (See Further Reading, page 134, for a selection of books that will introduce your child to birth.) By all means read aardvark books. But do not let them be your first child's only introduction to labour.

CHILDREN AT THE BIRTH | Your mind may be made up on this already ('no way') but if it is not, there are some basic things you should ask yourself before you make a decision about whether your first child should be at the birth. If you are scared of birth your child probably will be too. If your child is under seven, she is going to become restless and bored unless her sibling emerges pretty fast. She may also be anxious about the hospital equipment, or about the midwife touching you. If your labour is not quicker this time, what is she going to do in a hospital for 36 hours? Does your partner want her there? It is common sense to discuss these things thoroughly before making your decision.

Expert opinion is divided on whether 'sibling-attended birth' is a good idea. Some believe that under the right circumstances children can benefit greatly from watching their little brother or sister come into the world – they can feel included and may bond instantly. Many, however, say that children under the age of five or six cannot completely comprehend the birthing experience (and may be alarmed by it). There is also a strong argument that a sibling-attended birth is better handled at home (the familiarity of the surroundings help to make the situation more normal and your child will be able to sleep, or watch TV).

Women with more than one child will tell you that getting time alone with either child is a rare and special thing. You may want this birth to be just about you and your new baby. It can be nice to have time away from your other child after the birth; time when you can just hold your newborn and count his tiny little fingers, recover from the birth, and bond with him without worrying about how jealous the sight of all this is making his big sister.

TIPS FOR SIBLING-ATTENDED BIRTHS

- Have someone there whose only job is your child.
- Make sure the babysitter is not scared of labour, and that they understand the emotional and physical stages you will be going through.
- Prearrange how your child will leave (and where to) if you need him to.
- Prepare your child extensively for witnessing the birth. Take him to each midwife visit, let him hear your questions and note his reactions to your midwife's actions. Prepare him for the fact that there will be BLOOD. Many children are really scared by the sight of this (usually the 3rd stage when you're delivering the placenta). And remember that when children say they are bored, often they are feeling apprehensive.

- You may want to go to sibling preparation classes and/or have a special appointment with your midwife just for her to talk with him about birth. Older children may benefit from seeing birth photos (videos with sound and 'blood' can overwhelm them) with the midwife explaining each one.

Three present-buying tips for your first child:

Get a present for your child to play with while you are in labour – a new toy or game. It will help her feel special.

Get a present for your first child 'from the baby'. Give it to your firstborn when she meets her sibling for the very first time. This can smooth the way marvelously.

Also, go shopping with your first child for a present for him to give to the baby – just something small like socks. This, in some sense, gives your first child an emotional 'stake' in the baby.

A final word on preparing for this birth.....

If you are worrying about repeating your difficult first experience, then pull out the list of ten positive things about second births (see page 114) and stick it on your fridge. Read it when you feel panicky. But do not assume that all you have to do is pitch up in the labour room and become another nice, happy statistic. You have a high chance of doing this (especially if you prepare now) but you do not want to be bulldozed should any complications or challenges arise.

Many women fall into the trap of thinking second births are a doddle, and so fail to prepare themselves adequately.

But what exactly should we do? The whole notion of 'preparing' for a birth is particularly difficult for those of us who did months of diligent reading, yoga breathing and birth classes first time round. And still had a nightmare. I certainly look back on my weeks of 'preparation' and ask myself what on earth I was achieving. The problem was that even though I knew the **textbook version** of birth, I didn't really know the basics about **real first-time labours,** which can differ radically from that text book – why fear matters; why it is important to eat, drink, walk, move around to get things going; how to plan for the unexpected. No wonder most of my 'preparations' proved useless when my body did not behave in an obliging way.

I am not the only woman in Britain to feel 'cheated' by this. Many of us feel this way first time then conclude that there is no point in preparing for the second birth. For some of us, any risk of a repeat performance is a risk too far. However, if you're tempted by an elective caesarean, don't forget that there is a vast array of options between a repeat trauma and surgery. Second timers are very different from first timers. Most of Julia's clients are second-time parents and she takes them on because she likes the 'challenge'. There is no way to scientifically 'prove' whether first births are harder than second ones though in general this seems likely. You cannot control what happens in childbirth this time either (this even holds true for a planned caesarean). But you can stack the odds in your favour. And – as you have seen – they are good odds. You **will** influence how you cope in labour, if you're prepared to work at it. A good place to start is by making meaningful, active choices about this birth. The next chapter will get you started.

• •

FIND OUT MORE

Further reading

Two good, general books on second children
Twice Blessed: Everything You Need to Know About Having a Second Child – Preparing Yourself, Your Marriage and Your Firstborn for a New Family of Four by Joan Leonard (St. Martin's, US, 2000) A nice introduction to the whole subject of second babies, with some general discussion of second births too.

Three Shoes, One Sock & No Hairbrush: Everything You Need to Know About Having Your Second Child by Rebecca Abrams (Cassells, UK, 2001) Not much on birth itself, but good for getting your head around being a mother of two, and coping techniques once the baby arrives.

Four books to read to your first child
Welcome With Love by Jenni Overend illustrated by Julie Vivas (Kane/Miller, UK, 2000) Somewhat idealistic (a gentle, natural homebirth on a windy night: not what most of us will have), but still it has great coverage of all the issues: a fantastic way to introduce your child (around 1–7) to the idea of birth (without it being scary).

These three books, which go together, have no words, just pictures and are great for discussion with your child about the pregnancy, birth and what it will be like to have a new baby:

Waiting for Baby Frank Endersby, Annie Kubler (Child's Play International Ltd, US, 2000)

My New Baby illustrated by Annie Kubler (Child's Play International Ltd, US, 2000)

There's a House Inside my Mummy by Giles Andreae and Vanessa Cabban (Orchard Books, UK, 2002)

Online

Childbirth educator Sheila Kitzinger runs **Birth Crisis** which offers support to women who have had traumatic or difficult birth experiences (see above, page 126, for helpline details). Go to www.sheilakitzinger.com for more information and articles.

www.mothers35plus.co.uk contains lots of general information and support for 'older' mothers.

Online breech support group: www.groups.yahoo.com/group/breechbirth/

www.birthstories.com has a 'second or more' section where people post their stories.

Chapter Five: Your options

'I had four children in the 1950s and 60s and never questioned the process. My family doctor gave me an approximate due date and told me what to eat, and that was it, until the deliveries. I went into each birth blindly – the system was foreign and scary. Dilation, effacement, transitions... I learned about those things 30 years later when my grand-children were born. I didn't know I had the option NOT to have drugs. It is with great sadness that I think back on what giving birth could have been like for me, if I had had the information my daughters have today.'

MEREDITH, 70, MOTHER TO FOUR GROWN DAUGHTERS
AND THREE GRANDCHILDREN

Knowing your options – and using them – will make a huge difference to how this birth turns out.

You can choose:

1   **Where and with whom** you'll give birth.

2   **To be informed:** the information you need is at your fingertips; how much you find out is your choice.

3   **How you'll cope with labour:** from the positions you use to the pain relief you'll have; if you know about it, you can make the choice to use (or ditch) it.

4   **To be involved in decision making.** You have the right to be consulted on ALL decisions made during the birth and to consent – in a genuinely informed way – to anything that happens to you and your baby.

5   **To be taken seriously:** these days your health care team is trained to consult and respect you. You can ensure this happens.

Options? What options?

Most of us spend more time choosing where to go for our summer holiday than we do when deciding where, how, and with whom we'll give birth to our babies.

When it comes to this earth-shattering, once in a lifetime, fundamentally crucial event we are, in general, a bunch of fatalistic, ill-informed chancers. When you think about it, this is probably a little ill-advised.

Most of us (particularly first time around) trot along to the GP when we get pregnant and trundle obediently through the 'system'. What we get there depends on largely on our postcode and circumstances. This is not surprising, really. It's hard to have an opinion if you haven't seen the inside of a maternity ward since you came out in one, so going wherever the GP sends you and accepting whatever care is arranged for you is certainly the easiest thing to do.

It isn't necessarily the wisest.

Maternity care is subject to exactly the same variable standards as any other kind of health care in Britain. Hospital policies vary. Staff attitudes, motivation and outlook can be radically different from unit to unit. But within this seemingly concrete system lurk a wide range of options for childbirth. If you are well-informed you can make the sort of choices about, and during, labour that will help you handle it fantastically wherever you are, whatever happens and whatever health care professional is with you.

This chapter will show you what your options are. It's time to start making some serious choices about this birth.

A WORD ABOUT CONFIDENCE | If you walked into Jigsaw, stood there while the shop assistant bossed you around, squeezed you into a dress you hated, told you that no, you couldn't have the one you wanted, then sent you packing after painfully separating you from a large amount of money you'd feel pretty dissatisfied, if not distressed, about the whole thing. Now, childbirth, of course, isn't shopping. It's nothing like shopping. But it's astounding how we'll abnegate responsibility for birth in a way we'd never *dream* of repeating in any other area of our lives.

This isn't about personality. Or even self-confidence. You may be a red-blooded demon in the boardroom and the most assertive shopper ever to darken the door of Harvey Nicks, but when it comes to making decisions about who'll do what to your body and baby during labour, you could well crumple if you're not truly informed.

Part of the problem here is the tendency many of us have to be self-effacing when it comes to medical matters. It's like they're totally beyond us. Nothing to do with us. Scarily difficult. Absolutely not our responsibility. Julia encounters this attitude a lot. Her clients often don't want to rock the boat during pregnancy; they don't want to tie up their midwife or doctor with too many questions, or appear to think of themselves as a 'special case', or presume to 'interfere' with the doctor's job. Psychologists have found that feeling respected by staff and treated as an individual during childbirth are crucial factors in deciding how we feel about it later. But there's no way you can be an active participant if you don't have the first clue about what you're doing.

'*I was so disempowered during the birth*,' writes Tanya, mother of Amelie (2). '*I never felt that I could make any decisions of my own despite a good degree, a career and birth preparation etc.*' Part of the problem here is that it's not easy to be assertive with a baby bearing down on your perineum. This is why you have to make the bulk of your decisions **before you are in labour.** Understanding your hospital and having a birth partner who can really support you, as well as a good grasp of what might happen and what you're going to do about it, will all help you feel 'empowered' – even when you're on hands and knees grunting like a wildebeest.

A WORD ABOUT SAFETY | You probably assume that going for the hospital closest to home is the only 'safe' or 'reasonable' option for this birth. It isn't. You probably assume there's no point in making choices about how you'll cope in labour because you don't know what it will be like, and anyway, the medical staff will tell you what to do. This is not the case. You may believe that making active choices about where, how and with whom you'll give birth is possibly risky and almost certainly futile. It isn't. Trusting your health care team, feeling comfortable and safe in your hospital (or at least understanding why, if you don't) and feeling genuinely informed about what's happening are the foundations of a good experience of childbirth. If you ignore this stuff and bumble along doing what you're told, things **may** turn out OK on the day. But then again, they may not. Do you really want to chance it?

**MAKING PROPER CHOICES: SOME QUESTIONS THAT
NEED ANSWERING**

1   **Where** will I give birth?
2   **Who** will be with me when I do it?
3   **What** will I do during labour? (This includes anything from pain relief to how you'll push your baby out.)

Your options second time around

If this is not your first baby, you'll be tempted to skim this chapter or skip it completely. Fair enough: you certainly do know a lot more than you did last time. Studies have shown we are generally better at coping with childbirth if we've done it before. But this does not mean you should stop making choices. No two births are the same. If a strategy didn't work in your last birth, it may well work in this one. I didn't touch the birth ball during Sam's birth but spent my entire labour leaning on it with Ted. (I didn't even know what a birth ball was with Izzie.) Whatever you do, don't narrow your options through ignorance or apathy.

Tip for second timers:
Make a list of the choices you made in your last birth then rate your own satisfaction with each.

- Did you say yes to something for reasons that still aren't clear?
- Would you have liked something you didn't get?
- Did you get something you didn't like?

Take this list to your midwife (and to Chapter 7 to turn it into your birth plan) and discuss (and research for yourself) alternatives to the bits you didn't like, or ways to handle them. This will help you make active, meaningful choices, not knee jerk or pointless ones.

Control freaks beware. Our message here is subtle, but vital: **you can't control this birth completely** no matter how many excellent choices you make. Your baby (or body) may have different ideas on the day, and you'll have to deal with the unexpected. You can, however, **feel** more in control – and at least influence events for the better – if you're making good choices. Your options, then, start here, and are ON GOING.

Why bother?

It all sounds like a lot of work. But many women report that a feeling of 'helplessness' was one of the most upsetting aspects of giving birth. Professor Josephine Green, a psychologist specialising in women and childbirth at Leeds University, has studied the psychological effects of women's sense of control during childbirth[1]. *'Our studies have found that feeling in control – particularly about what staff are doing to you – is a major factor in how good women feel about the birth afterwards.'* Since how you feel afterwards has been linked to post traumatic stress disorder and postnatal depression (both of which will affect how you mother your infant), it's not some middle-class indulgence to care.

Keeping an open mind

You may think you want to give birth with only endorphins for company, then end up choosing a buttock full of analgesia. Or you may decide to get an epidural at the first twinge only to end up coping brilliantly without a needle in sight. *'I thought I wanted a water birth,'* says Janet, 33, mother of Clea (3) *'I fought so hard to get it (I have herpes and my doctor wanted to give me a caesarean). But on the day I'd rather have cut off my own hand than get into that pool: I gave birth on the hospital bed without having so much as dipped my big toe in the water I'd fought so hard for.'* Many of us, largely through nerves, become shackled by preconceived ideas about the way we want things to go ('I simply WILL not allow anyone to break my waters/give me drugs/operate on me'). Try not to do this. Instead, see your options as **a process** that will be on-going throughout pregnancy **and labour**.

HOW TO MAKE MEANINGFUL CHOICES

1 **Understand** your options
2 **Discover** what your natural inclinations are (for example, are you scared of white coats or comforted by them? Squeamish or blasé? Anxious or confident?)
3 **Work out** how to maximise your chances of having the kind of birth that matches these inclinations.

Ultimately, the choices you explore in this chapter will become a flexible birth plan. We cover how to write one in Chapter 7: Expect the unexpected.

Will it work?

'Trying to control birth is futile: you can't control it. Trying to do so just sets you up for failure,' says Jessica, mother of Tyler (2) and Bea (1). Jessica is not alone in thinking this. And she's also right – up to a point. Going with the flow is vital during childbirth. But going with the flow blindfold, possibly in a panic, alone, in pain and fear and at the mercy of a hospital system you don't understand is clearly not your best strategy. You may not be able to change medical events, but how you handle them can make the difference between a horrifying ordeal and a series of decisions and coping techniques. One study[2] in 2001 found that the main factors that influenced how we feel about labour are:

- Support from our partners
- Positive attitudes of the midwives caring for us during pregnancy and labour

- Information given to us during pregnancy and labour
- Being able to make and be included in decisions during labour.

You can influence all of these things.

What do to before the birth

One thing women repeatedly said about their first births, when we spoke to them for this book, was 'If I'd known then what I know now...'. You might think it's sensible not to think too much about the details of birth. We're all tempted to do that. But ignorance, when it comes to childbirth, is **not** bliss. Here's a run down of the things you should be making active choices about right now.

1. Location, Location, Location

Even if you have no intention of going anywhere other than your local hospital, a bit of research will help you understand the ethos of the place: if you know the beast, you can plan how best to handle it.

HOSPITALS | Most of us think we're doing this when we diligently traipse around on the 'hospital tour', pretending to listen while trying to blank out the unfamiliar smells and lurking medical equipment. Here's how to use your tour effectively.

Tour tips:

- **Be self-aware**. What are your instincts about the kind of birth you want (medicalised, drugged, natural, somewhere between the two?). Does this hospital *feel* like it'll accommodate you? Are you scared or reassured, unnerved or calmed by the tour?

- **Be conscious of your specific needs**: if you're having triplets you may want and need different things than if you dream about giving birth in a Yurt in Oregon. Is this hospital likely to meet your needs? Will you need to compromise or negotiate?

- **Ignore the décor**. Most NHS hospitals are pretty shabby but this has little or nothing to do with the kind of care you'll get. You can bring things to make the room feel more comfortable and 'homey' anyway.

- **Think about how you could improve the room:** The National Childbirth trust did a national survey of 2,000 new mums in 2003[3] and found that your birth environment can influence your birth experience. Factors that influence a better birth, they found, include easy access to a toilet, use of bean bags, pillows and mats and being able to control things like the temperature of the room. You can't do much about the location of the loo, but you can ask for more pillows, bring a fan, ask if they have a mat for the floor and birth balls or a bean bag (or simply bring these with you if they don't). Birth balls, by the way, are just oversized 'exercise' balls, available from Argos or sports shops. This may seem like overkill, but you're likely to cope better with this birth if you feel safe, comfortable and manage to stay mobile (not flat on your back in bed) during labour.

Irritating things to ask on your hospital tour:
- **What other facilities are available?** e.g. does it have the water pool you want? If so, how often is this pool actually used? The facilities can tell you a lot about a hospital's general approach. Do the midwives use aromatherapy? (Yes, really, the midwives at the John Radcliffe Hospital in Oxford, for instance, carry aromatherapy kits and are trained in aromatherapy for labour at home or in hospital.) Or it is all talk of epidurals and resuscitation equipment?

- **How flexible are they about your individual needs**? Good questions include:
  - Can I move around/eat and drink/give birth in upright positions?
  - Can my baby be monitored with a hand-held fetal heart monitor unless there's a reason to use an electronic one?
  - Can I bring stuff from home to make the room feel more familiar?
  - Are there any time restrictions on how long the different stages of my labour can go on for and are these at all negotiable?

- **What are their caesarean and vaginal-birth-after-caesarean (vBAC) rates**? A high caesarean rate is anything over about 20 per cent. A genuinely low rate would be something like 15 per cent. However, be aware that different kinds of hospitals will have different rates because of the kinds of cases they get (a big hospital that deals with lots of complicated or high-risk pregnancies will have a higher caesarean rate) – so don't panic if yours seems high. Do, however, use this information to understand more about your hospital's approach in general – will they, for instance, be more likely to offer medical intervention where it might not be strictly necessary?

Changing hospitals: You actually have a legal right to choose where you will give birth. Ultimately, if you are really not happy with the hospital you've been referred to, you don't have to lump it. Switching to a different hospital, investigating a home birth or going to a birth centre (see below) are not radical things to do as long as you have thought them through carefully and listened to any medical concerns the midwives or obstetricians have. As midwife Jenny Smiths puts it: *'It's really important to choose a hospital where you feel comfortable and secure and can trust the medical professionals to work with you. Switching to a different hospital is not always straightforward, but many people can do this if* *they try.*' If you can't switch to a different hospital (perhaps because there isn't one in your area), make sure you understand yours well, and are aware of any particular challenges you may meet there; this way you can plan how you will tackle them.

Switching hospital tip:

If your GP is unable (or unwilling) to refer you to a different hospital, talk to your Primary Care Trust (PCT). The best person to ask for your local PCT address is your GP's practice manager.

> **Further reading:**
> **Dr Foster's Good Birth Guide** (Vermilion, UK, 2002). Written in consultation with the Department of Health, the Royal College of Midwives, and the Royal College of Obstetrics and Gynaecologists, has the facts and figures about every maternity unit in the UK (also online at: www.drfoster.co.uk).
> **You're Pregnant!** is a localised magazine in 100 editions (available from your GP or midwife) which gives local information about maternity services in many areas of the country (try the information line 08701 555 455 if you can't get hold of a copy).
>
> **Online:**
> **www.birthchoice.co.uk** has information on hospitals across the country, ranging from facilities to caesarean rates.

MIDWIFE UNITS | Sometimes called 'birth centres', 'midwife units' or 'GP Units', these will generally take you if you're having a low-risk pregnancy. They tend to have a lower intervention rate than many hospitals and usually don't have facilities for caesareans (so you'd be transferred to the hospital should you need one). They can be attached to a hospital, or in a separate building on site, or they may be in a different location entirely, but are usually relatively near a main hospital (in case of emergency). The facilities vary, but many are smaller and more 'homely' than hospitals. It's worth having a look at your local one if it still exists (some units are facing closure because of midwife shortages). At one of these units you are more likely to be encouraged to walk around during labour and have access to a birthing pool than you are in a hospital: again, things that maximise your options for the birth. You will also probably have more control over your privacy in a midwife-led unit, than in a hospital. Having said this, some women say they didn't get the 'woman-centred' approach they'd hoped for by going to a midwife-led unit. It's also worth knowing that according to the latest NHS caesarean guidelines for health professionals, being in a midwife-led unit does not reduce your likelihood of having a caesarean.[4] Units, like hospitals, vary. So ask the same kind of questions you would on any hospital tour.

PRIVATE BIRTH CENTRES | These are not common in Britain but they can be a great option **if you've got the cash.** They tend to focus on natural birth, are nice and plush, have extremely supportive and encouraging midwives and very low caesarean rates. But you'll pay through the nose for this (still, some would argue that this is a better use of your money than that holiday in Barbados). At a London birth centre, for instance, a full package birth might set you back about £4000.

Where to go for help:
www.babycentre.co.uk has articles and information on birth centres in the UK.

GIVING BIRTH AT HOME | Only just over 2 per cent of British women have their babies at home. But these numbers mask some pretty hefty regional variations; in some parts of the country as many as 20 per cent of us give birth at home, in others, less than 1 per cent do. Much of this comes down to the attitudes of health professionals. Some doctors are reluctant to agree to home births and some midwife teams find it hard to cover homebirths because of stretched resources. If you decide you want to give birth chez vous – providing there is no compelling medical evidence that this would be a bad idea – you need to get the support of your midwives. If you give birth at home you want the best medical care available: experienced, trained midwives.

Lots of women say the first reaction of their midwife or doctor to their request for a homebirth was knee-jerk discouragement (with a hefty dose of scepticism). Often this will change when they realise you're serious, reasonable and informed. If you end up (God forbid) having to fight for a homebirth, it's worth knowing that you have a legal right to give birth at home (or indeed, anywhere you fancy).

Homebirth used to be a matter of necessity – hospitals were reserved for illness not childbirth. Then, with the early women's movement, came the drive towards birth in hospitals. *'It was a safety issue. To go from giving birth in your home to delivering in a clean doctor-run environment felt like a huge step in the right direction,'* says retired nurse Gloria Fleischer. *'Back in the 1950s and 60s home birthing women were seen as crazy. We were even trained to strap the "natural birth" women down – to keep the other women from getting upset.'* Today homebirth is not the defiant option it once was. Research has shown that for a healthy woman having a straightforward pregnancy, homebirth is as safe as hospital birth. Many midwives are highly experienced at homebirth and will encourage it, where appropriate. They bring with them medical equipment including gas and air (for pain relief), equipment to resuscitate the baby in the unlikely event that something should go wrong, and a suturing kit, to give you any stitches you might need when the baby is out – unless your tear is severe, in which case you'll need to go to the hospital.

Neither are the practicalities of a homebirth as daunting as you'd think. Your midwife gives you a list of things you'll need for the birth, including plastic covers for the carpet and things like towels and food for you to eat in labour. You call the midwives when you go into labour and one will come out and see you.

Homebirth certainly isn't for everyone, but if you are 'low risk', confident and live within easy reach of a hospital (should you need to transfer to one), your home can be a very reassuring place to give birth. As Sarah, 36, mother of Leo (born in hospital) and Harry (born at home) puts it: *'Being at home made me feel in control and relaxed (once we had dispatched the builders!) and helped the birth to be straightforward. Harry was born in a pool in the living room. I was so comfortable in the water that my contractions quickly became very strong. The last ten minutes with no pain relief were absolute agony but delivering him and keeping him in the water were beautiful. The three of us got into our own bed afterwards – it felt so much more civilised than being in a noisy, dirty hospital ward.'*

Wot, no epidural? You can't get an epidural at home. If this is worrying you, you may not be the best candidate for a homebirth. Though you can get a prescription for injected analgesia such as pethidine or meptid (see page 167), some midwives will tell you that if you think you are going to need drugs in early labour then you shouldn't go for a homebirth.

Is it safe? There are some scenarios in which hospital births are certainly your best option, such as if you're having twins, a breech baby, or if you or the baby have certain medical complications. Your own inclinations are also important. If you're scared of birth, think it's inherently dangerous or risky and worry about medical safety issues or getting hold of drugs, then hospital may be the place for you. But if you believe that birth is a safe, normal event, feel comforted and safe in your own home, trust your midwives, don't have any medical complications and live relatively near the hospital then it might be something to consider.

How to make up your mind about homebirth Homebirth isn't a panacaea and your birth can be fantastic regardless of your location, as long as that location suits you. Some women choose homebirth out of bitter defensiveness, often after a bad first experience ('I'm not letting those evil doctors anywhere near me this time'). If you feel this way, and you end up having to transfer to hospital again, you're not going to be exactly calm and reconciled.

IF YOU'RE THINKING ABOUT HOMEBIRTH ASK YOURSELF:

- Do I feel safe in my home?
- Do I think of birth as normal and safe and do I feel confident that I can do it?
- What appeals to me about homebirth?
- Am I prepared to cope with pain using largely natural methods?
- How far am I from the nearest hospital if it becomes necessary? (More than about 20 minutes or half an hour is probably not ideal.)
- Can I cope with an emergency transfer to hospital? (See also Chapter 7.)
- Am I choosing home birth because I am avoiding something? (This is fine, as long as you're aware of what that something is and what you'll do if you CAN'T avoid it, i.e. you end up transferring to hospital.)
- How does my partner feel about homebirth? If it worries him, will he support me anyway or will he be lurking resentfully throughout?

- Do other people I care about (i.e. friends, family) support this choice, and if not, will it really matter to me in the end?

Remember you can always plan and prepare for a homebirth but then decide, on the day, to go into the hospital. Nobody is going to penalise you for changing your mind.

Pressure from others NOT to have a homebirth From the moment you suggest you might like to give birth at home you'll start hearing alarmist stories. Julia has seen this on many occasions: '*One of my clients had a mother-in-law who was a retired nurse. Every phone call or visit the mother-in-law would tell long gruesome stories about babies that would have died if not for the miracles of medicine. Pregnancy is a time when we are sponges – especially for emotional issues. Consider just keeping your birth plans between you and your partner. Nobody needs to know where your baby will be born, and after the fact nobody will care.*' The only thing that really matters is that you make a sensible, informed choice after serious thought and discussions with medical professionals.

Where to go for help:
Association for Improvements in the Maternity Services (AIMS) offer information about your rights and publish a leaflet *Choosing a Homebirth*. www.aims.org.uk or call AIMS 0870 765 1433.

Further reading:
Birth Your Way: Choosing Birth at Home or in a Birth Centre by Sheila Kitzinger (Dorling Kindersley, UK, 2002). An updated book about making confident choices beyond your local hospital.
Homebirth – Information to help you decide (2002), a booklet published by the National Childbirth Trust. Available from NCT Maternity Sales. 0870 112 1120 Email: sales@nctms.co.uk. www.nctms.co.uk.

Online:
Our website has more on homebirth (www.bloomingbirth.net)
Homebirth Reference Site has lots of information – www.homebirth.org.uk
You can also find peer support in 'Homebirth meet up groups' around the country. www.homebirth.meetup.com.

2. Your health care team

It's impossible to overestimate how important your health care team will be to this birth. A midwife can become a god-like presence for you in labour: your mother, sister, guru, spiritual leader, teacher, professor rolled into one pragmatic, competent bundle. It is important that you're able to discuss your worries and concerns openly with the midwife you see most during the pregnancy, and feel she's listening to you (Chapter 3: Fear and Pain spells out why). But she probably won't be with you during the birth itself.

There are many different types of midwife care in this country, and it's a really good idea to understand how your care is organised so you can get the best out of it. Get your midwife to explain exactly how her team works (and write it down for yourself, or you'll forget the minute you walk out of her office).

THREE DIFFERENT TYPES OF MIDWIFERY/HOSPITAL CARE | Yours may not work exactly this way so ask for an explanation.

1. Shared care: a community midwife and your GP see you during pregnancy and a midwife at the hospital (you may not have ever met her) will attend the birth. You may have a check up or two at the hospital, and will go there for any scans. If you take a violent dislike to your community midwife (and feel this is jeopardising things for you) first talk to her about why you're finding it difficult, then ask to transfer to another team or speak to the senior midwife in charge of community midwifery. Don't just grin and bear it.

2. Team midwifery: a smallish team of midwives will see you during pregnancy and labour and you have a greater chance of getting to know the midwife who'll end up attending your birth.

3. Domino scheme: a midwife you've seen during pregnancy actually attends your birth.

MIDWIFE SHORTAGES | The Royal College of Midwives estimates that Britain is short of around 10,000 midwifery staff. One of the main effects of this is that you may not be cared for by the same midwife during the whole birth (shift changes happen) and those you do see in labour are likely to be strangers to you. They'll also probably be somewhat overstretched. Some midwives say that on a full moon (yes, really) bedlam descends on the maternity unit. But even if the moon is not full, the chances are that your midwife will be looking after at least one other woman (and sometimes more) at the same time as you during your labour. Usually, she'll time things so that she can be there for you when your labour is hotting up (and, obviously, for the delivery itself). But many of us do have relatively long periods of being left alone with only a midwife popping in from time to time to make sure we're OK.

'OK' is, of course, a relative term when you're having contractions. What may seem fine and normal to a trained medical professional may appear extremely unreasonable to you. One recent study[5] found that 13 per cent of women who'd given birth before, and 16 per cent of first timers, said they were left alone in labour at a time when it worried them to be alone. This is a pretty convincing reason to have some other form of support sorted out (see Chapter 9: The Love of a Good Woman). It can get lonely, worrying and dispiriting if it's just you, your contractions and your increasingly knackered partner rubbing away helplessly at your back.

Bedlam tip:
'Try and become part of the team rather than a frustrated outsider,' advises midwife Jenny Smith, 'Don't be afraid to ask questions and find out basic information about the

facilities on offer. But try to remind yourself that she's not "abandoning" you – she has to look after other women and their babies just as she has to look after you and yours. Her biggest concern, on really busy days, is simply the safety of every woman and baby in the unit.'

A WORD ABOUT CONSULTATION... | There's a lot of talk these days about how you should agree to, and understand, what's being done to you by doctors and midwives. But even the most gung-ho among us can feel distinctly disempowered when juggling anxiety, pain, medical jargon and an expert who may not have a PhD in tact. If you're facing a genuine medical emergency, full consultation might not be possible (they'll be too busy helping you or the baby to check that you're ok with this). But as a basic guide, don't agree to any treatment, test or intervention, until you've had answers to the following questions:

CONSULTATION AT-A-GLANCE

When a test is suggested ask:
- Why? What problem are we looking for?
- What will the test tell us?
- How accurate or reliable are the results?
- What will happen next?

When a treatment or intervention is suggested (during pregnancy or labour) ask:
- What are the benefits, risks and alternatives to the procedure (including doing nothing)? Of course, in the heat of labour, you (and probably your partner) may not remember to ask systematic questions, weigh up facts or quibble about statistics. But as a basic rule do try to make sure you understand WHY this intervention has to happen right now and whether anything else would do instead. This will help you cope both while it's happening, and afterwards, when you look back on the birth.

PERSONALITY CLASHES | If you are having 'personality differences' with the midwife try to resolve things (or get your partner to do this on your behalf). *'If you feel your midwife's approach is dramatically affecting the way you labour–for the worse–get your partner to pop out and ask to speak to the person in charge (this will be the coordinating or senior midwife),'* advises midwife Jenny Smith. *'Be polite. Say something like, "I think we have a bit of a personality clash–would you please help us to sort it out?" Often it can just be a case of misunderstanding, and with good communication I have known women who have been extremely happy continuing with their original midwife after an initial hiccup.'* If, however, the problem really is your midwife, it's not a good idea to press on, fretfully, feeling bullied or unsupported once attempts to sort things out have failed. You can, ultimately, get your partner to ask if you can swap to a different midwife. *'My midwife was a* *harridan,'* says Katherine, mother of Millie (1) and about to give birth to her second baby. *'I found out later that she was famous for it. She bullied me, pushed me around - quite literally - and said many unhelpful things. I feel she made the birth unnecessarily scary. This time I'm going to ask for a different one if I get her: no question. I feel much more confident about doing so as a second time mum. I wish I'd known I could ask for someone else first time round.'*

AN UNFAMILIAR PAIR OF HANDS | Most women, after they've given birth, use superlatives when talking about their midwives. I still have dreams featuring the wise, comforting figure of Penny who attended Ted's birth. But if you are worried about being attended by a stranger during childbirth talk this over with your midwife beforehand. Choosing to have another woman (friend, relative or doula) with you during labour means you - and your partner - will be with someone you trust, even if you won't know your midwife.

You can also call the Head of Midwifery at your hospital and discuss your worries with her. It's not unheard of (resources providing) to be allotted a smaller 'team' of midwives, who you can get to know, and one of whom will do their utmost to attend the birth. Midwives want to help you give birth in the way that's best for you. They can be surprisingly flexible. But be realistic: these are overworked women fighting staffing shortages and they can't work miracles.

And incidentally, your midwife may be a 'he'. At the end of 2002 there were 93 male midwives in the UK.

INDEPENDENT MIDWIVES | If your concern about not knowing your midwife is acute, if talking to the hospital was fruitless and if you have the readies, this is certainly an option. An independent midwife is not cheap (they can cost somewhere in the region of £2000). They are basically freelancers, fully trained by the Nursing Midwifery Council, as are all NHS midwives. Many have opted out of the NHS simply because they want more human interaction and continuity from their jobs. They can be fantastically supportive and committed. Some will do hospital births - they may have a contract that allows them to attend you in your local hospital. Many, however, restrict themselves to homebirths (but will stay with you if you have to be transferred to hospital). If you hire an independent midwife she should see you throughout pregnancy for all your antenatal checks and be there for the birth. It's worth knowing, though, that independent midwives may not be insured (because of the high cost of insurance). You should consider this when weighing up whether to hire one.

Where to go for help:
Independent Midwives Association, 1 The Great Quarry, Guildford, Surrey GUI 3XN 01483-821104 Email: information@independentmidwives.org.uk
www.independentmidwives.org.uk

Options for your baby and body

There are many things about birth that may seem like hitches or horrors, but are actually a series of choices for you to make if you know how. Here are some common labour challenges and what to do about them.

Your baby's position

A baby that isn't lying right is one of labour's biggest challenges. A vast proportion of difficult labours (particularly first time) happen because the position of the baby's head makes it hard for him to move smoothly down through your pelvis. This slows labour down and can make it more painful. This is one of the most common reasons why women have a caesarean first time around. Sometimes, when you are in the last stages of pregnancy, a midwife may be able to feel your baby's position (with her hands, and by locating your baby's heart beat). If your baby is not in the ideal position, there may be things you can do to change the way he's lying: spending time on hands and knees is one approach commonly suggested to mothers-to-be. There is, however, some debate in the medical community about whether these approaches really work or not. Still, if something might possibly help your baby to get into the ideal position for this birth, and it's not painful or unsafe to try, then it's surely worth a shot.

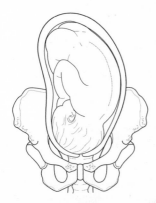

Left occipito anterior *The most usual way for a baby to lie, i.e. facing more towards your spine, with the narrowest part of his head pressing on your cervix.*

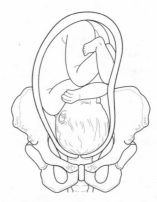

Right occipito posterior *The baby is lying in a 'posterior' position, i.e. facing upwards. Can cause problems in labour.*

GOOD POSITIONING IN A NUTSHELL

During pregnancy, particularly the later stages:

- Spend about half an hour (or more) a day doing tasks that make you lean forwards on hands and knees: for instance, cleaning the other side of the bath or scrubbing the floor.

- Sit, when possible, upright with your hips above your knees, leaning slightly forward.
- When watching TV or whatever, sit upright, as above, lie on your side, sit on a birth ball or bean bag (or lean forward on one) but whatever you do, do NOT slouch or lie on your back.
- Walk around on hands and knees a lot (you're probably doing this anyway if you already have a toddler).

> **Where to go for help:**
> *Sit up and take notice: Positioning Yourself for a Better Birth* by Pauline Scott (National Childbirth Trust, 2003). Available from NCT maternity sales 0870 112 1120 www.nctms.co.uk

Breech baby

A baby is breech when instead of being head down, her bottom, foot or feet – instead of her head – want to be born first. About three to four per cent of babies are breech at the end of the pregnancy. Finding out your baby is breech is the sort of hitch that plunges many pregnant women into a panic. But it's important to stay open minded about your baby's bottom. Throughout most of your pregnancy it's fine for her to be hanging around facing any way she fancies. But by about 36 or 37 weeks she probably should be thinking about turning head down. Some babies stay breech until the last minute – some even turn during labour – but you may not want to leave it this long. In 2003, researchers concluded[6] that having a planned caesarean rather than a planned vaginal birth reduces the chances of your baby dying or becoming seriously ill during or after the birth if she is breech. However, several options for attempting to turn a breech baby (see below) are worth trying before you schedule surgery.

Turning the baby: natural options

BREECH TILT | This is something many doulas would suggest. It's harmless and some women say it worked for them.

1 Lie on your back with your knees bent, feet flat on the floor. Raise your pelvis and put a couple of cushions under your bum so that it is about 15 inches above your head (or try lying head down on an ironing board or similar flat board that you've tilted up by putting one end securely on a low chair, the other on the floor).

2 Stay in this position for about ten minutes three times a day when the baby is active. Try to relax your abdominal muscles and breathe deeply. Expect your baby to wriggle around.

LURING THE BABY | Penny Simkin, in her book *Pregnancy, Childbirth and the Newborn* (see further reading), suggests something that may seem wacky in cold blood. You shine a light up your vagina several times a day, hold a radio playing softly at your vaginal opening/pubic bone or get the baby's father to talk to the baby from there. As Simkin puts it: *'We know that the fetus can hear very well and responds to sound coming from outside the womb. We think that if the fetus hears pleasing sounds coming from low in the uterus, he might move his head down to hear it better. While not always successful, numerous women who have tried this technique have reported that their babies turned.'*[7] There's a certain logic to this and, again, it won't hurt to try.

ACUPUNCTURE | A technique called Moxibustion has been used for centuries in China to turn breech babies. Limited trials in the West have also shown it may work, but there's no conclusive clinical evidence. Many women also believe acupressure (there's a point on your little toe called 'Bladder 67') helped turn their baby. Talk to your midwife before you go to an acupuncturist. Try the British Acupuncture Council, 63 Jeddo Road, London W12 9HQ 020 8735 0400 www.acupuncture.org.uk

EXTERNAL CEPHALIC VERSION (ECV) | A lot of research has been carried out to show how safe this technique is and it has excellent success rates. All hospitals should now offer this to you, at around 37-38 weeks, and if yours doesn't you can ask to go to one that does. You may be given a drug to help relax the muscles of your womb. The doctor will work out your baby's position using an ultrasound. She'll then press on your abdomen to turn the baby into the head down position. If the baby shows signs of distress she'll stop. Sometimes ECV works completely, sometimes it works but the baby turns back later and sometimes it doesn't work at all. ECV is more likely to be successful if:

- this is not your first baby
- there is a normal amount of water round the baby
- the baby's head is not engaged

ECV can be pretty uncomfortable (this isn't a euphemism - it shouldn't be actively 'painful'). Women have described it as 'a huge rummage', and this, for most of us, can be hard to handle (mentally as much as anything else), so use your relaxation techniques and take someone for moral support. It's pretty counter-intuitive to have anyone pushing at your abdomen when you're heavily pregnant and it's easy to tense up. But remember that this is a common, safe procedure and it may well work.

Breech baby coping tip:
If your baby does stay firmly breech this does not mean the birth is now out of your hands. It is perfectly legitimate to discuss vaginal breech birth with your obstetrician and to get a second opinion if you want. You will feel much better about having a caesarean if you are completely convinced of the reasons why it

is advisable. If you choose a caesarean don't give up on your preparations for this birth: you can make the surgery FEEL like a birth rather than a scary op, by reading Chapter 6: Surgical Birth.

> **Where to go for help:**
> **Breech Birth: A Guide to Breech Pregnancy and Birth** by Benna Waites (Free Association Books, UK, 2003) A comprehensive book, written by the mother of a breech baby, addresses the whole experience of breech from causes to turning techniques to the options for birth.

Overdue baby

If your baby is hanging around past her due date, you're not alone: only 58 per cent of women have actually produced a baby by the time they are 40 weeks pregnant[8]. Around 20 per cent of us end up having our babies induced by doctors or midwives (see below for methods)[9]. If you don't go into labour within 10-14 days of your due date, your hospital will probably offer to put you out of your misery by inducing the baby. They may present this as a *fait accompli*, but, like all else, it is a choice you can make by weighing up the pros and cons. The usual concern is that if a pregnancy goes on too long, your placenta may begin to work less effectively, putting your baby at risk. Studies show that the risk of stillbirth increases from 1 in 3000 for women who are 37 weeks pregnant, to 6 in 3000 for women who are 43 weeks pregnant[10].

Grey areas

That's not to say ALL overdue babies are 'at risk'. Some hospitals have a policy of inducing all babies when they are ten days overdue, some at two weeks. If your midwife or obstetrician mentions induction, consider this an opening gambit. Discuss the pros and cons. If your baby is more than two weeks overdue and you still do not want to induce, doctors and midwives should monitor you closely (usually this involves the baby being monitored in hospital every other day). Having said this, most women, by 42 weeks, are begging the doctors to get labour started.

On the begging front – here's a note of caution: in the US (and it's not unknown in the UK) there's a trend towards women scheduling inductions for convenience. They're sick of being pregnant, they want to time the birthday to a certain date and so on. It is worth knowing, if you're tempted by this, that while induction can be a blessed relief, it isn't necessarily much fun. Studies show it is likely to result in more medical interventions (e.g. ventouse, forceps and caesarean) and many women describe their induced labour as more painful than their 'natural' one. Of course, if your baby has to come out (but doesn't seem keen to) you may not have the option of turning down induction. Don't give up on the birth though. There are tons of things you can do to ensure a safe and positive experience of induced labour.

Induction: your 'natural' options

SEX | It may be a grim thought at this elephantine stage but having sex is an excellent way to induce an overdue baby. Sperm contains prostaglandin, the hormone that softens the neck of the womb (which will help it to open). If you can orgasm, your body will also release some oxytocin (responsible for womb contractions too). If you're not, perchance, feeling like a sex goddess just grit your teeth and think of England. And do this as often as you (and your partner) can bear to (well, at least a couple of times anyway) in a 24-hour period. Don't expect to go into crashing labour immediately one single act is over. It might be a few hours before anything begins to happen. And it might not work at all.

SOME OTHER NATURAL WAYS YOU COULD TRY

- **Nipple stimulation**: by your partner's tongue, fingers – his or yours – or a breast pump. This will stimulate the release of oxytocin (a hormone that works to contract your womb). You may have to do this for a while, so don't expect it to be fun, necessarily, for either of you.

- **Massage/acupressure**: 'spleen 6' may be just the thing. Make sure you are at least 40 weeks pregnant. Measure up your leg, 4-6 fingers above your inner ankle bone (the pressure point called 'spleen 6'). Press the inside of your shin bone here firmly for ten seconds, then rest (3-6 times). It should feel like you're pressing a bruise. I did this for my second and third babies and went into labour the next day which could of course be mere coincidence. Trained massage therapists and acupuncturists may also have other methods for inducing labour.

- **Spicy foods/laughter/meditation**: anecdotal, but some women swear by this combination. Eat your vindaloo in front of *Will & Grace*, then have a rest. Again, no major hardship here.

- **Walking:** for 30 minutes or more, as briskly as you can.

- **Homeopathic/herbal:** a homeopath or herbalist may be able to help your labour to start. Some say they work, others scoff: there's no conclusive clinical evidence either way. Make sure you check with your midwife before taking anything.

- **Castor oil with concentrated orange juice**: somewhat controversial, but the castor oil 'cleans you out' (you poo like crazy and make way for the baby). Julia did this when overdue with Larson and it seemed to work. It can give you 'flu symptoms, so do this only with the guidance of your midwife.

- **Reflexology**: some women swear it helped to kick their contractions off.

- **Visualisations** (see Chapter Four): self-hypnosis might help you to relax and feel less miserable about your enormity. You can try to visualise your baby coming and feel your body open to make way for her. Why not?

A word of caution. Always make sure your midwife apporoves whatever you're trying. If your baby isn't ready nothing will happen. But if he just needs a little prod things can go fast.

Medical induction

This shouldn't really be a singular noun. Medical induction can mean many things, ranging from the midwife breaking your waters ('artificial rupture of membranes' or ARM) to getting hooked up to a drip of synthetic hormones for the duration of labour. Each of these methods has pros and cons so discuss all the angles with your midwife/doctor before you agree to anything. It's also best to see induction as a possible series of events rather than a fixed date at which you'll have your baby.

CERVICAL SWEEP | This can be done from around 40 weeks. The midwife puts a finger into your cervix and swirls it around the edge. You get to go home after this and it may take 24–48 hours to work. **Good because**: it's minor and you can then labour without intervention if it works. Studies show that it prevents one in six inductions. **Drawbacks**: like any internal exam, it can be uncomfortable. **How to cope:** Talk to your midwife about what to expect and tell her if you are nervous. Ask her to explain what she's doing as she's doing it. Agree with her that you can say 'stop' at any point. Help yourself by lying with your hands under your bum, as this will bring your cervix forward. Focus on staying calm and relaxed using slow breathing, and have your partner with you. Try visualisations to distract yourself and remember it's a quick procedure.

PROSTAGLANDIN GEL | This is sometimes – though not always – used along with a cervical sweep. Prostaglandin is a hormone that gets labour started. The midwife will put a pessary or gel up your vagina so that it's next to your cervix. You'll stay in hospital from now on. Your baby will usually be monitored with an electronic fetal monitor before and after the pessary goes in. You'll probably then be asked to rest in bed (at the hospital) for an hour then get up and walk around but you won't be allowed to go home after this. After six hours, if nothing has happened, you can have another pessary. Three pessaries are usually the most you'll be offered. **Good because**: it involves little intervention, does not hurt and may not involve any further interventions **Drawbacks**: might not work or it might stimulate your womb to contract too frequently ('hyperstimulation') which can distress the baby.

BREAKING YOUR WATERS ('ARTIFICIAL RUPTURE OF MEMBRANES' [ARM]) |

The medical words sound scary (anything with 'rupture' in the title, at this point, can seem unpalatable). But ARM should not be hard to handle. The midwife breaks the bag of waters surrounding your baby by hooking and puncturing them through your cervix (they don't have nerves in them so this should not be any less fabulous than a basic internal exam). After ARM you'll be advised to walk around for a few hours, before being checked again. Often ARM is used after prostaglandin. Sometimes you'll be offered ARM if your labour stalls part of the way through. There are other options to get a stalled labour going again, though, see page 162 below. **Good because**: it isn't particularly painful and may not involve any further interventions. **Drawbacks**: once your waters are broken most hospitals will have a policy that the baby needs to be out within 24 hours to avoid 'infection'. This is a 'no going back' step.

Julia has seen women lose all sense of control because of an induction:
'*Raiza was an assertive woman who wanted natural childbirth. We worked for the weeks before her birth on positions for comfort and natural methods for moving the baby along. The baby was very overdue and Raiza agreed to have a syntocinon drip to get things moving. She then became a woman I didn't know. She lay passively, allowing the attending doctors to speak over her to her partner about her progress. She took the induction as defeat and not as a choice she herself had researched and approved. She had little joy in the vaginal delivery of her little girl and told me later that no matter how many times I'd told her to expect the unexpected, she thought it wouldn't apply to her. A thoughtful acceptance of medical interventions, or a quick choice due to medical necessity should never be seen as defeat. You are still giving birth, and many elements of your birth plan (see Chapter 7) can remain, if you keep making those choices as you go.*'

Induction tip:
'Aromatherapy can help induction,' says Penny Green, an Oxford midwife. *'Clary sage, rose, jasmine or lavender can be used before any medical intervention or an hour after ARM to get things going.'*

SYNTOCINON DRIP | Syntocinon is the artificial form of oxytocin, the hormone your body gives off to start labour. This is the most major induction step. The doctor prescribes syntocinon and the midwife gives it to you, following a strict protocol as to the rate/speed of the drip (the drip starts slowly and is gradually increased so that your womb is not over-stimulated which would distress the baby). You'll usually be in bed for this, hooked up to a drip and your baby will be monitored using an electronic fetal monitor (a band around your waist attached to a machine by wires). This kind of induction can make contractions come hard and fast. Sometimes a 'whiff' of syntocinon can start your labour off brilliantly, and you will be able to come off the drip and labour on your own. Some people react quicker to syntocinon than others because of the stage of labour they are in, or their readiness to labour if they are being induced. However, particularly if this is your first baby, you may need to be hooked up to the syntocinon throughout labour. You are more likely, if this is the case, to want an epidural (be realistic about this possibility – syntocinon really can make labour harder). **Good because**: it really will get labour going once and for all. **Drawbacks:** contractions can be more painful, and it raises your chances of having other interventions such as epidural, ventouse, forceps or caesarean.

Drip coping tips:
Don't panic: this procedure might just kick things off for you.

Discuss all risks and benefits in advance. Understanding it properly will help you cope if it's tough.

If at all possible, opt for a mobile epidural: this way you can still walk and pee with your syntocinon IV tagging along (see epidurals, below, page 169). Your birth partner can manoeuvre the IV pole and tubing so you won't notice it. You can stay mobile, and use gravity to minimise the chances of further interventions. (Even sitting upright in a chair is better than lying flat on your back.)

> **Where to go for help:**
> **When Your Baby is Overdue**, a MIDIRS 'informed choice' leaflet is good for presenting all the issues (see Find Out More). Download it free from www.infochoice.org.

The Birth

There's a baby in there and it's got to come out – you've no choice about that. But you have many options when it comes to the details. I remember when I was pregnant the first time, a mother of three in my yoga class advised me to 'read up on everything to do with birth'. This was somehow meaningless to me. I had no idea where to start or what to read. Apart from handling pain, I didn't know what I should be concerned about. So I read one (very medical and thorough) popular childbirth book. I went into that birth in a quivering state of ignorance that did me no favours when the going got tough and I had to make decisions. Many women have this experience first time, and vow never to be like that again.

CHOOSE TO MOVE | It's simple: you should move around and, as much as possible, stay upright during labour. If you think you might forget this, have it tattooed in fluorescent foot high letters on your belly **right now**. Don't rely on the medical staff to remind you about positions during labour. The National Childbirth Trust (NCT) says that up to 40 per cent of us are currently not advised to stay upright and move around during labour and instead lie on our backs, even though research shows that upright positions and movement can be very beneficial. In other words, it's up to you – and your birth partner.

Midwife Jenny Smith is unequivocal on this one:

'It is always best to be in an upright position rather than lying on beds. The best way to encourage your womb to work in the most proficient way is for you always to adopt a sitting, standing or kneeling position during labour. This will maximise the opening of your cervix and help your baby to descend through your birth canal. It will also ensure that the blood flow from you to your baby is good. If you lie on your back during labour, you may compress a large vein called the vena cava. This can impede the blood flow to your baby, which can reduce the oxygen available to him and then cause "fetal distress".'

You don't, of course, HAVE to move if it doesn't feel right. You can choose to stay very still if this is what your body is telling you to do. But if you do feel like lying down (as opposed to being told to lie down by someone else), **don't lie on your back for any length of time unless you have to** (for instance, if you're having an internal examination). Instead lie on your **left side,** as if you are asleep in bed, sit up against pillows, or lean over a birth ball (see page 171 for positions).

> **Where to go for help:**
> **The Active Birth Centre** is helpful on positions 020 7281 6760
> www.activebirthcentre.com
> The **NCT** also has good information on movement and positions for labour.
> Try the NCT 'Guide to labour' available from NCT maternity sales 0870 112 1120
> www.nctms.co.uk.

Some common labour challenges

Monitoring the baby

FETAL DISTRESS

What is it?
Mostly, 'fetal distress' is used to mean changes in the baby's heart rate tracing. But the term is subjective, and there is no universal medical definition. This is why the American College of Obstetricians and Gynecologists now urges American doctors to say 'non-reassuring fetal heart rate tracing' instead of 'fetal distress'.

What are some possible signs of fetal distress?
- 'Bradycardia' – when the baby's heart rate dips **below** 110 beats per minute (bpm)
- 'Tachycardia' – when the baby's heart rate goes **above** 160 bpm
- Presence of meconium (baby's first poo) in the amniotic fluid (waters)
- Decelerations – when the heart beat dips with or after contractions, but then returns to its previous normal level in between.

What do these signs mean for you and your baby?

- Everything may be fine. Sometimes changes to the heart-rate tracing are not serious: they can be caused by normal events in labour (like the baby's head coming through your pelvis).
- But sometimes they are serious because they mean the level of oxygen in your baby's blood is starting to fall. If this happens, then the cause needs to be reversed (for instance, by reducing the level of a hormone drip if you are having one to speed up labour). Or the baby needs to be delivered quickly.

Listening devices

Listening to your baby's heart rate is the best way for the midwife or doctor to tell whether or not your baby is becoming 'distressed'. This may be done using either one or all of the following:

- A hand-held monitor (usually a 'doppler' or 'sonic aid')
- An electronic fetal monitor (EFM), sometimes called a 'cardiotocograph' or 'CTG'
- A scalp clip (sometimes called a 'fetal scalp electrode'). Used occasionally.

HAND-HELD MONITOR | Hospitals have different policies and approaches to monitoring the baby's heart rate. The most recent recommendations from the National Institute of Clinical Excellence (NICE) say that if you're healthy with a trouble-free pregnancy then about every 15 minutes (and about every five minutes towards the end of labour) the midwife should simply listen to your baby's heart using a hand-held device. She should listen to your baby before, during and after a contraction to see how he copes with the squeeze of the contraction. According to NICE there should be no need for electronic monitoring unless there is genuine concern about how well your baby is coping. However, many hospitals will ask to hook you up to the EFM when you arrive, so that they can get an initial picture of how your baby is doing. This is your choice. If you decide you'd rather the midwife used a hand held device, you should say so (and put it in your birth plan).

ELECTRONIC FETAL MONITOR (EFM) | There are many reasons for the hospital wanting to monitor your baby using an electronic fetal monitor (EFM). These include certain pregnancy complications (such as diabetes or pre-eclampsia), a twin or multiple pregnancy, an induction or epidural and any concerns about your baby's heart rate during labour. If you agree to an EFM, the midwife will attach a couple of elastic belts around your belly. One belt monitors the contraction, and on the other the sensors pick up the baby's heart rate and transmit it to the electronic monitor which 'traces' the heartbeat on a print out (called a 'trace' or 'CTG').

EFM isn't, however, necessarily your best choice if you have no complications. *'You'd think continuously listening to the baby using an electronic monitor would be an excellent idea,'* says obstetrician Lucy Chappell. *'But the benefits of EFM are not so straightforward. EFM was introduced with the aim of reducing deaths and cerebral palsy in babies. But it has not actually been shown by studies to improve these outcomes over hand-held monitoring in a low risk birth. In fact, there can actually be disadvantages to having EFM (such as more medical interventions) unless there are medical reasons to do so.'* One issue is that *'interpreting the CTG is more imprecise than you would imagine. Human error – both in how the print out is interpreted and what happens next – can happen'*. Occasionally doctors or midwives might not recognise a problem, might not act on the information they have in front of them or might act too soon, intervening unnecessarily.

It is, then, a really good idea to talk to your midwife before you are in labour about the pros and cons of EFM. This way you won't have to make any stressed, sudden decisions and also you will fully understand any risks you are taking either way.

Once the monitor is on, remember that you do not have to become the 'patient'.

You may have to be lying on a bed while the belt is being attached but there is no reason why you should be forced to lie on your back while the monitoring is actually going on. Although your range of movement will be limited by the wires which are attached to the machine, you can sit in a chair or on the bed, upright with pillows and the bed back up, or you can rock on your birth ball, stool or beanbag. Again, you might want to put this in your birth plan so you don't have to quibble about it at the time. Even if you have a drip in your arm, you can do all of these things.

EFM devices tip:
A few hospitals have mobile EFM devices – they work by 'telemetry' – and you can wander around happily while the monitoring is going on. There are even devices which work in water. You can at least ASK about these options before you are in labour: if they have these kinds of monitors – particularly if you know that you will be having EFM – you can plan to use them.

FETAL SCALP CLIP | Occasionally, if there are some concerns about your baby, the doctor may want to put an electrode on your baby's head to pick up her heartbeat directly. This is a kind of clip, attached to your baby's scalp (via your vagina) and connected to the monitor. If there's real concern from this, they have to act. They may want to deliver your baby quickly (instrumentally or by caesarean), or they may decide to take a couple of drops of your baby's blood from her scalp ('fetal blood sampling') to test the oxygen levels (to find out for sure whether she is 'in distress').

AND YOU! | *'One of the very best monitors of your baby's well being, during labour, is you – the mother,'* says midwife Jenny Smith. *'If you feel the baby's movements have stopped or slowed down, tell your midwife straight away. Your baby is probably just resting, but your instincts, and your relationship with the baby inside you, can tell us a lot about how your baby is coping during labour.'*

Where to go for help:
The Active Birth Centre offers information on staying mobile in labour.
020 7281 6760 www.activebirthcentre.com
National Institute for Clinical Excellence: MidCity Place, 71 High Holborn,
London wc1v 6NA 020 7067 5800

Further Reading:
Monitoring Your Baby's Heartbeat in Labour: A Guide for Pregnant Women and Their Partners (National Institute for Clinical Excellence, 2001) This is the official advice on fetal monitoring.
Full Clinical Guideline on the Use of Electronic Fetal Monitoring, published by the Royal College of Obstetricians and Gynaecologists is more detailed. Both available from www.nice.org.uk
Listening to Your Baby's Heartbeat During Labour (MIDIRS, 1996). A Midwives Information and Resource Service (MIDIRS) 'informed choice' leaflet (see Find Out More). Download it free from www.infochoice.org.

'Failure to Progress'

The vast majority of first time caesareans (not to mention other interventions) happen because of 'failure to progress'. Basically, this is when your labour takes too long or stalls entirely. Usually this happens because the baby's head is not in the best possible position for birth. To lower the chances of your labour stalling:

- Stay upright in labour, use movement and positions outlined below.
- Prepare yourself mentally for feeling demoralised, exhausted, bored and frustrated at times during labour. These are all common, normal challenges, particularly first time.
- Minimise interruptions: dim lights and privacy may help your labour to progress. If you find yourself in a room with the lights on, and strangers coming and going, talking loudly, get your birth partner to act assertively.

Where to go for help:
The Labour Progress Handbook: Early Interventions to Prevent and Treat Dystocia, Penny Simkin and Ruth Ancheta (Blackwell Science, UK, 2000) is quite technical, but a great resource for anyone concerned about failure to progress.

'Back Labour'

If your baby is head down, but facing upwards with his spine against yours (instead of his face towards your spine) this is called 'back labour' or a 'posterior' baby. This position can slow labour up, and make contractions ridiculously painful. But don't give up all hope if this happens to you. Sometimes a baby will turn into a better position during labour. Some midwives say being on your hands and knees as much as you can in labour will encourage this. The methods below can all help to relieve the backache that usually comes with a back labour. Some are going to sound silly, but if you've had back labour once, you'll try anything to help it the second time.

Water: a jet of water on the lower back works as 'counter pressure'.

Tennis ball: counter-pressure again – your partner can roll a tennis ball on the sore bit during contractions. A cold coke can or a bottle of frozen water will also work.

Rice sock (see Chapter 9, page 278, for what it is and how to make one): put it on your lower back or on top of your pelvis.

Double hip squeeze: again, counter pressure focusing on the hip area. Your partner presses one hand on each of your hips during the contraction, pushing them gently but firmly together.

Rolling pressure: the cold can or bottle or even a rolling pin.

Cold pack/hot pack on your lower back: again, if it feels right, then do it.

Hands and knees: just getting onto hands and knees and staying there for a while helps to get the baby off your back for a breather. It may even encourage the baby to turn a bit.

Group B Strep (GBS)

Group B streptococcus (GBS) is a common type of bacterium carried by about a third of women. It can come and go which makes screening controversial and possibly not as helpful as it might be. You wouldn't know it's there and it doesn't do you any harm, but it is the most common cause of bacterial infection in newborn babies in the UK (though it's still rare: about 1 in 1000 babies develop GBS – that's only about 700 babies in the UK a year). It can make a baby get very sick, or even die, which is why some hospitals are now screening women during pregnancy for GBS. If you are found to be GBS positive you will be advised to have intravenous antibiotics when you go into labour. These should be given at least four hours before the baby actually comes out, and involve being connected to an IV tube and pole for 15–20 minutes every four hours.

Again, probably the biggest challenge here is how to avoid suddenly feeling like a patient (having an IV in your arm can make you feel like something out of ER if you've not thought it through first).

Tips for coping with an IV in labour:
Discuss your plans to move freely/use water with the midwife: there is no technical reason why you can't be in a tub with an IV in your arm providing you keep the arm out of the water, but your midwife may take a little persuading.

Get your birth partner to take charge of the IV: moving the pole if you want to move, keeping you from having to think about it at all.

Remember that you are still healthy and strong and more than capable of giving birth: the IV is nothing but a safeguard.

> **Where to go for help:**
> **Group B Strep Support**, PO Box 203, Haywards Heath, West Sussex RH16 1GF.
> They have an excellent leaflet called **GBS and Pregnancy: preventing GBS infection in babies**. Helpline 01444 416176 or online www.gbss.org.uk

Instrumental birth (ventouse and forceps)

An instrumental birth is where the baby needs to be 'helped' out, in the final pushing stages, by a suction device called a ventouse or by tong-like instruments called forceps. This might happen if the doctors judge that your baby needs to be delivered quickly (if, for instance, your baby is in distress or you are exhausted and have been pushing for a very long time with no progress). A ventouse looks a bit like a small hat with a tube coming out of it. The doctor puts this on the top of your baby's head to pull as you push. Sometimes, after ventouse, your baby's head might be temporarily (and harmlessly) 'cone' shaped, or have a red mark where the suction was put on. Forceps look like a large pair of spoons. The doctor puts them round the baby's head to pull as you push. Again, sometimes your baby's head might be marked or bruised by this – but not permanently. Ventouse is more commonly done in British hospitals as it is considered gentler and you do not usually need an episiotomy (a surgical cut to your perineum that is stitched after the birth under local anaesthetic). But forceps often involve an episiotomy.

YOUR CHANCES OF INSTRUMENTAL BIRTH

If you think all this won't apply to you here are the facts:

- You have more than a one in ten chance of having an instrumental delivery.
- You are more likely to have a ventouse delivery than a forceps one (about 65 per cent of instrumental deliveries are ventouse).
- You have a 14 per cent chance of having an episiotomy .

If you are making the right decisions – before and after the birth – you really are going to reduce your chances of having an instrumental birth. But you won't eliminate them entirely. This sort of thing may sound unpalatable but there are many ways to cope if your baby needs a bit of help to emerge. Instrumental births can be a huge relief from an exhausting pushing stage. But if you're totally unprepared, they can also be upsetting. Julia has seen women really distressed by the use of ventouse or forceps, largely because they took the 'never thought it would happen to me' stance (so tempting, for all of us). It's a good idea, then, to look instrumental delivery in the eye now, so that if you end up staring down the barrel of a suction cap, you will cope fabulously. This is particularly true for first-time mothers: you are more likely to have an instrumental delivery first time around, than if you have had a vaginal birth before.

One of Julia's clients, Topanga, 29, mother of Sean (2) describes her forceps delivery like this:

'The forceps looked like salad tongs or farm equipment. I had been pushing for quite a while and my midwife explained how and why they were needed. I had an epidural and also a local anesthetic in my perineum, so I really didn't feel anything at the time. The metal sticks looked scary. But, oddly, I was fine. I felt pressure on my back as Sean was born, but at the time it was only odd, not painful. I couldn't have really prepared my body for the forceps, but I did speak with my midwife before Sean's birth about instrumental births, so mentally I sort of knew what was coming. Sean was fine, but had three small bruises over and around his eye. He was watched for jaundice and his head looked a little pointy for a bit, but within 24 hours he was fine. My recovery was harder, I was sore, couldn't really sit up and in hindsight, I should have taken every pain reliever they gave me. Everyone around me acted like I should be elated to have had a vaginal birth, not understanding the special recovery I needed.'

HOW TO LOOK INSTRUMENTAL BIRTH IN THE EYE | Talk to your midwife about instrumental delivery before you are in labour (and don't be brushed off with 'oh, that won't happen to you' type of response).

Ask her:
- When might ventouse or forceps be used?
- What other things can we try before ventouse or forceps are needed?
- What kind of pain relief can I have before they are used?
- Can you talk me through what happens in a ventouse/forceps delivery?
- If I had an episiotomy how might it change my recovery?

If you've done this, then should you have an instrumental delivery, you will know the answers to these questions and will be able to hunker down and deal with the process, accepting that you've done everything you can to avoid it. (See 'Ways to cope' below.) Finally, as with every other aspect of birth, don't be tempted to see instrumental birth as some kind of failure. If you have prepared, made active decisions and feel genuinely informed and consulted about these procedures they can be totally manageable (even a blessed relief: they'll get that baby out once and for all, and labour will be OVER).

Instrumental birth pushing tip:
'You can make a huge difference by making these the best pushes of the whole labour: really give it your all. This way the obstetrician has to use less effort, which is much better for you and your baby.' Obstetrician Lucy Chappell

Choosing pain relief

When I had Izzie, my first baby, I was convinced that only drugs would really work when it came to 'proper' labour pain. I had an epidural followed by various interventions. Second time around, I gave birth in hospital with no medication, and third time around, I had Ted on the living-room floor using gas and air. There is no 'right' or 'wrong' way to handle pain of childbirth. But there are mistakes you can make if you're ill-informed. I made a classic with Izzie: I had an epidural because I was scared that it might GET too painful - not because it actually WAS so at the time (though it was no picnic). If I'd had a clue about alternative ways to relieve the pain, I wouldn't have considered the epidural at that early stage. I had no idea that an epidural might lead to more interventions (such as the syntocinon drip I was then given to keep labour going). I just thought it would stop the birth from hurting. If you'd asked me back then whether I thought things like massage, relaxation, positions, movement or water could really work against labour pain I'd have laughed. Now I've actually used these methods all the way through, I honestly believe that as long as the birth is going smoothly (and this is a **big** caveat), these woolly-sounding methods of pain relief work wonders.

The large US survey *Listening to Mothers*[11] highlighted how little women actually use alternative (i.e. not pharmacological) methods of pain relief, but how highly we rate them when we do. If you want to avoid medical intervention where possible, the trick is to try everything - properly - before you dismiss it as hippy nonsense. Our capacity for guilt and self-blame when it comes to childbirth is apparently boundless. If you've tried lots of ways to cope with the pain, and you fully understand the pros and cons of each choice you make, then you're more likely to be reconciled to events.

Pain relief tip:

Jenny Smith says, '*It's vital to practise these natural methods of pain relief (with your partner) BEFORE you go into labour, so you know how to do them – so they're second nature to you both – when you need them.*' You may, of course, feel absurd squatting in your loved one's arms breathing deeply while pretending to give birth but it's worth doing.

A WORD ABOUT THE PAIN RELIEF POLICE | There's a certain tyranny out there about pain relief - a knot of fervent birthers who'll give you the impression that it's somehow morally BAD to have an epidural or that you're a failure or 'not woman enough' if you turn to the anaesthetist. This is claptrap. Childbirth hurts. If it's hurting too much and nothing is working, you should surely not be suffering traumatic pain if you can do something about it.

No two labours are alike, and no woman can tell another what she should, and shouldn't do about hers. There is, however, certainly an argument that we're so woefully unprepared for handling the pain of normal childbirth that we panic when it hurts and think that drugs are the only option. Drugs are AN option. And thank the Lord they are. But they're not without their drawbacks, and they're certainly not your ONLY option. The best place to start, as always, is with the least risky approach to pain relief, working your way up a scale that runs from yogic chanting to general anaesthesia. This way, if someone suggests you are selfish, weak or ill-informed for having an epidural you can deck them there and then, with a clear conscience.

A WORD ABOUT TENS MACHINES | The 'transcutaneous electrical nerve stimulation' machine (you can hire one from Boots 0845 070 8090) fixes onto your back with sticky pads, and sends electrical pulses which stimulate the release of your body's natural painkillers (endorphins). This has no effect on the baby. It's most likely to help if you're having a long, slow early labour. Some women say it doesn't work well enough to make a difference, others say it was great – an early labour lifesaver. Studies into whether TENS really works have been inconclusive.

Most common forms of medical pain relief

1 **Pethidine:** a morphine-type drug injected in early labour to dull (but not eliminate) pain.
2 **Gas and air:** inhaled any time in labour to take edge off pain.
3 **Epidural:** anaesthesia injected by anaesthetist into your spine. Blocks pain.

Pethidine (or other opioids)

The most commonly used pain relieving injection for women in labour is pethidine. Pethidine is an opioid, a bit like morphine, and it sedates you (basically, so you care less about the pain). You may even go to sleep. It does, however, have well-documented adverse effects on babies. It crosses into the baby's bloodstream and can make a baby sleepy and slow to feed, which can be a genuine problem in the first few days. It can also give the baby breathing problems. A fair number of women say they hated pethidine – it made them throw up and feel sleepy and disorientated. Others say that feeling 'out of it' helped them through the long, painful early stage. One study in 1996[12] concluded that labour pain is not sensitive to injected morphine or pethidine and that the drugs only cause heavy sedation so shouldn't really be offered as pain relief to women in labour. You may, then, want to think about other forms of pain management (TENS, positions, breathing etc.) instead of pethidine.

N.B. Some hospitals use 'meptid' for this kind of injected analgesia because there is a lower incidence of respiratory problems in newborns. But this drug can also make you sick, sleepy and spaced out, as above.

Gas and air (Entonox)

This is a mixture of nitrous oxide and oxygen, inhaled through a mask or mouthpiece to take the edge off the pain. Many women find this a fantastic source of pain relief and some use only gas and air in labour. Rarely, it can make you a bit hysterical. But then again, so can childbirth. You can use it at any stage of labour, with any other form of pain relief. I had gas and air in the final stages of Ted's birth and though I don't think it made many inroads on the pain, the ritual of grabbing that mouthpiece and breathing deeply when it really hurt was amazingly helpful. There are no known adverse effects on you or the baby.

Epidurals

You've probably met women who grip your arm and hiss 'get an epidural' the minute they hear you're pregnant. This is understandable. Epidurals can be fantastic. But they are also linked to other – less fantastic – interventions. And you may not be able to get one the minute you want one. Understand the issues, here, and you will make real choices about pain relief, not pretend ones.

About a quarter of us will have an epidural. This can be genuine blessing – if the pain really becomes unmanageable, or if medical interventions are needed, or if your labour is long and arduous and you are exhausted. But an epidural is not without some drawbacks.

A recent study[13] examined eleven trials involving over 3,000 women and found that while epidurals provide better pain relief than non-epidural methods, they are associated with: longer first and second stages of labour, an increased incidence of fetal malposition (when the baby's head is not in the best position for birth) and an increased use of oxytocin (a drip to speed up or strengthen labour, which can lead to fetal distress which in turn can lead to other interventions to deliver the baby, including caesarean). An instrumental vaginal delivery (see above) is nearly twice as likely with an epidural. Of course, there is a bit of 'chicken and egg' going on here: it is hard to distinguish in studies whether the epidural itself actually caused these interventions or whether the labour itself was becoming complicated and therefore led to the need for stronger pain relief (and interventions to get the baby out). All doctors can really say for sure is that there is a 'link'. Studies have shown, incidentally, that having an epidural does not directly affect your chances of having a caesarean. Finally, women who have an epidural tend to report lower satisfaction levels with the birth, despite saying they had good pain relief.

How do epidurals work?

CONVENTIONAL EPIDURALS | The anaesthetist injects local anaesthetic (bupivacaine) through a tube that has been inserted into your lower spine. This completely removes all sensation from the lower part of your body: you are immobilised, and, once the anaesthetic takes hold – usually this takes about 15 minutes – you should feel no pain at all. The tube is left in your spine so that the anaesthetic can be 'topped up' (about every 90 minutes) by the midwife. Often, the midwife will allow the epidural to wear off when you reach the pushing stage, because this can help you push more effectively. For some women, this means being catapulted into pain again (how much pain will depend on how much of the epidural is allowed to wear off). You might want to discuss – before you go into labour – the advantages and disadvantages with your midwife of letting the epidural wear off for pushing. *'There is a fine balance when it comes to the pushing stage,'* says Jenny Smith. *'You certainly do not want the mother to feel acute pain but you do want her to feel pressure so that she can work out how to push effectively.'*

N.B. Some hospitals use a 'combined spinal' epidural, where the anaesthetist injects the anaesthetic directly into your spinal fluid. The resulting pain relief is the same, but it works more quickly (in about five minutes). You might be given this kind of epidural if you need one quickly (for instance, if you are going to have an emergency caesarean).

MOBILE EPIDURALS | Nowadays, most (though not all) hospitals offer 'mobile epidurals'. These combine a local anaesthetic with another pain-relieving drug called fentanyl. The addition of fentanyl means that you can have a lower dose of the numbing local anaesthetic. This 'low dose mixture' keeps you pain-free, but lets you move around much more than a conventional epidural. A mobile epidural can either be administered the same way as a conventional epidural, but using low dose mixture (this should take about 20 minutes to work), or it can be administered using a 'combined spinal epidural', where the anaesthetist injects the anaesthetic directly into your spinal fluid and at the same time puts in an epidural tube so you can have future top ups. This technique works in about five minutes and might be used if you need pain relief very quickly.

A mobile epidural lets you feel your legs, walk about, and feel the urge to push (all without pain if the epidural is not allowed to wear off). You may feel a tightening in your abdomen with each contraction, but it shouldn't hurt. The best thing about a mobile epidural is just what it says – you're mobile. You can therefore move, use gravity and positions that may keep labour progressing, and help you push the baby out more effectively. If you have a conventional epidural, you can't, for instance, squat to push, thereby using gravity in your favour. Having said this, if you need very frequent top ups of the mobile epidural to manage your pain, you may not be able to walk around, but you can still stay upright in a chair or on a birth stool for the pushing stage. Studies have found that having a mobile epidural means you are less likely to have an instrumental birth than you would if you had a conventional one. One major study[14] concluded that: *'The proven efficacy of mobile epidurals and their beneficial impact on delivery mode make them the preferred techniques for epidural pain relief in labor.'* Finally, if you have a mobile epidural you're more likely to feel in control, and less likely to feel like a 'patient': which is certainly going to help you to feel as if you are coping well with the birth. There are no special medical indications for whether you should have a mobile or a conventional epidural: the only question is, which kind does your hospital offer?

There are some other advantages for choosing a mobile epidural over a conventional one. With a conventional epidural you may need a urinary catheter, but with a mobile one you may be able to pee unaided (if you have a long labour with lots of top ups this might not be possible). With a conventional epidural, your baby's heart rate will be monitored continuously, using an EFM (see above page 160 for the pros and cons of this), but with a mobile one, you might only need to be monitored using an EFM intermittently. Again, this may reduce your chances of having further medical interventions.

SIDE-EFFECTS OF ALL EPIDURALS

1 **You might get localised backache** where the needle has been, which settles quickly. Studies have shown that long-term backache is no more common after epidural analgesia than after other forms of pain relief.

2 **You might get a persistent headache** after the birth. One per cent of women who have epidurals get this and need medical treatment for it.

3 **Your blood pressure may drop,** making you nauseated, dizzy or shaky. This may also cause changes to the baby's heart rate (which may lead to further medical interventions). These are less likely with a mobile epidural.

4 **You might shiver** (quite dramatically) as the epidural starts to work.

5 **You might itch,** if you have a mobile epidural. (This is a side-effect of the drug fentanyl.)

6 **You may face other medical interventions,** such as ventouse, forceps, episiotomy, to get the baby out.

What women say

Most women find their epidurals helpful, sometimes immensely so. But they may not always be quite as straightforward as you'd expect.

Julia experienced the simple good side of a conventional epidural with her first birth: *'I laboured for days and sobbed when the anaesthetist walked in. My midwife put her face to mine and said calmly: "Let it go." I ate, dozed and waited for Keaton to be born. I had no side-effects of the epidural and it was a very positive experience, completely blocking the pain.'*

Lissa, 35, mother of Phoebe (3) and Esme (1) had a mobile epidural with Phoebe: *'The pain, which was horrific even though I was only at 4 cm, just stopped. I could barely feel the contractions after that – just a faint tightening round my belly – and I could walk around normally. I even had a sleep, which was weird. I remember thinking "I'm supposed to be in labour, and I've just been asleep". When they let it wear off, for pushing, though, it was really tough: I was catapulted from nothing, into horrible pain and I pushed for two hours. This was a big shock.'*

On rare occasions, an epidural may go a bit wrong:

'I had two epidurals,' says Michelle, 30, mother of Joey (7) and Justin (4). 'The first one "missed" and I just felt a cold tingle. The second one took but I felt "shocky" and cold. I developed a whopper of a headache immediately. I was crying, shivering and eventually my blood pressure crashed. It was a nightmare. Everyone acts like the epidural is just what you do, but for me, it was the worst possible choice.'

Epidurals may not, then, be a simple matter of getting a needle in your spine and settling down with *Hello!* until the baby comes out. Perhaps the most important thing to remember, however, is that even if you decide you will 'definitely' have one, you will still need all the pain-relief methods you can learn because epidurals are not instant. If you go into labour spontaneously, you've got to get to the hospital and, once there, it can take a couple of hours for an anaesthetist to get to you. You need some coping mechanism while this is happening. You may also have a labour that is zipping along so fast that there is no time for an epidural.

An epidural may be your salvation. But don't rely on it alone to get you through the pain of giving birth.

Ten pain relieving positions

START HERE when labour starts to hurt
Don't get hung up on the small print here – they're just ideas. The basic rule is MOVE and STAY UPRIGHT. If nothing else, make this your mantra.

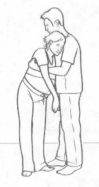

1 **WALK, STAND, LEAN** | Most doctors and midwives will want you to stay at home until your labour is really going (half an hour to an hour of contractions every 3–5 minutes lasting about a minute that you can't talk through). During this time it's a good idea to walk around. When you are walking, and a contraction comes, lean on your birth partner, who might naturally sway slightly during the contraction, inadvertently helping you to stay mobile. **Why do it?** You are using gravity, it helps if you are having a backache, it may make contractions more productive and it feels better than just standing. If you're hooked up to an EFM and need to be next to the bed, you can still lean on your partner during contractions.

2 **BOUNCE ON A BIRTH BALL** | A birth ball is just an oversized 'exercise' ball (available from shops like Argos or sports shops or some baby shops). Sitting still on one is virtually impossible. **Why do it?** Your gentle hip sway, bouncing up and down and just the act of holding yourself

on the ball all work with gravity to help keep your baby in a good position. You can also rest on your birth ball during labour: it will keep you moving very gently.

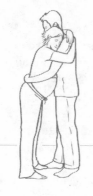

3   **SLOW DANCE** | Wrapping your arms around your partner's neck, rest your head on his chest or shoulder, his arms around your waist, fingers locked behind your back. It's like being 14 at the school disco all over again only this time your moans are more than teen anguish. If you have back pain, he can put pressure to the small of your back ('counter pressure') to relieve it. **Why do it?** All the advantages mentioned above, but the movement of your 'dance' also causes changes in your pelvic joints, encouraging the baby's rotation and descent. Being embraced by the bugger who got you into this mess may be comforting, and if you are listening to music you may also feel calmer.

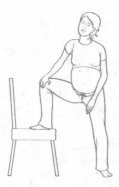

4   **LABOUR LUNGE** | Stand with a chair on one side of you. Put one foot on the chair seat, knee bent, and make gentle sideways lunges during a contraction – each lunge should last about five seconds. You should feel a stretch in your inner thighs. Lunge in the direction that is most comfortable, or in the direction your midwife recommends (depending on baby's position). Your birth partner can support the chair or you can put the chair against the wall to prevent it moving. This can also work on a hospital bed, if it lowers far enough. **Why do it?** It widens your pelvis and encourages your baby's head to get into a good position.

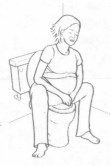

5   **SIT ON THE LOO** | Every good doula knows that an effective way to get a woman to push with gusto is to move her to the toilet. Your partner can also press on your lower back or rub your shoulders during contractions. **Why do it?** Gravity: this may help relax the perineum for a more effective pushing stage. Pooing or peeing while you are there may also help move your labour along, and will most certainly make you feel more comfortable; fear not, your midwife will make sure your baby isn't delivered into the toilet. There's also a kind of Pavlov's dog effect; you're used to 'letting go' here and if you're worried about pooing on the labour bed you may feel less inhibited. Finally, you may feel more private and safe in the loo.

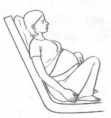

6   **SEMI-SITTING** | By turning the hospital bed into a 'chair' (the top portion all the way up) you can be upright but resting. **Why do it?** Better than lying on your back, this uses gravity, to some extent, and is an effortless position (doesn't require the muscles of the birth ball for instance) if you're knackered.

7   **ROCKING CHAIR** | Just rock yourself in an old fashioned rocking chair when you're having contractions. **Why do it?** Gravity again (you're fairly upright), plus many doulas think rocking speeds labour up. It keeps you moving while resting and the movement can be hugely comforting.

8   **LEAN FORWARD (STANDING OR KNEELING)** | Put the arms of the hospital bed up and the bed back up almost to the chair-like position. Put a birth ball, pillows, or bean bag on the bed. Kneel on the bed and during each contraction, fold your body over the birth ball (the bed can be made high or low to accommodate your height). **Why do it?** It can help backache – your partner can apply counter pressure during the contraction or just give a gentle backrub. You can do this with the ball/bean bag on the floor. You can also straddle a chair and lean on its back to get the same effect.

9   **HANDS AND KNEES** | Simply go down on your hands and knees, on a hospital bed if you want, with a towel under your hands if your wrists are sore. **Why do it?** It gives the baby more room and, if you are having 'back labour' (see page 162 above) this position may be your salvation. It can also be a good pushing position. N.B. *If you have high blood pressure your midwife may not recommend this, or she may just want to make sure you don't stay in that position for too long.*

10   **THE DOULA HULA** | This is simple: just a hip-swaying movement that many women instinctively do – whether sitting on a birth ball or standing – to cope with contractions. **Why do it?** Particularly with a squat, this can really open your pelvis and make room for baby to descend.

Three good positions for specific points in labour

1   **LYING ON YOUR SIDE** | Just lie on your left side as if you're curling up to sleep, supported by pillows or partner. **When?** It's a good resting position,

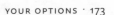

a good place to be while getting an epidural or a vaginal exam and a good pushing position. **Why do it?** It helps lower elevated blood pressure and can be used with an epidural. It takes the pressure off your pelvis without drastically slowing your labour down. In the pushing stage it can work the other way, and help slow things down a bit if things are moving too fast (this can help minimise tearing). Your partner can stand at your front and hold your leg up while you push.

2   SQUATTING | The word 'squats' may conjure up images of gruelling aerobic classes but fear not: squatting in labour can be done leaning (over the birth ball, bean bag, chair) supported in your partner's lap (birth partner sits in a straight-backed chair, you straddle them, arms round their neck, and allow your bum to dangle: great for a pushing stage) or between your partner's legs (your partner sits on a chair: you face away from him and dangle between his thighs into a fully supported squat. **When?** This is good for pushing, or getting ready to push.**Why do it?** It can help backache (it's making more room for baby to drop), uses gravity, widens your pelvis – helping many things, not least the often gargantuan effort of pushing. It may help the baby to descend in a difficult birth. It can bring on an urge to push and allows you to move too.

3   THE LABOUR BAR/SHEET/CHAIR | Your hospital may have a bar that hangs from the ceiling for you to grab while pushing, or an upside down 'u' shape that fastens onto the end of your bed. You grab it, pull it, and push your baby out. You may also move the bed to a sitting-up position, and put your feet up on the bar as counter resistance. You can also use a sheet, twisted like a rope: you sit on the bed and pull your end of the sheet, a sturdy person pulls back on the other end, and the effort somehow helps you push the baby out (this is how I pushed Sam out in my first vaginal birth – it felt very empowering). Ask your midwife about these techniques if she doesn't offer them up. Some hospitals now have birthing stools: an odd looking low plastic chair that allows you to lean, rest and be supported in just the right position for pushing the baby out. Ask your midwife if the hospital has these. **When:** pushing stage. **Why do it?** These positions and techniques can really help you push your baby out more effectively.

Breathing, relaxation and visualisation

These techniques should be a vital part of your pain relief armory. We cover them in Chapter 3: Fear and Pain. I'd say – and this still sounds as improbable to me as it may to you – that breathing and relaxation above anything else are what got me through the pain of Sam and Ted's births. Go back to Chapter 3, page 108 and practise these like a swotty schoolgirl hell bent on an A grade. They may not work for you, or work only for a while, but they're certainly worth knowing about.

Other labour options to consider

Food

If your birth will be in a hospital make sure you understand exactly what they will allow you to ingest and why. In the UK fewer than 5 per cent of hospitals have a policy of letting you eat and drink whatever you want in labour, because of fears of complications should you need general anaesthesia (which are rare). The evidence of this is controversial. And surveys have found that it goes against our instincts.[15] Graze – little and often – throughout labour if you feel like it. If you can't, prepare other ways to fuel yourself: take sports/energy drinks, wholemeal crackers if allowed, and fruit juice. If you go into labour slowly, at home, try eating light but slow-burning food (see below). This kind of food will give you sustained energy for the hours ahead.

Fuel tip:

Avoid sugary food or food made with refined white flour that will give you an energy rush, then a crash when you need it least. If you choose wholegrain foods they'll sustain you for longer. Things like wholemeal toast and marmite or if you feel like a meal, something like wholemeal pasta or a brown rice salad. But don't eat large meals (you might just throw up – your stomach does not have room for lots of food while those big contractions are going on).

Water

Drink it, lie down in it, run it over you, sit in it, think about it, spray it gently on your skin: in whatever way it is used, water can be a major source of comfort in labour. Research has confirmed that using a birthing pool can really help you cope with labour pain.[16]

IS IT SAFE? | You might balk at the idea of giving birth in tubs or pools, thinking it's the preserve of earth mothers and hippy chicks. It's not. When waterbirth was first popularised by Dr Michel Odent in the 1980s knives were drawn in the medical establishment, but the method is now supported (so long as proper precautions are taken) by both the Royal College of Obstetricians and Gynaecologists (RCOG) and the Royal College of Midwives (RCM). Around half of all our hospitals and maternity units currently offer waterbirth facilities (the ones that don't are generally hampered by hospital finance rather than medical reservations). This does not mean that half our infants are swimming into the world like Jacques Cousteau. Only 0.6 per cent of births in the most comprehensive study to date[17] actually occurred underwater (9 per cent of these were home births). Most women use the tub for pain relief during contractions then get out (or stand up) to actually deliver the baby. The main safety worry with water birth is that – rarely – a baby can gasp as it is born and inhale water into its lungs. Other possible 'risks' of water birth, according to the RCM, include unrealistic labour expectations, restricted mobility and infection. However, the RCM say: *'Women experiencing normal pregnancy, who choose to labour or deliver in water, should be given every opportunity and assistance to do so.'*[18]

A word of caution. Getting into a birth tub or deep bath and staying there from very early in labour may actually slow your contractions. A bath can help in the early stages, but it's probably not wise to stay in there forever unless it's helping your labour to genuinely progress. Most midwives say it's best to wait until you are having good, established contractions before getting into water. Your midwife should have the instincts and experience to know whether water is helping you or not, so trust her judgment on this one.

You can hire a birthing pool for home or hospital use. Talk to your midwife about bringing a hired birthing pool with you to hospital. Don't think this is extreme: many women do this (it cuts out the uncertainty about whether you'll get access to the hospital's only pool or not and maximises the chances that you'll be attended by a midwife who is experienced using water tubs). Try Splashdown Water Birth Services 020 8422 9308 www.waterbirth.co.uk or The Active Birth Centre 020 7281 6760 www.activebirthcentre.com

> **Where to go for help:**
> *The Use of Water in Labour and Birth* (RCM position paper 1a) is available online at www.rcm.org.uk
> *Labour and Birth in Water: How and Why You Might Use Water* (NCT 2002) is available from the NCT maternity sales 0870 112 1120.

Your labour; your way

You may want to give birth surrounded by a huge team of medical professionals or just a midwife. You may want jokes and rallying. Or you may want reverential darkness and aromatherapy oils. You may want to howl like a wolverine or sit in spooky silence. You may not know what you want until you get into labour. But the crucial thing is if you want to do it, do it (and get everyone else to respect your desire to do it). Julia says the women who have the best time are the ones who aren't afraid to do their own thing: *'One couple I had practised bible verses during labour. While she was pregnant he'd read scripture to her each night. In labour they did the same, and she seemed to be doing well. Then he went to the bathroom and she grabbed my arm and hissed "Get him out of here!" So I asked him to go and get his wife a sandwich. The woman dilated fully while he was gone, moaning in low, animalistic tones. Sometimes what we plan for is not what we need on the day.'*

> **COPING WITH CONTRACTIONS**
>
> Midwife Jenny Smith encourages her women to cope with contractions like this:
> - **Focus** when the contraction begins.

- **Breathe** deeply and slowly while it is happening, visualise your baby's head coming down.
- **Relax** your body as much as you possibly can while it is happening.
- **Release** when it is gone scan your body to be sure you have released all tension, let a long breath out.

Once the baby is out: your options in immediate postpartum

Managed third stage
In some hospitals it is routine to offer you an injection (usually of 'syntocinon' – the synthetic form of the hormone oxytocin; or 'syntometrine': a combination of the hormone oxytocin and the drug ergometrine) to help you deliver the placenta. This is to speed things up and minimise the risk of haemorrhage. There are pros and cons to this and it's a choice you can make, so do discuss it before the birth with your midwife.

Vitamin K
Extremely rarely, a newborn baby may start to bleed internally for no reason. Vitamin K given soon after birth stops this from happening. The Department of Health (DoH) says that vitamin K is not harmful, but some studies in the early 1990s raised concerns about a possible link between injected vitamin K and childhood cancer (these studies have not been confirmed). Some parents choose to give their baby vitamin K orally rather than by injection. Some parents avoid it entirely. Again, discuss it with your midwife before your baby emerges, when you are unlikely to be thinking clearly. There's a good DoH leaflet on vitamin K available from your midwife (*Vitamin K: Information for parents-to-be*) or www.doh.gov.uk or fax 01623 724 524.

Perineal tear: to stitch or not to stitch
If you have a minor tear because of a vaginal delivery you have a choice about whether or not to be stitched up. Some obstetricians assume that any tear must be stitched, but others believe that it is better to leave some tears to heal by themselves. You might want to discuss this with the midwife if you have a minor tear and she's wielding a needle.

Handling your new baby
You can make choices about whether:

- You'll be the first to hold or touch your baby (evidence shows that if possible, the best possible thing for a new baby – and you – is for the baby to be placed **skin to skin** on its mother).

- Whether you want to have your baby, skin to skin, **before** she's taken for a check over by the midwife (if she's healthy, all check-ups/weigh-ins/wiping off etc. can wait).
- Whether your partner will be the one to cut the umbilical cord.
- Whether you'll breastfeed straight away (when the baby's ready).

These are just things for you to discuss in advance.

FINALLY, A WORD ABOUT 'HIGH RISK' BIRTHS | If you're told you are 'high risk' (see Chapter 1, page 48), it's easy to feel your options shrink rapidly. Julia has seen many clients panic when they hear these words, and it's surprising how many people accept, but do not understand, the 'high risk' diagnosis. (See Chapter 2, page 56 for more on the 'high risk' diagnosis.)

- Get specific answers, and second opinions if necessary.
- Ask what exactly are the risks? What can I expect? What options do I have?

It's surprising how many people accept, but do not understand the 'high risk' diagnosis. You may still have many choices about how you give birth, even if you are 'high risk' in some way.

••

FIND OUT MORE

Comfort check list

Get your partner to use this when you are in labour
Have I tried:
- walking
- standing
- bouncing on my birth ball
- standing while leaning forward
- slow dancing
- labour lunges
- sitting with a straight back
- sitting on the toilet
- semi-sitting
- rocking
- leaning forward
- peeing
- the doula hula

- drinking water
- using water: shower, tub, cloth
- pampered extras: aromatherapy, massage, foot/hand rubs etc.
- eating/drinking for energy

Birth basics

There are many 'philosophies' of how you should give birth and you may want to explore them a bit. You should not assume that because a childbirth class, book or website tells you one way is best it will be best for **you** (or, indeed, achievable). Everyone out there seems to have their agenda about how you should give birth. We've got one too: we want you to give birth the way that's BEST FOR YOU. Your birth, then, may be a mixture of all sorts of approaches: you may be Hypnobirthing® one minute, active birthing the next, with a bit of yoga breathing or whatever, on the side. Only you will know what appeals to you.

NATIONAL CHILDBIRTH TRUST (NCT) CLASSES | Used by many first-time parents. Good at giving you an overview of issues and solid information, and for putting you in touch with other people in your area who are having babies. The classes are a way to help you make informed choices and aim for a positive birth – they're not an 'ethos' and your teacher should support you whatever and however you choose to give birth. **For more information:** The National Childbirth Trust, Alexandra House, Oldham Terrace, Acton, London W3 6NH. 0870 770 3236 Enquiry Line: 0870 444 8707 www.nctpregnancyandbabycare.com

HOSPITAL CLASSES | These can vary but tend to concentrate on basic medical information. Good for basics. Contact your hospital maternity unit.

BIRTHING FROM WITHIN | Again, a relatively new childbirth education programme that was devised by Pam England and Rob Horowitz and written up in their book *Birthing from Within: An Extraordinary Guide to Childbirth Preparation* (Partera Press, US, 1998). It does a lot of exploring feelings and often uses artwork as a medium to discover unconscious emotions and beliefs. This is one of the few classes which systematically addresses emotional as well as physical preparation. **For more information** on Birthing from Within go online to www.birthingfromwithin.com and click on the 'find a teacher near you' section.

HYPNOBIRTHING® | Hypnosis can help you overcome your birth fears, help you to cope with pain and build your confidence. It can also help you, on a practical level, to relax and stay calm during contractions. I did a Hypnobirthing® course (for a magazine article) when pregnant with Ted. There were claims in the literature that it could make my birth *pain free,* which frankly was codswallop in my case, although the relaxation and breathing certainly HELPED with the pain. I'd cautiously recommend Hypnobirthing®: a course will give you fantastic coping skills, but do beware of assuming it will lead you to a dream-like, swift, painless birth. Courses normally run over an intensive weekend, with resources – CD and book – to take home afterwards). **For more information:** www.HypnoBirthing.com

ACTIVE BIRTH | Created by author Janet Balaskas, who founded the Active Birth Centre in London. The basic idea here is solid and sensible: you can be an active participant if you are fully informed and have useful skills for coping in labour. They generally expect you to aim for a natural birth, with no unnecessary interventions. **For more information:** Active Birth Centre, 25 Bickerton Road, London N19 5JT. 020 7281 6760 www.activebirthcentre.com

Directory of alternative therapies

Aromatherapy Organisations Council Holds a database of fully registered, qualified and insured aromatherapists around the country. Some midwives now use aromatherapy for pain relief in labour and the promotion of good contractions. 0870 7743 477 www.aromatherapy-regulation.org.uk

Association of Reflexologists Reflexology is a treatment that uses massage to specific areas in the feet and hands to treat the body as a whole. It may help induce labour (and there are claims that it can help labour go smoothly too). 0870 5673320 www.aor.org.uk

You can also try the **British Reflexology Association** Tel: 01886 821207 www.britreflex.co.uk

British Acupuncture Council The UK's main regulatory body for the practice of acupuncture. Can provide a free list of qualified, registered acupuncturists in your area, plus a leaflet on acupuncture. A few areas of the UK – Oxfordshire for one – even have 'Acupuncture for Childbirth' Teams. Ask if there's one in your region. 020 8735 0400 www.acupuncture.org.uk

Society of Homeopaths Homeopathy is a therapeutic system which treats 'like with like' and claims to be helpful during labour (and afterwards). Online searchable register of qualified homeopaths, articles, and online leaflets. 0845 4506 611 www.homeopathy-soh.org

Also try the **British Homeopathic Association** 0870 444 3950 www.trusthomeopathy.org

The British Wheel of Yoga Yoga is thought to be a good exercise to prepare your body for birth, and also gives you good movement/breathing skills for coping with contractions. 01529 306 851 www.bwy.org.uk

General Osteopathic Council Can provide details of registered osteopaths. Osteopathy may help prepare your body for labour. 020 7357 6655 www.osteopathy.org.uk

The Hypnotherapy Association Professional organisation of psychotherapists using hypnotherapy to help people investigate and resolve their emotional problems. They should be able to put you in touch with hypnotherapists in your area who specialise in birth. 01257 262124 www.thehypnotherapyassociation. co.uk

Institute of Complementary Medicine Information on complementary medicine and can help you locate a reputable, registered practitioner. 020 7237 5165 www.icmedicine.co.uk

National Institute of Medical Herbalists Can help you to locate a qualified, registered herbalist near you. Some people say herbalists can help you go into labour, and labour effectively. 01392 426022 www.nimh.org.uk

Two more useful resources:

The Coalition for Improving Maternity Services This is worth a look. It's American, so not all issues will be familiar, but it includes 'Having a baby: 10 questions to ask' which you might find useful. www.motherfriendly.org

Disability, Pregnancy & Parenthood International A great resource for disabled parents and parents-to-be. National Centre for Disabled Parents Unit F9, 89-93 Fonthill Road, London N4 3JH Freephone: 0800 018 4730 www.dppi.org.uk.

Further reading

Pregnancy, Childbirth, and the Newborn, revised and updated: The Complete Guide by Penny Simkin, Janet Whalley, Ann Keppler (Meadowbrook Press, US, 2001).

Obstetric Myths Versus Research Realities: A Guide to the Medical Literature by Henci Goer (Greenwood, US, 1995)

The Thinking Woman's Guide to a Better Birth by Henci Goer (Perigee, US, 1999)

Birth Rights: A Guide to Getting the Best Possible Care for You and Your Child by Pat Thomas (The Women's Press, UK, 2002)

Am I Allowed? by Beverley Lawrence Beech (AIMS, 1991) This lays out your options and rights through all the stages of pregnancy and birth. Available from Association for Improvements in the Maternity Services (AIMS) Publications, Manor Barn, Thurloxton, Taunton, Somerset TA2 8RH or online from www.aims.org.uk.

Keep looking

Your specific issues may not be covered here, or not in enough detail, so it's up to you to keep researching. You can often borrow books from local branches of the NCT or from NCT teachers (Local contact details can often be found in local telephone directories or from the national NCT enquiry line on 0807 444 8707). It's worth checking out the **Midwives Information and Resource Service: MIDIRS,** 9 Elmdale Rd, Clifton, Bristol, BS8 1SL Tel: 0800 581 009, which has a range of 'informed choice' leaflets, also available online at www.infochoice.org. And the Association for Improvements in the Maternity Services (AIMS) is another good resource for a vast range of maternity issues: try their website www.aims.org.uk or call: AIMS Helpline 0870 765 1433.

Chapter Six: Surgical birth

'I never thought I'd have a caesarean.
I thought it was something that happened
to other women, the sort who had
"complications". It was profoundly shocking
to me and I still don't understand why
it happened.'

CLARA, 36, MOTHER OF TAMSIN (7) AND GRADY (2).

'My caesarean was a blessing. I thought
my baby was going to die. The operation
saved him and I will always be thankful
for that.'

DANA, 29, MOTHER OF RAOUL (6 MONTHS).

1   **It's not just for the person sitting next to you in your childbirth class:** it's for you. All pregnant women should know about caesareans whether they think they're low risk or not. You need information, information, information – about all aspects of birth.

2   **An unplanned caesarean that you are unprepared for can be hard to handle** – physically and emotionally.

3   **You may not be fully informed:** your doctor, midwife or childbirth teacher may not have talked about many of the issues we cover here.

4   **You are having a planned caesarean.** You might think that because your caesarean is scheduled you won't need support, postpartum information or to consider what the surgery itself will be like. But knowing about these things can make a huge difference to this birth, your recovery and to any future experience of birth you might have.

5   **Your partner may not understand caesareans,** so you need to highlight the important parts and make sure he understands what to expect and how to help you.

6   **A caesarean is a birth, not just an operation:** this chapter will show you how to make it a positive experience, not just a clinical (or possibly scary) one.

SIX COMMON CAESAREAN MYTHS

1   It's safer for you than vaginal birth
2   It's easier than vaginal birth because you don't have to push a baby out
3   It will stop you being incontinent later in life
4   It's the only safe option if you've had one caesarean already
5   Most caesareans are a genuine emergency
6   Most women who choose caesarean do so because they're 'too posh to push'

The reality of a caesarean

If you are considering skipping this chapter, don't. You may feel perfectly healthy. Your pregnancy may have been utterly straightforward. You may see no reason why anything should go amiss in the birth. But you still have, statistically, almost a one in four chance of greeting your baby for the first time on the operating table.

I am a classic first-time caesarean mother. After a healthy pregnancy, I went into labour on my due date. I spent a long day in pain on hands and knees in a soulless, brightly lit hospital room and by the end of it I was exhausted. My cervix had not dilated any further than 4 cm. I'd had nothing to eat or drink for 16 hours and no sleep the previous night (I was too excited when I realized I was going into labour, to lie down and even rest). So I had an epidural and the midwife broke my waters to try and 'speed things up'. I was then given a syntocinon drip to strengthen my contractions. Eventually, after several more internal examinations by a series of complete strangers, I was advised to have a caesarean. I was wheeled into surgery and, bulldozed by medication, my shell-shocked husband next to me in a mask and gown, I had my operation. I remember thinking, clearly, when I held Izzie the next day: 'I have a baby, but I don't know what it's like to give birth.' Of course I **did** know what it's like to give birth: after all, this is how 22 per cent of British women do it these days.

The emotional fall out was what surprised me most. Like around half of first-time caesarean mothers, the three-word reason I was given for my operation was '*failure to progress*'. In the months after the surgery the word 'failure' stuck. I began to feel I'd somehow chickened out of giving birth properly, that I'd missed some important 'rite of passage' by not pushing out my baby and even – weirdly – that I'd disappointed my husband (who in reality didn't give a damn how our daughter got out as long as we were both safe). Nobody was more surprised than me about all this. Before having Izzie, I'd thought caesareans sounded like a good idea – pain-free, private parts intact, all nice and safe and time-limited and under control. My post-caesarean emotions seemed to me, at times, hysterical and silly not least because I didn't **believe** any of these things rationally. But I couldn't stop feeling this way.

In the months afterwards, in an attempt to pull myself together, I began to do some reading. Despite my antenatal yoga, childbirth classes, and diligent reading of *What to Expect When You're Expecting*, I'd managed not to **really** understand that walking around, resting or eating and drinking in early labour can help your contractions get going. I didn't know that my fears about labour (and they were big) might possibly get in the way of how my labour progressed. I didn't know the basics about any of the things I agreed to: and above all I didn't have any idea that a caesarean was a realistic possibility **whatever I did right** in my birth preparations, and in the labour itself. Consequently, I was totally unprepared for surgery: my childbirth teacher never discussed caesareans in any detail (even though, in the end, half of our group ended up with one) and it genuinely never occurred to me that I'd give birth that way.

I'm actually very lucky. My caesarean wasn't traumatic. I was never seriously worried for my baby, I didn't have to have any other major interventions first, like ventouse or forceps; the doctors were kind, I had pain relief early on and my recovery was OK. But to say the experience was 'easy' would be a lie. It was disempowering, scary and undermining – largely (I think) because I was totally unprepared for it.

A caesarean can be a perfectly manageable experience and, as obstetrician Michel Odent writes in his book *The Caesarean*[1], it really can be a 'magnificent rescue operation'. Women who feel fully informed and in control while this is going on generally don't have a problem afterwards. '*I'd planned a home water* birth,' says Dea, 38, mother of Scarlett (4), *'but she became distressed and I was transferred to hospital. There was no doubt for me that this was the right thing. Every step was explained to me, and I was consulted the whole way. I was just relieved, in the end, that she was safe. I stayed calm during the whole thing and I never felt bad about what had happened afterwards.'*

A caesarean can also be a blessing if you have been genuinely traumatised by a bad experience of a previous birth. Jennifer, mother of Miles (5) and Louise (2) says *'Miles' birth was a nightmare. He ended up in intensive care and I was traumatised by the whole thing. This time I just wanted them to extract a healthy child from me in a safe, medical environment whatever that took.'* She got an epidural early on, felt in control throughout the labour, and the caesarean she ended up with was, she says 'empowering'.

Giving 'birth from above' is, then, neither inherently bad nor good. But it should certainly be something that every pregnant woman thinks and learns about – before she goes into labour. Caesareans carry certain risks and you should understand these **before** you are offered one. There are also many ways to minimise your chances of giving birth by caesarean. Should you have one – and you might well - you should know that there are ways for you to make your operation feel more like a birth; there are ways to make it calmer, more joyful, less scary and clinical. This should help not only your own recovery, but your ability to bond with your baby and move on into motherhood totally reconciled to what happened.

What's all the fuss about?

Caesareans are becoming increasingly common. These days most major health bodies, including the World Health Organization (WHO), are trying to reverse this trend. The WHO recommends that no more than 15 per cent of births should be by caesarean because of the unnecessary risks it can pose to both mother and baby. But the numbers keep rising. In the UK you are now five times more likely to have your baby surgically than you were in 1970 (around 24 per cent of first births are now by caesarean).

Your chances of giving birth surgically depend on tons of factors, not all of which will be obstetric. One is where you live. According to NHS statistics[2] some maternity units have a caesarean rate lower than 5 per cent, while others perform the operation on over 30 per cent of mothers. Some of this may be down to what kind of hospital yours is (a large regional unit that takes special cases may have a high surgical birth rate because it sees more mothers with complications). But equally some of this may be down to a more 'interventionist' ethos. There is certainly an increasing fear, among medical professionals, of litigation: if something goes wrong with a vaginal birth you don't want to get sued, so you'll operate 'just in case'. In other words, the reasons why a caesarean might be performed are not always straightforward or obvious.

WHAT ARE THE RISKS OF CAESAREANS?

A caesarean is major abdominal surgery, whether it's planned or not: in fact, it's actually more risky – for you – than giving birth vaginally.

- **Caesareans tend to involve more blood loss** than a vaginal birth.

- **There is a higher risk of thrombosis** (the leading cause of maternal death in the UK) than there would be in a normal vaginal birth.

- **Other possible complications include** transfusions, bladder and bowel injury, anesthesia complications and a very slightly increased risk of hysterectomy (these risks will be higher if you have any existing medical complications, and lower if you are perfectly healthy).

- **There is a risk of re-hospitalisation due to surgical complications.** About 2–3 per cent of women overall experience medical complications that require hospital treatment more than two to three days after the operation (the risks are higher if you have an emergency caesarean, lower if your caesarean is planned).

- **A caesarean increases your risk of having serious complications in subsequent pregnancies** such as problems with the placenta (e.g. placenta praevia and placenta accretia).

- **You can also get complications from scar tissue adhesions** which include pelvic pain and bowel problems (then again, a vaginal birth can leave you pretty painful down there too).

- **Your odds of having a future miscarriage** may also rise when you have had a caesarean.

- **You are more likely to suffer from infertility** when you next want a child ('secondary infertility').

- **Babies born by caesarean** (almost always when it is an elective caesarean) are more likely to suffer from respiratory problems.

- **A tiny proportion of caesarean-born babies will be cut** or nicked by the surgeon's knife during the birth.

- Having a caesarean **can make breastfeeding harder to establish** (it can reduce your chances by about a third).

Clearly, virtually every woman would be prepared to risk all of these things if it meant saving her baby.

A WORD ABOUT EXTREME RISKS | Whether or not you are more likely actually to die during a caesarean is debatable. The International Cesarean Awareness Network (ICAN) says that you are two to four times more likely to die during a caesarean than a vaginal birth. However, the Confidential Enquiry into Maternal and Child Health, which looks at the reasons for maternal death in this country does not list caesarean section as a risk factor. Basically, it's a complicated issue because it's hard to disentangle the effect of the operations from the reasons for it. Perhaps all you need to know is that the risk of you dying – whatever way you give birth – is absolutely minute in Britain today.

Emotional fall out

The emotional after effects are rarely talked about, in childbirth classes, with other caesarean mothers, or really at any point after the event. Friends or family can be reluctant to engage in your emotions, feeling understandably that the only thing that matters is that 'you and the baby [or babies] are OK'. Your partner may genuinely not understand what you are going on about, for the same reason. Of course having a healthy baby **is the most important thing of all**. No birth 'experience' could possibly matter more than this. But this doesn't mean you're not *feeling* some other stuff. It can be distinctly isolating to be told that what's upsetting you is selfish, irrelevant nonsense.

This gets worse if you are genuinely traumatised by your caesarean. Caesarean birth (like traumatic vaginal birth) has been linked to post traumatic stress disorder and postnatal depression: some women report feeling 'violated' by their operation, others – many of whom encountered frightening, emergency situations – will have flashbacks, panic attacks and nightmares long after the event. Women who have had a caesarean (particularly an emergency one) can be very frightened of giving birth again and this is something that many medical professionals don't fully acknowledge.

> **Where to go for help:**
> If you feel traumatised or panicky because of a past caesarean you need to get help and support from professionals. Start by talking to your midwife or GP and asking for help. You can also try these support groups:
> **International Cesarean Awareness Network:** www.ican-online.org
> **Birth Crisis:** an organisation set up by childbirth educator Sheila Kitzinger which offers support to women who have had traumatic or difficult birth experiences. Helplines: 01865 300 266/ 0207 485 4725/ 01380 720746/01454 299449

What actually happens in a caesarean?

Yes, this section is for you: don't skip the description below out of squeamishness or fear. It is far better to have an idea, in advance, of what could happen, than to be shocked and upset by it if it does. (Even if you don't have a caesarean, someone you know might.)

What happens during a caesarean will depend on why you are having one. Some caesareans are planned – you are usually asked to go into the hospital in the morning, and are not allowed to eat and drink for 12 hours before the operation. Unplanned caesareans, on the other hand, may feel more panicky. Some – if you do not have an epidural already in place and need to get the baby out immediately – will involve a general anaesthetic (this is relatively rare). Others, though they happen in labour, are not really an emergency, and there'll be time for you to have a spinal anaesthesia (this is like an epidural) before you go in. In most caesareans, there's a bit of a run up as interventions begin and the baby begins to look distressed. Most women, by the time they get to the caesarean stage, have already been given an epidural, which then just needs 'topping up'.

Whatever the circumstances, when it becomes clear that you are going to give birth surgically, you'll be asked to sign a consent form. The top part of your pubic hair will be shaved. An intravenous drip and a catheter will be inserted (your bladder needs to stay empty). Your blood pressure will be monitored with a cuff on your arm. Your jewellery (except your wedding ring, which will be taped down) will be removed. Your nail varnish will be taken off. If you already have an epidural in, the dose will be increased so you are completely numbed from the waist down. If not, you'll be given spinal anaesthesia and when the anaesthetic is fully working, the surgeon will paint your abdomen with antiseptic. You'll be shielded from seeing anything by a kind of screen that starts at your chest.

Your partner will usually be allowed in with you, wearing scrubs. Some surgeons might allow a doula, or another female birth partner, to come in too (the only issue, really, is space). If you know in advance that you're having a caesarean, this is something you may want to request and negotiate about. You can also put in your birth plan that you strongly want both the baby's father and a female birth partner in surgery with you (see Chapter 9 page 266 for why you might want a female birth partner too). They won't have to see anything gory (they'll be standing at your head).

The surgeon will make an incision – which you definitely should not feel – and the birth begins. Mostly, you'll feel tugging and pulling and pressure. This doesn't hurt. But it can be surprisingly weird and uncomfortable. Some people describe it as 'someone doing the washing up in your abdomen'. Not a nice idea, but you get the picture: there's lots of disturbing rummaging. This is when you need your relaxation/visualisation techniques for distraction and calmness.

Your baby will be lifted out – and, in most cases, you can see and touch her right then (the surgeon can drop the screen so you actually see her being born if you want). If she is in good shape you should ask for her to be placed on your chest – skin to skin – as soon as she is out. There is usually no reason why this can't happen (though the staff may not be used to this request). A paediatrician will only be in the room if the doctors know there may be a problem with the baby. When you are ready (unless it's an emergency), your baby will be taken to a corner of the room to be checked over. If she needs more help – oxygen or resuscitation, you won't be able to hold or touch her first. Her APGAR scores will be taken (see Chapter 2, page 75). Then she'll usually be wrapped up, and given to your husband to hold as you'll still be on the operating table, and at least one of your arms may be immobilised by your drip. (See below for better ways to have contact with your new baby.)

Repairing your womb and abdomen (these are both stitched up, one then the other) takes about 30 minutes. After this, you and your baby will be wheeled into the 'recovery room'.

A WORD ABOUT ANAESTHETISTS | The anaesthetist can be your greatest source of comfort and reassurance in a surgical birth and will talk you through the process when it's happening. Mine talked calmly to me throughout my caesarean, and made a vast difference to what was, for a hospital-phobe like me, an essentially terrifying experience. Of course, you can't choose your anaesthetist but if he or she is reticent, ASK for reassurance and information. Most will be glad to give it to you.

Watching your surgeon tip:

When the surgeon was rummaging about, I was freaked out to see sweat on her forehead, assuming (in some horror) that it was because of the physical effort of opening my womb and pulling out my baby. This is not the case. Your surgeon may perspire but not because of the physical strain: the operating theatre is hot, the plastic aprons they wear under gowns are hotter, and the longer they are in the room the more they will sweat.

The necessary caesarean

Clearly all of this messy stuff – physical and emotional – is worth it if your baby's life (or your own) is at stake. Absolute indications for having a caesarean are really quite rare, but they certainly do exist.

What are definite reasons to have a caesarean?

Usually pre-labour:
- **Placenta praevia** (where, in late pregnancy, the placenta is blocking or partially covering the cervix, so the baby can't get out) or other serious problems with the placenta.
- **A 'transverse' lie** (i.e. the baby lying sideways in your womb).
- When the baby is in **any other bad position** for birth e.g. breech.
- **Eclampsia** or severe pre-eclampsia (if induction is risky).
- True **cephalopelvic disproportion** (where the baby's head is too big to fit through your pelvis – very rare).
- When there are problems with your baby's health; for instance your **baby is not growing properly**.

- **Genuine emotional reasons:** a traumatic first birth or unresolved sexual abuse may both make you want a caesarean. If counselling and support are not working for you, a caesarean might, indeed, be the right choice for you.

Usually in labour:
- **A prolapsed cord** where the umbilical cord begins to drop down through your cervix, into your vagina.
- First ever outbreak of active **herpes** at the onset of labour
- True **fetal distress**
- **Uterine rupture** (when a scar from a previous operation, or simply the womb, begins to come apart – again, very rare).

The grey areas
Here are some reasons that are often given for caesareans, which may not be straightforward.

LABOUR NOT PROGRESSING/BABY IN WRONG POSITION | About half of all first caesareans are performed because of 'dystocia' – this means either labour stops progressing, or the baby seems to be 'stuck' in some way. The most common reason for this is that the baby – though he is lying head down – is still in the wrong position for birth (see Chapter 5, Your Baby's Position, page 151). If the wider part of the baby's head enters your pelvis first, this part of the baby's head does not press down efficiently on your cervix to dilate it with each contraction of your womb. The upshot is that although you are getting strong, painful contractions your cervix dilates unevenly and very slowly.

When this happens, and the baby does not shift into the right position (a baby can turn at any time in labour), it's common for a 'cascade' of medical interventions to ensue. The baby can then become 'distressed' and – ultimately – you end up with a caesarean. Many childbirth experts believe that if our births were managed in a more 'woman-centred way' (where we feel safe and confident rather than scared or panicky, and where we keep moving, upright, hydrated and supported during the course of labour) the incidences of caesarean for 'dystocia' would decline.

Here are some things you can do to minimise (though by no means eliminate) your chances of having a caesarean for dystocia:

- **Fetal positioning during your pregnancy**: the way you sit and move in pregnancy may help get your baby into a good position. See Chapter 5: Your Options, page 152.

- **Moving and staying upright in labour**: this can help your baby descend and your cervix to open.

- **Conquering your fears and staying relaxed** (see Chapter 4: Fear and Pain).

- **Having a female birth partner**: for encouragement, reassurance and to keep you moving and upright (you might forget if left to your own devices). See Chapter 9.

Second timers' tip:
It is much more common for the head of your first baby to be in a difficult position for birth, than it is for subsequent ones. If you had a caesarean for 'dystocia' first time around, you are very likely to give birth vaginally next time.

> **Where to go for help:**
> *The Labor Progress Handbook* by Penny Simkin ed. (Blackwell Science, UK, 2000)
> While a bit technical, this book will tell you all you need to know about dystocia.

BABY'S HEAD TOO BIG | Although a fairly common reason given for a caesarean, 'cephalopelvic disproportion' is actually an extremely rare condition in the UK and is usually associated with a pelvic deformity or an incorrectly healed pelvic break.

BABY TOO BIG ALL OVER (MACROSOMIA) | It is actually unusual for a woman to grow a baby that is genuinely too big for her body to push out. And the way that doctors can estimate a baby's weight is very inaccurate (see Chapter 1, Fear of having a big baby page 36). *'I have seen several cases in which women choose to have a caesarean with no trial of labour because they are told the baby is big,'* says Deanna, a doula. *'I've heard things such as "My baby was over 9lbs so there was NO WAY I could have had her naturally if I had tried". But I have seen many babies, way over 9lb, born with no complications.'*

PROLONGED SECOND STAGE | Sometimes women are hurried through labour because of hospital protocols that dictate that you should dilate at 1 cm per hour and not push for more than one hour. The main reason for limiting your active pushing stage is that your baby's condition can deteriorate if pushing is not going well. For ways to help your pushing stage, see Chapter 5: Your Options, page 171. Many doctors and midwives say it is actually less traumatic to have a caesarean if the baby genuinely is 'stuck', than to have a difficult instrumental birth.

A PREVIOUS CAESAREAN | We talk about vaginal birth after caesarean (VBAC) below; see page 204.

Why NOT to debate these grey areas during labour
The labour room is NOT the place to start debating these issues with doctors and midwives. Once you are in labour, have chosen your hospital, your midwives and your birth partner(s); once you've made out your birth plan and understood the basic risks and benefits of various procedures you should never find yourself

arguing between contractions over whether or not you are experiencing true dystocia, or whether your baby's head is, really, disproportionate to your pelvis. Ultimately, you have to do all you can to minimise your chances of having an unnecessary caesarean, then **trust your health care team** to keep you fully informed and consulted. You can certainly ask questions, or negotiate on certain points. But if you are being told categorically by an obstetrician that your baby will be damaged if you don't have surgery – and you are given good solid medical reasons why this is the case – then you really do have to **take their word for it.** Caesareans are not necessarily 'traumatic'. And doctors are not evil monsters lurking with scalpels to get you when you're vulnerable. Indeed, obstetricians don't want to see you in surgery unless you really need to be there.

A WORD ABOUT TWINS | Having twins certainly increases your chances of having a caesarean, but in itself it is not a reason to schedule one. 'Multiple pregnancy' is the primary reason behind 1 per cent of caesarean sections and, overall, 59 per cent of twin pregnancies are delivered by caesarean (37 per cent elective and 63 per cent emergency). Having a caesarean to deliver the second twin after giving birth to the first baby vaginally happens in 3.5 per cent of twin births.[3] However, a normal twin pregnancy – that is, one where the babies are healthy and the first twin is head down (cephalic) – is not in itself a reason to schedule the operation. The National Institute of Clinical Excellence (NICE) Guideline on caesarean section (CS) says that in otherwise uncomplicated twin pregnancies there is always a slightly increased risk to the second twin at birth. But *'the effect of planned CS in improving outcome for the second twin remains uncertain and therefore CS should not routinely be offered'*.[4] If you are having identical twins, however, the obstetrician might advise you to have a caesarean because your twins share a blood supply through the one placenta. Discuss the risks and benefits with your obstetrician before you make any decisions, and don't be bullied into something you are not comfortable with. Keep asking questions until you feel happy with any decisions you have to make.

TEN WAYS TO AVOID AN UNNECESSARY CAESAREAN

Many caesareans are unavoidable, for many different reasons. But there is much you can do to maximise your chances of having an uncomplicated vaginal birth.

1   **Read and educate yourself:** make sure you understand the process of birth, how you can influence the position of your baby and what the risks and benefits of routine and emergency procedures are. Start with Chapter 5: Your Options.

2   **Understand your birthplace/midwife/doctor fully:** understand the unit's caesarean rate and any policies they have about how long you are allowed to labour for without interventions.

3   **Write a detailed, meaningful birth plan** in consultation with your midwife (See Chapter 7: Expect the Unexpected for how to do this).

4   **Talk to your midwife/childbirth group about your fears** in advance, or, if you find talking too difficult, work through these fears using Chapter 4: Fear and Pain so that you are as relaxed and confident as possible during labour.

5   **Have a female companion in labour:** studies have shown that continuous emotional support from a woman reduces your chances of having a caesarean (see Chapter 9: The Love of a Good Woman).

6   **Stay at home as long as possible** when labour starts. Walk around in early labour and change positions frequently. Eat and drink lightly, if you feel like it. When you get to hospital, if the midwife says you are still in the early stages of labour, walk around the hospital or go home and rest.

7   **Try to stay healthy,** well-fed and rested during pregnancy so your baby and your body are in good shape for birth

8   **Be aware that having labour induced** increases your chance of caesarean section – particularly in a first labour.

9   **Request intermittent electronic fetal monitoring (EFM)** or the use of a hand-held monitor, unless there are specific medical reasons to have continuous EFM (for instance, meconium in the waters, an epidural or a syntocinon drip). Research has shown that continuous EFM may increase the risk of caesarean but does not actually improve the outcome for you or the baby if you are 'low risk'. (See Chapter 5: Your Options, page 160)

10 **If your baby is breech,** ask your midwife or doctor about ways to turn the baby (see Chapter 5: Your Options, page 152).

The elective caesarean

More of us are asking for caesareans than ever before. Doctors put the rise in 'elective caesareans' down to anything from an increased fear of birth to our modern obsession with celebrities: *'It has become a sexy operation,'* obstetrician Yehudi Gordon, known for his natural approach to childbirth, once told me in an interview. *'People see celebrities like Liz Hurley or Victoria Beckham having planned caesareans and think it must be the best option.'* 'Too posh to push' makes great copy, but it's not the reality for most women who elect to have a surgical birth. Most do so because of medical reasons, after discussions with midwives and obstetricians and usually after quite a bit of soul-searching.

Medical reasons to plan a caesarean

There is no complete consensus among obstetricians about absolute indications for having a planned caesarean. This means that if a planned caesarean is mentioned to you, it's important to discuss the subject fully with your doctor and midwife. Before you agree to the surgery, make sure that you have fully understood:

1 What exactly the condition is that means you should have one.
2 What the risks and benefits are if you don't have one.
3 What the risks and benefits are if you do have one.
4 What you can do if the situation changes.

If you don't feel happy after these discussions, it is fine to ask for a second opinion, and, if you are tactful about doing this, your doctor should not be offended.

The myth of 'informed consent'

In theory, 'informed consent' means you have surveyed all the available information, talked to people in the know, explored your options and made up your mind to have the caesarean (without pressure). Many doctors are very careful about this. But some are more fixed in their views. In practice, informed consent may mean you are informed by one doctor who has given you the information *they* want you to have but it may not be the full picture. You then consent, thinking you know all sides, but with a gnawing sense of doubt (or regret) in your gut about what you have agreed to do.

True informed consent involves:

* questions answered
* emotions explored
* a sense of resolution

If you don't get the resolution you need, ask for a second opinion. Bear this in mind when discussing whether to schedule a caesarean.

Emotional reasons for a planned caesarean

There's a lot of talk these days about the modern woman wanting to schedule the baby's arrival around her board meetings, or hair appointments or something. This is largely a media fantasy. Currently only 7 per cent of caesareans in England and Wales are carried out because of maternal request alone[5]. As one midwifery text book[6] puts it: *'There is much evidence to support the fact that very few women actually request caesarean section in the absence of medical indications.'*

Most women who request caesareans, when they are not medically indicated, do so for powerful emotional reasons (often fear-related) that might stem from things like past sexual abuse or a previously traumatic vaginal birth. Studies have shown that if women requesting caesareans because they are afraid of vaginal birth are given proper counselling, they are likely to withdraw their request.

Some women feel they might prefer a caesarean because they are reluctant to subject their vaginas to the stretching necessary to get a baby out. The truth is that every woman is different. But normal vaginal birth is unlikely to leave you permanently damaged, particularly if you do your pelvic floor exercises afterwards (see Chapter One, page 30). Vaginas are made to stretch and contract again and most of us do not feel we've permanently stretched out of all proportion after giving birth. Women also say things like 'a caesarean will stop me being an incontinent old lady'. This isn't strictly true either. Studies have shown that caesarean birth will not necessarily protect you from incontinence pants later in life because pregnancy alone can weaken your pelvic floor. Pelvic floor exercises, done regularly for the rest of your life, are the best way to reduce your chances of incontinence.

If you *are* considering a caesarean for non-medical reasons, don't beat yourself up about it. But do talk it over fully with your midwife or obstetrician and if your fears are driving you towards that scalpel, consider asking for a referral to a counsellor. You may end up feeling that you still want the caesarean, and **this may indeed be best for you**. But you do want to be informed, reconciled and ready for it.

Planned caesarean tips:

Try and make it feel like a birth. If your caesarean is planned, you may be in an even better position to make it feel more like a 'birth' than a scary operation (see below).

Beware waiting times: *'Be prepared for a long wait!'* says Astrid, 38, mother of three caesarean-born children. *'I was told to come in at 7 a.m. on the day of my caesarean, having consumed nothing for 12 hours beforehand. I didn't get into the operating theatre until 5 p.m. that day (still with no food or drink). It was nerve-wracking. Because you're not the emergency, if it's a busy day you're going to be bumped down the list repeatedly. Bring plenty of distractions: magazines, books, games to play with your husband – anything that'll take your mind off your situation. And be mentally prepared for a long wait. The worst thing is the expectation.'*

Prepare your partner. Don't make the mistake of thinking that because it's a planned 'operation' you won't need support. There are quite specific things your partner can do during a caesarean, and he needs to know about them, and to understand caesareans so he's not freaked out. Get him to read this chapter.

If you were considering having a female birth partner too, she can still be a huge help (see Chapter 9: The Love of a Good Woman) but you may have to negotiate with your obstetrician about whether she'll be allowed in. Do this in advance (see Julia's story below).

If possible, make sure that you are more than 39 weeks pregnant: the likelihood of your baby having breathing problems after a caesarean is higher if you are less than 39 weeks pregnant.

Talk to an anaesthetist: you might get the chance to meet an anaesthetist at your pre-booking appointment so use this to build up a picture of what the operation will be like: ask lots of questions, no matter how silly they may be.

How to make your caesarean a birth

On the wall of the maternity unit at Queen Charlotte's hospital in London are black and white pictures of a caesarean birth. In one, the mother, baby and partner are snuggled together in a blissful moment: the baby is lying on the mother, skin on skin, their heads are all close together, marvelling at each other. Behind this beautiful image you can just see the surgeons, finishing up the operation. This is how caesarean birth can be – if it is handled well.

One of the most disturbing things about a surgical birth is how clinical the whole thing can feel. Lying immobilised on a trolley, awake, while surgeons operated on me certainly put me *way* beyond my comfort zone – and I'm sure these feelings contributed to my sense that I'd undergone an operation, rather than a birth. Of course, if you are being rushed in during a dire emergency, you're not going to be caring about aromatherapy but there are many simple things you can do to make your caesarean feel like a birth. You can also ensure that you don't feel like an inanimate object, being unzipped, and having the baby 'extracted'. This is your body and your baby's birth. You can 'normalise' it, even in the most 'abnormal' circumstances.

Julia was once hired for a planned caesarean:

'Melinda's baby was breech so she planned a caesarean. She then hired me. We used my 2–3 pregnancy visits to talk about caesareans and she did a lot of on-line research into surgical birth. We all met early in the morning at the hospital. She was very nervous. It can be very unsettling to get into a hospital bed, have physical exams, an epidural and an IV put in when you are a healthy person. I spoke reassuringly to her while this was going on. Many women are also terrified that the epidural won't work and they'll feel something. Throughout the operation my head was near hers, reassuring her, until she asked me to take photos. My role in making it a birth was simple: I called it a BIRTH about a million times and I told Melinda again and again how well she was doing (she used her relaxation techniques to calm herself). Together we normalised that birth. Melinda asked to have the baby put on her chest, and then kept him with her constantly – he was totally healthy so this wasn't a problem. After a caesarean, many women feel upset by things that are, in fact, normal parts of surgical birth. If those women had known about caesareans, they wouldn't have been so shocked at the procedure. This – the physical reality of being operated on – is a big part of post-caesarean distress for many women. If a pregnant woman educates herself on all forms of birth then she'll know what to expect from, and hopefully how to get, a fantastic caesarean birth.'

WHY BOTHER? | The main reason is that a negative caesarean experience can affect mother-baby bonding. Most people would say that just getting the baby out is all that matters when it comes to surgical birth, and sometimes there just isn't the time, or opportunity to make the experience more positive for the mother. Clearly safe baby, safe mother is the number one priority. But a caesarean is not always, by any means, an 'emergency', even when it is done during labour. As midwife Jenny Smith says, *'Part of the problem is that when things do go amiss, the birth quickly becomes a medical procedure. Many women say to me that in those first few days after the surgery they felt somewhat unconnected to their baby. This can be very damaging.'*

This emotional fallout can also affect your confidence in your body. Many women feel it hasn't worked properly. And there is a link between caesareans and postnatal depression and post traumatic stress disorder where women have panic attacks, flashbacks or nightmares about the birth (this can happen with a traumatic vaginal birth too).

Though some women will, unavoidably, end up with a difficult or scary emergency caesarean, surgical birth for the rest of us simply does not have to be this way. The psychology of caesarean birth is often overlooked by health professionals who are, understandably, focusing on delivering a healthy baby. There is huge scope for improving our experience of caesarean birth. *'Even surgical birth can be magical,'* says midwife Jenny Smith. *'While all medical precautions need to be taken, it's important that, for instance, you should be able to hold and touch your baby straight away – skin to skin – if possible in the operating theatre. You should also stay with the baby afterwards, in the recovery room. The moment when you first meet your baby is really the miracle of birth. You can never get that back and as professionals we should do all we can to help women have these profound first few moments of being together.'*

HOW TO MAKE YOUR CAESAREAN A BIRTH

Before the operation:

- **Prepare your partner:** even if you have not scheduled a caesarean make sure he understands that you might need one unexpectedly, and what this will involve. Having someone with you who can encourage you, keep you calm and keep the operation feeling like a birth is invaluable whether your surgery is planned or not.

- **Understand who will be there, and what will happen should you have a caesarean.**

- **Consider having a female birth partner too and** make sure that in your birth plan you write that should you have to have an emergency caesarean, you want her in the operating room (see above). This can be perfectly possible, depending on the attitude of the staff, and the space in the operating theatre.

During the operation:

- **Remind yourself continuously that this operation is quick.** In five to ten minutes from the start of the operation you will see your baby for the first time.

- **Use your breathing** and relaxation to stay calm during the operation.

- **Consider asking the surgeon to narrate** what he or she is doing: this can make you feel more connected to the birth.

- **Try to focus on your baby, not the sensations of the operation.** Your anaesthetist will be making sure that you can feel no pain. Remind yourself you are about to see your baby.

- **Create an atmosphere of birth.** Some women say the medical staff chitchatted away to each other over their abdomen during the op, making them feel 'dehumanised'. Many doctors do this not because they're blasé, but because there is a feeling that silence is much more frightening for the woman they are operating on. But if you actually *want* silence, ask them to stop talking (or get your partner to ask).

Taking photos tip:

Ask if your partner can take pictures during the surgery, if you (and he) want. *'Instead of sitting near my head, my partner was next to the surgeon, with his camera,'* says Patty, mother of twins. *'I love those photos – they make me feel really connected to the birth.'* (If you have a digital camera, this can be really useful if the baby has to be taken off for special medical attention: you can look at the picture straight away.) Michelle, chair of International Cesarean Awareness Network (ICAN), Seattle says, *'Black and white photos can be better than colour ones – they show the beauty of the baby born with less of the graphic elements of the surgery.'* Matt finish tends to be better than gloss for the same reason.

Clinical smells tip:

Smell nice smells not surgical ones. This sounds bonkers, but if your caesarean is not a dire emergency (i.e. you have time to think about this sort of thing) you might want to use a drop or two of essential oil (like lavender) on a handkerchief next to your face or dabbed onto your neck, to counter the surgical smell, particularly if you're scared of hospitals. Aromatherapy is unlikely to be at the forefront of your mind if the operation is an emergency, but your birth partner might be able to do this for you.

When the baby is out

- **Seeing the birth**. You can ask for the screen to be lowered when the baby's actually coming out, so you see the moment of birth. The baby will be bloody.

- **The sex**. If you don't want to be told the sex, but want to look at your baby for yourself, make sure the surgical team know this so they don't shout out 'It's a boy!' as soon as they see the baby.

- **Skin to skin.** At no point does the baby need to be separated from you unless she requires resuscitation at birth. Often babies are whisked off for checkups, or wrapped up before they are given to you. Unless there's a pressing medical reason for this, it should **not** happen. Ask to have your baby put on your chest, against your skin, lying across your body, with your partner's hand supporting her back or bottom. If this is not possible for some (good medical) reason, have her cheek brought up to yours, or get your partner to hold her next to you so you can stroke and make eye contact with her. Talk to her. Look at her. Touch her. Keep her close to you as you would in a vaginal birth. As the National Institute for Clinical Excellence (NICE) guidelines put it: *'Early skin-to-skin contact between the woman and her baby should be encouraged and facilitated because it improves maternal perceptions of their infant, mothering skills, maternal behaviour, breastfeeding outcomes, and reduces infant crying.'*[7] **Nobody should be taking your baby out of your reach, unless you say it's OK, for any reason other than a pressing medical one.**

- **Stay in touch**. If your baby needs medical help, get your partner to watch and to tell you – if possible – how the baby is, what is happening. There is nothing more disempowering (or worrying) than lying pinned to an operating table while people crowd round your baby somewhere out of sight.

- **Stay together**. Keep your baby with you all the time in the recovery room.

- **Don't avoid pain medication after the operation.** Very little will pass to the baby. Being in extreme pain after the operation is not going to help you bond with your baby so take all pain killers they offer – even if you don't feel in much pain one minute, the pain can suddenly kick in.

- **Keep your baby's skin next to your skin** as much as possible in the next few days. This isn't airy-fairy advice: it can actually help your body to produce the right 'bonding' hormones and help to get your milk supply going.

- **Don't give up on any breastfeeding plans**. See below, page 203.

Post-caesarean tip:
It is common to get the shakes after surgery, so don't panic if this happens (though do call the midwife if she is not there). Warm blankets will help.

Postpartum caesarean care
For some women, recovering from a caesarean is straightforward, but for others it can be arduous. Much will depend on the kind of caesarean you had: if you have

an emergency caesarean after 24 hours of labour and are exhausted, you may take longer to recover than if you have a calm, planned surgery. Perhaps the most important thing about recovery is to remember that you have had **major surgery**. It's hard to think of another major operation where people would expect you to leap up and start caring for others just days after the surgery. Caesarean recovery can be unexpectedly painful and long-lived. Up to 10 per cent of caesarean mothers end up with an infection (usually of the wound, uterus or bladder). It is, then, worth being cautious, taking medical advice and making sure your partner understands that you need time to recover.

HOSPITAL STAY | Most women stay in the hospital for about three to five days after a caesarean, though many of us leave earlier (sometimes you just want to go home – wards can be noisy, hospital food is rarely nourishing, and then there's the fear of hospital borne infections...). It's worth thinking about your home situation before you discharge yourself though, and setting up extra help if you have other children. You also need to be totally sure that you are healthy and that going home will pose no risks. The community midwife team should know you are going home, and should visit you each day for about a week. After this, your health visitor will see you regularly.

YOUR BODY | **Post-op weakness:** Many women feel weak for a while after a caesarean. This may be because you have lost a lot of blood (blood loss can be higher than with a vaginal birth). **What to do**: rest, eat plenty of leafy green vegetables and take iron supplements (watch out for constipation though: drink plenty of water and eat fruit and vegetables). **Moving around:** you'll be encouraged by midwives to get up and move around very early on. This is not because they're fascist maniacs: it's to lower your risk of thrombosis (blood clots), the leading cause of maternal death in the UK.

YOUR SCAR | I've always been surprised at how unobtrusive my scar is. Most of it is below the pubic hairline and it has now faded to white. In the days after the operation you may find the scar shocking but by day two or three the incision should look all sealed up (though still very red). The midwives should remove your stitches after about five days: this is quick, but can be sore (see tip below). Don't leap on your treadmill just yet though: you do not want to strain or – God forbid – reopen the scar. When I got home from hospital after my caesarean, I was – I have no idea why – on a mission to prove to myself that I'd 'recovered'. I was out walking with Izzie in a sling within a week, bustling around, not resting, trying to squeeze into inappropriate clothing. I began to feel a very painful burning patch on my scar. I ignored it for as long as possible. Then, after a day or two, I reluctantly went to the GP. I had an infected stitch. Antibiotics are the usual treatment but if you leave it, you may need to have the infection surgically drained. So don't linger.

Your scar might seem, initially, to have a life of its own. It might itch or ache. It might be numb. It might feel as if it's permanently tugging your skin, or 'pinning you in'. You may have a complicated relationship with this scar for quite a while, particularly if you really wish it wasn't there. Some women describe feeling 'branded' by theirs. Others, meanwhile, see it as a badge of honour. How you feel about your scar will depend, of course, on how you feel about the birth. Your scar will enjoy a certain limelight at first: it will look quite dramatic; will be red, raised, possibly semi-obscured beneath an attractive fold of your post-baby flesh, initially exposed because the top of your pubic hair has been shaved. Most scars fade to a pale pink or white with time, and the uncomfortable feelings should disappear. But that scar is not going to go away (though when your hair grows back it may be harder to find). The best possible approach is to try and make friends with it: ultimately, it's a sign that you're a mother.

SCAR WARNING SIGNS

Call the doctor if you feel any of the following in your scar:
- Burning feeling
- Acute or sharp pain
- Foul smells
- Bleeding
- Any pus or other drainage
- Red patches on the scar

Stitches removal tip:
Take a couple of paracetamol half an hour to an hour before the midwife comes to remove your stitches.

Some scar care tips:
Follow the instructions you are given and take them seriously.

Lift nothing heavier than your baby for a minimum of three weeks and preferably longer.

Support your scar with your hand or a pillow before coughing, sneezing, or laughing.

You might want to pad your scar with a super-size sanitary pad: wear snug knickers and stick the sticky side of the pad to them, so that the pad runs the length of your scar, supporting it and keeping it comfortable.

Some women say that wearing a surgical support wrap around your belly also helps you feel comfortable. You can get one that has Velcro so as your belly shrinks, it shrinks with you. At a pinch, high support pants will work as well.

Don't scrub your scar in the weeks after surgery.

1 **Follow the instructions** you are given in hospital about how much exercise is OK, and what exercises are best. These really are important.

2 **Practise breathing.** Deep breathing – huffing, hissing, panting, deep yoga breathing –can help your scar (by increasing your circulation and oxygen supply). It can also help stomach pains you get from trapped wind – a real early days problem for many women who give birth by caesarean.

3 **Gentle walking.** Going for a short, gentle walk can also help the healing process by improving your circulation.

4 **Minimise your general tiredness (as far as possible).** Create a 'central zone' in your house to operate out of in the first two weeks (you might even want temporarily to move your bed downstairs). The main area would ideally be close to kitchen and bathroom. Have everything handy in this area, so you don't have to keep rushing up and down stairs all the time.

5 **Accept all the help you can get.** (See Chapter 10 for how to set up good postpartum help).

6 **Get a debrief on the birth.** When you are ready – this is not usually in the first 72 hours, when the hospital tends to do it – go through your notes with your doctor and midwife and make sure you understand what happened and why. Talk the birth through with your partner. Consider writing down what happened and how you feel about it. This can really help you become reconciled to an unexpected caesarean. It is also very helpful to get your hospital records and see exactly what was reported to have happened at the birth.

Breastfeeding after a caesarean

Some women find it hard to get breastfeeding going after surgery. Some say it took their milk a long time to 'come in'. Others say it was very uncomfortable at first, trying to manoeuvre the baby to avoid the scar. Medications that make you feel very tired and sleepy for a few hours after the birth can also make immediate breastfeeding harder. Your midwives should give you help and encouragement from the very beginning on this. But if they are not forthcoming, ask for help.

Breastfeeding tips:

A skin-to-skin connection between you and the baby starts the suckling/milk cycle, so taking your shirt off and putting baby onto your skin as much as possible in the early days can help.

Different positions work for different women: many women find they breastfeed best lying down on one side, or holding the baby under one arm, in a 'rugby ball' hold. Ask your midwife to show these positions to you.

Use tons of pillows to prop yourself and the baby up, and to protect your scar. A semi-circular pillow that fits round your middle can really help.

Vaginal birth after caesarean (VBAC)

There's an old adage 'once a caesarean, always a caesarean' which, though wildly out of date, seems to hold some unofficial sway even now in many hospitals. There is a small risk your scar might rupture if you experience labour when you have already had one caesarean. But this risk is really tiny, if you labour in the right – safe – conditions. Part of the reason for this outdated attitude to VBAC (pronounced 'veeback') is that caesarean incisions used to be vertical or ('classical') – running up your womb. This kind of incision can sometimes open ('rupture') – during labour, and this can be life threatening for you and your baby. Nowadays, however, most incisions are horizontal ('low transverse') – running along your bikini line. A bikini line incision in the womb is massively less likely to come apart under the pressure of labour. Doctors also now understand more about what can cause a scar to break open than they did in the past. All of this means that nowadays, if you labour in the right conditions with care from experienced staff, the risk of 'rupture' is minute. VBAC is now much safer than it ever was. This is why the official NHS guidelines given to doctors and midwives say: *'Pregnant women who have a previous caesarean section and who want to have a vaginal birth should be supported in this decision.'*[8]

Scar tip:
The slight complicating factor is that the scar you can see on your tummy does not tell you what kind of scar is on your womb. Doctors make two incisions to get the baby out: one to get to your womb and one in the womb itself. In British hospitals these days **virtually all** incisions in the womb are the 'bikini' kind. But in rare cases (for instance if your baby is extremely premature) the scar in the womb may be classical. This will be in your notes. If you are considering VBAC and are in any doubt about the nature of the scar on your womb, it is worth checking that it is a low transverse ('bikini') one.

Why attempt a VBAC?
It's quite simple. Studies have shown that VBAC is, in the majority of cases, a very safe option. And a repeat caesarean has its own risks.

The Royal College of Obstetricians and Gynaecologists, and the American College of Obstetricians and Gynaceologists, support VBAC under safe conditions.

In general, obstetricians are not concerned about whether you have the holistic birthing experience you've always dreamed of: they support VBAC because, under the right circumstances, it is not a dangerous thing to do. Indeed, according to the American College of Obstetricians and Gynaecologists, if you give VBAC a go, you have up to an 80 per cent chance of success.

The important thing is to get balanced information about the pros and cons, not emotive and off-putting comments. When I got pregnant with Sam, my obstetrician said I could have a 'trial of labour'. But there were 'conditions' under which I'd have to pop that baby out:

- early admission to hospital
- a drip in my arm throughout labour
- continuous electronic fetal monitoring (i.e. a certain amount of immobility, plus no use of a water tub for pain relief because their electronic monitors would not work under water)
- my cervix would have to dilate at 1 cm per hour
- I would not be allowed to push for more than an hour.

This is a common list for VBAC mothers, and there are some good reasons for many of the criteria. You may be happy to know that there are limits that will stop you from suffering unduly during this birth. But then again, you may feel that restrictions like these are off-putting. It might help to understand why such safety 'criteria' are given.

My obstetrician's explanations sounded terrifying: she talked about uterine rupture, scar 'dehiscence' (where the scar comes apart slightly), haemorrhage, brain damage to the baby, hysterectomy. Soon afterwards, I hired Julia. She was committed to getting me through this birth intact – both emotionally and physically – whether I had a caesarean or not. To do this, she knew I had to give VBAC my best shot in the safest possible conditions. Over the next six months, she helped me to better understand the reasons behind any safety measures (see below), work out how I would work with, not against, the ones that seemed restrictive or off-putting, and helped to build my confidence and knowledge about what to expect in a normal birth. She also encouraged me to plan what would happen should I end up in surgery again.

TRIAL OF LABOUR | You'll hear the term 'trial of labour' or 'trial of scar' applied to your VBAC. Don't be put off by this terminology. The idea is that doctors want to know that your labour is moving along well, so that there is little strain on your scar. The way they do this is to say that once you're in established labour your cervix should dilate by about 1 cm per hour. You usually wouldn't want to be in an active pushing stage for more than about an hour (as this may also put too much strain on your scar). If your labour does not seem to be progressing along these lines, doctors will then ask themselves why this could be happening, so you and your baby are not put at risk. They won't be hanging over you with a stopwatch, but they'll be aware of whether your cervix is, or is not, dilating. If the notion of being a watched pot concerns you, you should know that none of these limits are set in stone. If you are coping well in labour and there is no sign that your baby is in any distress, your doctor should not **force** you to stick to any rigid time limits against your will. As always, you can negotiate (talk to your obstetrician before you are in labour if the time limits worry you).

RUPTURE: THE FACTS | Uterine 'rupture' is a terrifying image for any pregnant woman to have in her head. But it is vital to understand the known risks. If your scar ruptures completely and you don't get to an operating theatre on time, you or your baby can indeed die, or be damaged. But no birth is risk free (indeed, even a uterus that has never been cut can rupture). The chances of you experiencing a life-threatening rupture in a VBAC are extremely low:

One in 200 VBAC mothers experience uterine rupture *of some kind*. Not all ruptures, by any means, are life-threatening.

This one in 200 statistic does not distinguish:

- Between a 'catastrophic' rupture (a life-threatening event where you need an emergency caesarean immediately) and dehiscence (where you may need an emergency caesarean, but are unlikely to suffer severe complications). Dehiscence can, in fact, remain totally undetected during or even after the birth.

- Between women who've had a VBAC under riskier circumstances, and those with excellent indications for success.

- Between types of scar ('classical' or 'bikini').

- Whether the woman has other 'contra-indications' to VBAC (e.g. if she is having twins, or has certain medical conditions such as placenta praevia or pre-eclampsia that make it less safe).

- Whether the woman was in labour under 'safe' conditions – i.e. with medically trained attendants rather than unattended at home.

- Whether the labour was induced with prostaglandin.

- Whether the labour was speeded up with a syntocinon drip.

You do, then, need to get that one in 200 figure into perspective. VBAC is something you should not dismiss until you really understand these risks and benefits. If you are giving birth with proper medical support, in – or close to – a decent hospital, your scar and baby will be monitored throughout labour and if a rupture happens, or looks like it might happen, you'll be whisked into surgery.

VBAC success is most likely:

- If you have a bikini-line scar in your womb and you did not have any medical complications with it last time.
- If you are carrying only one baby, head down.
- If you don't have any conditions like pre-eclampsia or placenta praevia.
- If you have had only one previous caesarean (the risk of rupture increases after more than one caesarean).
- If you go into labour spontaneously.
- If you feel safe and confident.
- If your hospital and medical team are supportive.
- If you've had a vaginal birth before (as well as your previous caesarean).
  N.B. Women have had successful VBACs with breech babies, twins, more than one previous caesarean and induced labour. But the risks do increase – sometimes very steeply indeed – with these factors. Incidentally, if you have already had one VBAC and want another your risks of rupture go down even further with your third baby.

Ways to have a safe VBAC

1 **HAVE ONE-TO-ONE CARE FROM AN EXPERIENCED MIDWIFE** | During labour you should be attended continuously by an experienced midwife who is used to VBAC. She will be alert to signs of a problem with the scar (e.g. bleeding from your vagina or the heart rate of the baby speeding up). Ideally, she (and anyone else in the room) should also fully support your VBAC endeavour.

2 **AVOID HAVING LABOUR INDUCED WITH PROSTAGLANDIN** | As we mentioned above, recent studies have shown that the use of prostaglandin to induce labour significantly increases your risk of rupture. This is particularly important thing to know when you are considering VBAC because women are sometimes offered inductions to stop the baby becoming 'too big'. Some hospitals will induce a VBAC but it may be safer to choose a repeat caesarean than have an induced VBAC. Discuss the pros and cons with your obstetrician if induction is a possibility. **What to do instead**: If you are very keen to try VBAC and need to be induced, it is possible to have a cervical sweep (see Chapter 5: Your Options) or your waters broken (at 41 weeks and above), possibly followed by a small amount of syntocinon some hours later to start off your contractions. The syntocinon will then be stopped when labour has kicked off.

3 **AVOID HAVING A SYNTOCINON DRIP ONCE LABOUR HAS BEGUN** | Syntocinon is sometimes used to strengthen contractions once labour is actually going. But having syntocinon during labour is a bad idea in VBAC as it

may put too much pressure on the scar. **What to do instead**: use upright positions, movement, and indeed any other strategies in this book to keep labour progressing well.

4   **LISTEN TO YOUR HEALTH CARE PROFESSIONALS** | Listen to any medical reasons you are given by your doctor or midwife that suggest VBAC may not be the safest option for you. Get second opinions and research these before you agree to anything. VBAC is not something to go for 'at all costs'. It's something to make an informed, confident choice about.

Things you can do to increase your chances of VBAC

THE TOP FIVE VITAL COMPONENTS OF A GOOD VBAC EXPERIENCE ARE:

1   **Communication:** with your health care team
2   **Support:** from them, and your birth partners
3   **Information:** understanding all aspects of birth, caesarean and VBAC
4   **Negotiation:** with your health care team on any possible restrictions
5   **Realism:** reconciling yourself to the possibility that you will have another caesarean (but only if it is really medically necessary).

TALK TO YOUR MIDWIFE | She is absolutely KEY to your VBAC success. You should talk to her about it early in pregnancy and ask for any VBAC resources she has. After 20 weeks you should also see your obstetrician and talk it over with her. You want to understand all the risks and benefits of your VBAC.

HAVE A FEMALE BIRTH PARTNER (IN ADDITION TO THE BABY'S FATHER) AT THE BIRTH | Studies have shown that having a trusted female companion lowers your chances of caesarean (and other intervention). If hiring a doula is a possibility this is a good idea: they can be invaluable in a VBAC.

WORK AROUND FETAL MONITORING | One of the best signs of rupture is the baby's heart rate speeding up and staying fast. (In about 70 per cent of scar ruptures, the first sign is a change to the baby's heart beat.) This is why most hospitals will insist that you are hooked up to an electronic fetal monitor (EFM) throughout your VBAC. But the last thing you want is to be immobilised on your back like last time, unable to change position, walk around or use a tub for pain relief. You are more likely to need an epidural if this happens, and studies associate epidurals with slower labours and more medical intervention.

Monitoring tips:
Ask if you can have EFM only once you are in established labour (so you can get labour going by moving around freely etc.).

You do not have to be on your back throughout the labour even if hooked up to a monitor. You can still move, sit upright, use beanbags, birth stools or birth balls, stand or rock.

Some hospitals may have monitors that use 'telemetry' and can let you roam free. Ask if yours has one.

NEGOTIATE ABOUT TIME RESTRICTIONS | Setting an artificial time limit on how long you labour for might lead to unnecessary interventions like ventouse or forceps. It is vital that you understand why any time restrictions may be imposed (see above). Talk it over with your obstetrician and come to an agreement with her that leaves you feeling confident and not under pressure to produce a text-book birth.

BUILD YOUR CONFIDENCE | Midwife Jenny Smith believes that '30 per cent of VBAC is confidence'. Many of us are told that the reason for our first caesarean might stop us having a VBAC. This isn't always true. Failure to progress or 'dystocia' do not preclude VBAC. Many women who were told first time that their pelvis was too small to let the baby's head through have gone on to give birth vaginally, often to even bigger babies. **What to do**: understand your previous birth fully and research any medical condition you had. If you had a caesarean during labour last time (even if your cervix did not dilate far) your womb is very likely to be much more efficient this time, even though you never got to push the baby out (my VBAC took 5 hours from start to finish).

AVOID AN EPIDURAL IF YOU CAN | Epidurals can also slow labour down – which may not be helpful in a VBAC, particularly if your hospital is twitchy about time limits. They can also limit how mobile you are, which is what you want to avoid as much as you can: movement and using positions that let gravity work can really help a birth progress. Lower abdominal pain between contractions can sometimes be an early sign that your scar may be having problems. An epidural can mask this. It is not a disaster if you have an epidural (particularly a mobile one, where you can stay upright), but do try and avoid it if possible.

FINALLY..... | *'Remember that you haven't failed if you have a second caesarean,'* advises obstetrician Lucy Chappell. *'Go into VBAC doing all you can to maximise your chances, whilst accepting that it's OK if it does not work out that way. You have done the best you possibly could, for you and for your baby.'*

Other VBAC concerns

OVERCOMING PRESSURE | When I was thinking about VBAC with Sam a few people said 'Why not just have another caesarean?' The implication was that it's somehow making things difficult for yourself by avoiding the 'easy option'.

People can make you feel selfish, masochistic, or hippyish when you say you want a VBAC. Often this is simply because they have no understanding of the issues. Remind yourself (and anyone who insists on questioning or criticising you) that a caesarean – even a repeat planned caesarean – is far from easy, is not safer for you, and that VBAC, **in the right conditions, with no contra-indications,** is considered by major medical organisations to be a safe option.

VBAC AT HOME? | Many women, having had what they see as one 'negative' hospital experience, are desperate to avoid replaying the same scene, so start to consider homebirth. If you are at low risk of uterine rupture (i.e. your scar is transverse and you have no medical complications) home VBACs are certainly possible (depending on why you had the first caesarean). But if you are thinking about homebirth consider what your home has that the hospital is not supplying, and find out if you can work around this with the hospital. It is crucial, if you choose to give birth at home this time, that you really have balanced the additional risks and benefits of this decision, that you live near a hospital (so can get to an operating theatre should a problem arise) and that you are attended by a **supportive and senior midwife with a lot of experience of both homebirth and VBAC**. This is vital.

MORE THAN ONE PREVIOUS CAESAREAN | It is still possible to have a VBAC, but most obstetricians will recommend that you have a repeat caesarean if you have more than one scar as your chances of rupture increase with each caesarean you have. Again, it's up to you to weigh up your risks.

UNSUPPORTIVE HOSPITAL | *'Your best shot at VBAC,'* says midwife Jenny Smith, *'is to find a hospital that will give you good informed choice and will be supportive of you.'* The NHS is certainly a lottery in this respect. According to the National Sentinel Caesarean Section Report (2001), in some hospitals as few as 8 per cent of caesarean mothers are even offered a 'trial of labour'. In this country the VBAC rate is currently only 33 per cent, but it ranges from 6 per cent in some hospitals to 64 per cent in others. **What you can do**: Ask your hospital what their VBAC approach is. If their answers are less than encouraging try to negotiate on individual points (see above). Ask if there are any pro-VBAC midwives who might take you on as a 'special case'. Swap to a different hospital or, if you can afford one, consider hiring an independent midwife who will fully support your VBAC.

Where to go for help:
Online:
We have more information on VBAC on www.bloomingbirth.net
Vaginal Birth After Caesarean website: www.vbac.org.uk
National Childbirth Trust: www.nctpregnancyandbabycare.com
Active Birth Centre: www.activebirthcentre.com
International Cesarean Awareness Network: www.ican-online.org

Ending up with another caesarean

It can be tough, if you have set your heart on a VBAC, to end up having a caesarean again. However, if you have done your research, sorted out supportive medical care and made conscious choices, and still you end up in surgery, you will – hopefully – be far more reconciled to it than you were first time around. You will also, if you follow our tips on making the surgery feel more like a 'birth' (see page 197), hopefully have a much more positive birth experience this time.

Julia knew one woman who planned meticulously for a VBAC. 'Carmen informed herself and understood all her options. The same complications happened with her second baby that had happened before, but with one difference: she was informed and involved at every step. By the time she chose to have the caesarean, she had walked the hospital halls, used water for pain relief, been given a nice amount of undisturbed labour time and space (she knew to ask for that this time), been massaged, tried every position in this book and kept herself calmly informed about her progress. The caesarean happened for reasons she understood and agreed with, and because she had worked hard on her fear of another caesarean, she wasn't panicked by the operation like she had been before. The birth was wonderful: Carmen didn't miss a thing, breastfed immediately and had all the postpartum help she didn't know to insist on before. She decided to call it an "EBAC" (Empowered Birth After Caesarean).'

Planned second caesarean

Would a caesarean be best this time?

If you have read the rest of this chapter, you will be able to weigh things up and make the decision that's right for you and your family instead of just taking the path of least resistance. If you are still uncertain, try this:

INFORMING YOURSELF

Questions to ask your doctor:

1 Do I have any medical condition that precludes VBAC?
2 What are the risks of having a VBAC given my medical condition?
3 Did my first birth leave me with physical (or emotional) damage that would suggest a caesarean is my best option this time?

Questions to ask yourself:

1 Was my previous birth extremely difficult, do I have flashbacks or nightmares that make me unable realistically to contemplate vaginal birth? If so, have I talked to a counsellor about these?
2 How will I feel if I don't try a VBAC?
3 How will I feel if I have a successful VBAC?
4 How will I feel if I try VBAC but end up with a caesarean?

5   Is the idea of another caesarean appealing? If so, why?
6   Do I fully understand the medical reason behind having a caesarean this time? (If not, do more research, go back to your doctor, discuss further: it's crucial that you are fully reconciled to this.)

How many caesareans can you have?

The risks associated with caesareans rise with each one you have, and increase more steeply after you have had about three. This is why most obstetricians advise women to stop having babies after three caesarean births. (Of course, in some countries women have seven or eight caesareans: it's all about balancing the increased risks of the operation against your fervent desire to procreate.)

Choosing a caesarean after a first vaginal birth

If your first birth was vaginal, and extremely difficult, you may be considering a caesarean because you see it as the 'easier' option. If there were problems with your first baby's health after the birth, you may also want a caesarean this time. Your reasons might be perfectly valid. But the decision does require serious thought. So, before you decide for definite, make sure you have really examined the risks and drawbacks of surgery against vaginal birth this time. And make sure you have got all the information about what to expect with a second vaginal birth (see Chapter 3: Second Time Around).

. . . .

FIND OUT MORE

VBAC checklist

Preparation

1   **Find out your hospital's VBAC rate** and any 'trial of labour' policy. If possible choose a hospital with a higher VBAC rate.
2   **If you can't find another hospital, remember you don't have to be part of the statistics**: you can have a VBAC even if most people don't.
3   **Get support**: Talk to the consultant obstetrician or the head of midwifery to ask how to find an experienced midwife who'll help you. Make sure your birth partner supports your plans. Consider hiring a doula or having a female birth partner who has had an uncomplicated birth (or VBAC) herself.
4   **Build your confidence**, read widely on VBAC and birth: confront your fears and believe you can do this.
5   **Talk to other women**, either online or in person who have planned/had a VBAC. This can help with your fears, and also build your confidence that it's

perfectly possible. ICAN (see Where to go for help, page 210) is a good place
to start).

6   **Eat well and look after yourself in pregnancy.**

During labour

1   **Work around continuous electronic fetal monitoring**. Make it work
for you not against you (upright positions, movement, peace of mind).
2   **Avoid induction with prostaglandin or a syntocinon drip during labour.**
3   **Let your waters break naturally** if possible.
4   **Make sure you're really in labour** before you are admitted to hospital
(regular contractions about every five minutes with effacement and dilation
of the cervix).
5   **Avoid an epidural** or other interventions if you can.
6   **Stay active**: stay mobile, upright if possible; create a 'safe' atmosphere
(dim lights, aromatherapy, music); make whatever noise you want, trust
your instincts.
7   **Have people with you who will give you great encouragement and
support**.

Resources

NHS **Direct** is a good place to get some really basic information. Phone NHS
Direct on 0845 46 47 or go to www.nhsdirect.nhs.uk.

Further reading

NICE *Caesarean Section Information for Pregnant Women* A clear booklet from the
NHS laying out basic issues, risks, benefits etc. of caesareans. You can get it from
the NHS Response Line: 0870 1555 455, quote reference number N0479. Or you
can download it from: www.nice.org.uk.

Caesarean Birth: Your Questions Answered by Debbie Chippington Derrick,
Gina Lowdon and Fiona Barlow (National Childbirth Trust, UK, 2004). Answers
questions that mothers frequently ask when they are told they may need a
caesarean, and gives the information you need to make an informed choice.

The Caesarean Experience by Sarah Clement (Pandora, UK, 1995) Written by a
psychologist, this book deals with caesarean emotions as well as the main issues.

The Caesarean by Michel Odent (Free Association Books, UK, 2004). Obstetrician
Odent is credited, among other things, with 'popularising' water birth. This

is an interesting look at caesarean issues today, including why so many of us have them.

Misconceptions by Naomi Wolf (Chatto & Windus, UK, 2001) American feminist writer Wolf, who had two caesareans, unpicks some of the politics and emotions of this way of giving birth.

The Thinking Woman's Guide to a Better Birth (Perigee, US, 1999) and *Obstetric Myths versus Research Realities: A Guide to the Medical Literature* (Greenwood, US, 1995), both by Henci Goer. We've already recommended these books in Chapter 5, but they are useful resources when considering caesareans too.

The VBAC Ccompanion: The Expectant Mother's Guide to Vaginal Birth After Caesarean by Diana Korte (Harvard Common Press, US, 1997) An American book, explaining risks and benefits of both repeat caesareans and VBAC. Also good on overcoming your fears.

Three books to build your confidence that your body knows what it's doing

Ina May's Guide to Childbirth by Ina May Gaskin (Random House, US, 2003)

Birthing From Within: The Extraordinary Guide to Childbirth Preparation by Pam England and Rob Horowitz (Partera, UK, 1998)

Birth Reborn: What Childbirth Should Be by Dr Michel Odent (Souvernir, France, 1994) OK, it's a bit dated, but this classic book really gave me a huge sense of hope, when facing my VBAC, that my body could do its job brilliantly under the right conditions.

Online

Caesarean birth and VBAC information: www.caesarean.org.uk

International Caeesarean Support Network www.ican-online.org

Chapter Seven:
Expect the unexpected...

'I planned to have a water birth in my local
hospital. I was convinced that it would all
go perfectly. I skipped the caesarean chapter
in my birth book – in fact, I think I skipped
a lot of chapters – and the birth was a maze
of confusion. I never expected it to be
so long, so hard or so lonely. The minute
the interventions started, my birth plan
went out the window and I sort of gave up.
Tao was born by caesarean and I've never
really understood why.'

JUNE (28) MOTHER OF TAO (1)

FIVE REASONS TO EXPECT THE UNEXPECTED

1 You'll cope rather than panic
2 You'll make good choices
3 You'll remember your preferences
4 You'll communicate well with hospital staff
5 You'll feel in control (even if, technically, you're not)

How do you prepare for the unexpected?

It sounds like a contradiction in terms, but it's possible. It's what this book is about, really. You have to inform yourself realistically about birth (Chapters 2, 5, 6), defuse your fears (Chapter 3), understand your preconceptions (Chapter 3), understand your options (Chapter 5), choose and prepare your birth partner(s) (Chapters 8, 9) and write a meaningful birth plan. In this chapter we show you how to write a Blooming Birth Plan: one that can actually help you cope when the unexpected happens; one that will get you through the whole birth, not go out the window when you hit your first speed bump.

Mind the gap: your expectations and why they matter

There is – to put it mildly – a significant gap between our expectations of childbirth and what actually happens (particularly first time around). In one survey[1], 45 per cent of mothers agreed in advance that 'giving birth is a natural process that should not be interfered with unless absolutely medically necessary'. Virtually all of them had some kind of medical 'interference' on the day.

The unpredictability of birth is, however, the one thing most doctors and midwives agree on. *'A first labour is like setting off to Scotland from London without a map or a car,'* says consultant obstetrician Jayne Cockburn. *'Your womb has not done it before and you just have to find a way to roll with this on the day.'* No matter how swotty you are about preparing for this birth, you'll never be truly prepared until you have accepted that your plans might be scuppered by a baby that lies in the wrong position, waters that break too early or a labour that just doesn't kick off. There are few things more disconcerting than expecting the birth to go in a certain way, then finding yourself haring off down some alien, unknown, painful route that you don't understand and can't control. Many of us lose it when this happens: we've been so focused on **what to expect** that we've failed to realise we should expect **the unexpected**.

You may be nodding nervously right now, saying to yourself: 'Right. Fine. I'll expect the unexpected.' But **how** will you do this? **Really**? The best way is to draw up a meaningful birth plan – a Blooming Birth Plan. You can start working on your plan as early in the pregnancy as you like, but the process will probably be most effective when you've done a few childbirth classes and the Herculean task of getting that baby out is starting to look decidedly real. This will probably be during the last three months or so of your pregnancy, when your worries are more concrete, and you learned more about how to handle them. A Blooming Birth Plan can help close this expectations gap and defuse your last fears.

Why bother?

If you've reached the stage where you view childbirth as normal, healthy and manageable this is superb. Confidence is a huge asset for any woman facing the delivery room. But it has to be confidence rooted in **realism**. Just assuming that the birth will be a joyous epiphany is not enough. You might, for instance, have weighed up your options and decided to give birth anaesthetised to the eyeballs. But what happens if you get to hospital and the anaesthetist isn't available? What happens if you have to wait two hours in hard labour until you get that epidural? If you only have Plan A (nuclear pain relief), and Plan B (a range of pain coping methods) is called for, you might be in trouble. Your Blooming Birth Plan will contain – in very general terms – **your Plan B**. It's your overarching plan for how you'll cope – generally – with whatever childbirth throws at you.

BIRTH REHEARSAL

A few weeks before their due date, midwife Jenny Smith takes her mothers-to-be through a 'rehearsal' of the birth, in a delivery room. *'I spend a half hour or so with the woman in a delivery room before the birth,'* says Jenny. *'This way she can visualise, more clearly, what labour will be like, and explore what would happen if the birth is not straightforward. You can try asking your midwife to do this with you: if you have done this, you will be far less worried should things not go smoothly on the day.'*

Pretend it's labour:

- Go round the apparatus in the room – the bed, beanbag, chair, birth stool while the midwife explores with you how you might use it in labour.

- Discuss your birth plan with the midwife while you are doing this: how would your plans work in this room?

- Go through what would happen if there was a problem with the labour or the baby: Jenny describes to her women exactly what she would do in this situation – everything from what her voice will sound like (quiet) to where the emergency bell is, what ringing it would mean and what would happen next.

But everyone says birth plans are useless....

'When eight women from our antenatal group met up with their babies, not one had experienced a delivery that went according to plan...Second time around, I didn't make a plan, and just hoped that the baby would be delivered vaginally..... If I'd written a birth plan, it would have been sheer fantasy.' Journalist Fiona Gibson, in 'Birth Plan: You're joking?' an online article.[2]

Breathe the words *'my birth plan'* in front of an experienced mother, and you'll probably encounter anything from a raised eyebrow to naked derision. First time around most of us write a birth plan because our childbirth teacher tells us to. At a bit of a loss, we write, in essence, 'I'll just see how it goes' (translation: 'please pretend to consult me, then make my decisions for me'). Because most birth plans are distinctly Utopian. Most of us don't write a birth plan that goes: 'I'll have a forceps delivery with some blood loss.' But this does happen and when it does, few of us have really thought about **how we'll cope**.

You'll also hear that 'no one reads a birth plan'. This isn't strictly true. A good midwife or obstetrician will. They'll even try to read between the lines to interpret how best to care for you when 'challenges' crop up. But you can't bank on this.

You should still write a Blooming Birth Plan

You should do this because the **process** of writing one can be immensely useful – for you. Even if you put your plan straight in the bin once complete, it would still be worth doing. In your non-gestational life, worry and pessimism are usually negative things but in pregnancy they can be really productive – if you tackle them constructively. Julia has seen many of her clients transform their worries into action while working on their birth plan:

'Lorraine was a 44-year-old first-time mother who worried obsessively about having a forceps delivery. She researched and took really good care of herself during her pregnancy, but the worry didn't go away. Working on her birth plan made her realise she had to speak to an obstetrician to tackle this lingering fear. The doctor mentioned her age six times in five minutes. He said a woman her age should be worried about many things as well as forceps (he gave her a list ranging from Down's syndrome to caesarean rates). After this meeting Lorraine swapped to a different hospital and a new obstetrician she felt understood her needs more. Her healthy daughter was born without the help of forceps or surgery. Lorraine's birth planning had led her in the right direction. The process can help you really zoom in on a worry, and can lead you somewhere you need to be.'

A BLOOMING BIRTH PLAN – OR, MORE ACCURATELY, THE PROCESS OF
WRITING ONE – CAN:

- Address any lingering worries
- Defuse any remaining fears
- Clarify all you've learned about your options (how, where, with whom?)
- Clarify your general preferences for the birth (i.e. silent and private/loud and reassuring/more natural/more medical...)
- Help you to understand your expectations and plan how you'll stay calm if they're not met
- Reinforce your overall confidence that you're going to cope – whatever happens

What exactly is a Blooming Birth Plan?

Really, 'plan' is a misnomer. A Blooming Birth Plan should really be called a 'strategy'. Instead of a task where you sit down for ten minutes and list the elements of your Utopian birth, then gripe afterwards about how pointless that was, think of it as a work in progress. It might take weeks to complete. It might change as you get nearer the birth, or as you find out more (about your options, fears, inclinations, or your pregnancy). The resulting document will be a brief but overarching **strategy** for how you'll cope during childbirth, not a shiny list of best-case scenarios. It will be flexible, succinct and most of all will answer this crucial question: *What will I do if this birth does not go the way I want?*

How to write a Blooming Birth Plan

We've divided it into four steps. But really, it's a process. You dabble in it. Think about it. Talk about it. Read. Research a bit more. Have another go. Leave it. Then come back to what you did before.

STEP 1: FACE YOUR WORST CASE SCENARIO | You need to get to the stage where your worst case scenario is no longer the threatening Yetti that it is now. Whatever it is – and yours will be uniquely horrifying to you – you need to look the beast in the eye and work out how you will overcome (or at least cope with) it.

How to do this:

- Quickly list your top five fears (you've worked these out by using Chapter 3, Fear and Pain) – the things that would make this a really difficult birth for you.
- Don't edit yourself, even if you thought you'd come to terms with a fear. If it springs to mind, write it down.
- Julia's birth clients often list: *fear of dying (self or baby), fear of being out of control, unbearable pain, unplanned caesarean, unplanned interventions, being abandoned in labour.*

STEP 2: IMAGINE YOUR DREAM SCENARIO | Step one probably didn't take you much time: you should by this time know those demons pretty well. Now you've got to work out your Utopia: the kind of birth you'd really dream of having.

How to do this:

- Quickly list five elements of a truly Utopian or dream birth.
- Don't let your left brain step in here, shouting 'that's just not practical'. Let your imagination take over, no matter how silly your scenarios seem.

When I did this exercise with Julia, before Sam was born, I found myself imagining giving birth in a stable – a place I associate with security, warmth and safety. Of course, in real life I have no desire to give birth like something out of the New Testament. But that equine moment told me a lot about my fundamental inclinations: I knew I'd cope best if I was allowed just to get on with it, safely but without any scary hospital equipment up my bum. When Julia asks her clients to do this bit, they often list: *being outside, being left alone (but feeling supported), being surrounded by women, having a fast labour. The vast majority of her second time mothers dream of giving birth at home or in water. One client, on the other hand, said a planned caesarean would be her ideal.*

STEP 3: START SHAPING YOUR PLAN | Look at your two lists. They may seem insanely different, but what actually happens to you on the day will probably lie somewhere between the two.

Worst case:
- baby or myself in danger
- panicking/not coping with pain
- husband not there
- unnecessary caesarean
- other scary medical interventions

Dream birth:
- outside under the stars
- in a warm lake
- in husband's arms
- calm and confident
- safe and secure

Now you start your first sketch of your plan, using these two lists. Take each fear from the **Worst case** list and work out what you are going to do about it. What have you done that lowers the chance of it happening? What will you do to cope if it still happens? As you do this, bear in mind how you will keep the *feeling* of your dream birth.

Here's an example of a first sketch, using the two lists above:

BIRTH PLAN SKETCH

- **I will be delivering at X hospital** (one you've chosen, understand and feel confident about). Fear tackled: *baby or self harmed.* Dream element: *desire for safety.*

- **For the pain, I will try** (list of all the methods you're hoping to use, your preferences etc.). Fear tackled: *panicking/not coping with pain.* Dream element: *desire for calm and confidence.*

- **Husband will carry a pager/mobile phone for two weeks before/after due date.** Fear tackled: *being alone/husband not there.* Dream element: *safe, calm, confident.*

- **I want to be fully informed about any signs that I may be heading for a caesarean, and consulted about each step.**

I want to understand the reasons and if I still have to have a caesarean, I want it to follow my caesarean plan (see Chapter 6). Fears tackled: *unnecessary caesarean/interventions/panic*. Dream element: *calmness/confidence/safety*.

- **I will use the birthpool if possible/bring a birthpool that I have hired.** Fear tackled: *unmanageable pain/unnecessary interventions*. Dream element: *warm lake*.

- **I'll use positions for pain relief that involve being physically held by my husband. During the pushing stage, I'll try a supported squat, held by him. If there are any interventions, he will hold me while I am coping with them.** Fear tackled: *unmanageable pain*. Dream element: *in husband's arms*.

- **I will cope with early labour by walking outside and I'll bring a nature sounds tape and pictures of nature to focus on during contractions later on.** Fears tackled: *unmanageable pain/unnecessary caesarean (mobility/uprightness lower chances of interventions and help manage pain)*. Dream element: *outdoors*. (Julia had one client who dreamed of giving birth 'under the stars' so brought fairy lights to the hospital – and why not?)

- **If I have to have interventions, I want to be fully informed of the reasons; I will have an epidural if possible and my husband and birth partner will be by my side, talking me through it. I will use all my relaxation techniques to stay calm, and will focus on my baby.** Fears tackled: *scary interventions*. Dream element: *secure, safe, calm*.

STEP 4: MAKE IT A DOCUMENT | Now distil your final plan into a succinct 'public' version that fits on one side of A4 and covers all your most important points. You will take this to the hospital and this is the version the midwives will read (see 'Your Blooming Birth Plan: a template' below).

A WORD OF CAUTION.... | Working on your plan might be tough, particularly if you've had one difficult birth (and are scared silly of repeating it). When I was Julia's client, I was so neurotic about having unnecessary interventions (including another caesarean) that even the thought of examining this for my birth plan had me in tears. Julia insisted that we isolate the elements that were frightening to me, then work out a plan for what we'd do about each one. This would, she said, stop the bad scenario being so frightening.

I was sceptical, but made myself break down, in a long email to Julia, the things that scared me most and what I was going to do about each one. By the time I hit the send key my fears were under control. I'd broken down my anxiety into specifics; reminded myself what I was doing to stop each one happening again, and planned how I'd cope with each if it did. This was the point at which I felt ready to handle Sam's birth whatever happened. With Ted, the process was much less detailed. I had far fewer fears and much more confidence. How much energy your planning takes will depend on all sorts of things. But if you are really anxious, you too may need a bit of help. Go through your worries AGAIN with your midwife, re-read any relevant bits of this book and do more research for yourself, using the information found at the end of each chapter. **Knowledge, when it comes to childbirth, really is power.**

This process should get you on the way to creating a birth plan that really means something to you. The next challenge is to get the people who are caring for you to read it.

FIVE TIPS FOR A BIRTH PLAN THAT WILL BE READ

1 Make it realistic, well-informed and really address your specific concerns.
2 Keep it to one piece of A4 paper or a card (front and back is fine), well spaced and clear to read. Headings can be useful as they help the doctor/midwife to navigate. If it's hard to read, or too long they might not bother.
3 Make it open and friendly. A contentious or aggressive plan will put people on the defensive and start things off on a bad note.
4 Show it to your midwife and discuss with her whether it's clear and realistic.
5 Staple it to the 'birth plan' section of your notes, or to the front of them, so the midwife/doctor can find it.

Why your plan can help even in an emergency

During labour, medical interventions can become genuinely necessary – often with little warning. Your plan can help you handle this. It can also help your medical team to have a 'flavour' of your inclinations, fears and desires for this birth, no matter what happens. If your midwife, and whoever else is with you at the birth, know that you are particularly anxious about a specific event, then – should this actually happen – they'll be aware that it's your nightmare. They'll be able to talk you through it, explain the process and reassure you that it is best for your baby, and you. This way, instead being plunged into your heart of darkness (the Horror!), out of control and scared, you'll be walked through it step by step, retaining some sense of control.

A few examples of final birth plans

Here (and on www.bloomingbirth.net) are a handful of birth plans used by Julia's clients.[3] (Remember, the process is more important, if anything, than the final result.)

SHORT AND SWEET (WRITTEN ON A 3X5 CARD) | **LaKenya and Adol**

I'm LaKenya Bollen, 22 years old, and this is my first child. I have no great fear of pain, so please don't offer me medication unless I ask for it. However, if an epidural is necessary I would like it to be mobile if possible. I will be supported by my husband and doula during the labour and birth. I would like to eat through labour, move around as I like and deliver where I choose. My baby will be set right on me, skin to skin with no cleaning, and I will breastfeed immediately if at all possible. Thank you.

'LaKenya's plan represents a long process of learning about birth and opening her mind to various possibilities. When she began to work on this plan, the only image of birth she had was one where she'd be anaesthetised with feet in stirrups, surrounded by doctors in masks. This scared her. She worked with me to isolate what she wanted for this birth and, by the end, had pinpointed the things that were most important to her. For instance, her older sister was not encouraged to breastfeed right away and regretted it, so LaKenya picked this out as a concern. Her labour took about 14 hours and was tough but triumphant: for the first part she moved, ate (until she didn't want to), drank and stayed upright. Later, she had a mobile epidural. She delivered the baby sitting on her hospital bed and was delighted by how the birth went. Her baby fed within the first two hours (with great help from the midwife).'

BUSINESS-LIKE AND TO THE POINT | **Polly and Kashen**

- Polly Sandra Isopolas
- age 37
- my second child
- hospital at sign of active labour
- epidural after 4 cm
- other medications or interventions only with discussion
- managed third stage
- baby's needs: yes to vitamin K. Other needs will discuss
- caesarean – only if strictly medically necessary
- breastfeeding – may need help

'Polly is a lawyer. This was her whole birth plan. But it said a lot about her. She's not overly emotional, and had a rough time with the pain of her first labour. She also had a haemorrhage after that birth, so decided to have a 'managed third stage' this time (an injection to speed delivery of the placenta, which can reduce risk of haemorrhage). She chooses to have an epidural once labour is established, but makes it clear that this will not be an open door for other procedures. She's active in this birth plan, there is room for change and even though it's brief, it's not defensive or off-putting. Polly agreed to have her waters broken when things were not progressing very well at the start, and labour then took hold quickly. She ended up without an epidural (she actually refused one when offered). Her pushing stage was challenging but she coped very well, deciding against an episiotomy when she was offered one. She pushed out

her 9lb 10oz son on a birth stool and says she felt she controlled what she could, and was able to relinquish control when she needed to.'

LONGER AND MORE EMOTIONAL | Kari and Allen

We do not believe that birth is a medical condition: Kari would like to give birth without unnecessary noise, distraction or invasion of privacy.

We agree to remain flexible about the birth of our son. We will stay at home as long as possible having notified you (*hospital 24-hour phone number*) that Kari is in labour. Our doula Julia (*phone number*) will be with us at home (*back-up doula is:name/number*). The maternity unit has already cleared use of a birth tub that we will bring with us.

Kari will be supported by Julia and Allen. Kari handles the unknown best if she can be as informed as possible. If you feel that intervention is necessary, those interventions are to be discussed as thoroughly as time will allow. She would like to be made a central part of the decision process, and should that not be possible, Allen and Julia will be her spokespeople.

Here is a list of Kari's desires:
- Labour at home as long as possible with Allen and Julia
- Transfer to hospital before it's scary
- Absolutely no vaginal exam without introduction, warning and explanation
- Free movement and eating and drinking as desired
- Kari's own clothes, pillows, music, slippers, aromatherapy oils etc.
- No EFM unless medically necessary – only a hand-held monitor
- If EFM necessary, Kari will stay in upright positions (not lying on back)
- Low lights
- Limited hospital staff (no coming and going)
- Tub ready for Kari to use if she wants
- Non-medical pain relief used
- No medical suggestions for pain relief offered until Kari asks about them
- Allen to be with Kari throughout the labour and birth
- When our son is born he is to be placed on Kari's chest, skin to skin
- Only necessary intervention for the baby
- Cord only to be cut after pulsating stops – unless there is a reason to do otherwise. Allen may cut the cord: please ask him
- Baby stays with Kari and breastfeeds
- Allen bathes the baby for the first time
- Vitamin K is OK

If it is a caesarean birth: Julia and Allen will accompany Kari throughout the birth and, if possible, the baby is to be put on Kari's chest skin to skin immediately after he's born.

'Kari's original birth plan was seventeen pages long and very, very inflexible. She quoted authors, used statistics and told stories of her childhood. That was a good start,

but definitely not a final birth plan. Kari and I went through those seventeen pages and saw that she was really just concerned with privacy and control – very common. She had been sexually abused as a child, but had had years of counselling, and her midwife was fully aware of her history. The four pages about her sexual abuse history from her first birth plan became one clear line about vaginal exams in her revised plan. It took us two hours to get her bullet points down to fewer than 20. As with most survivors of abuse, having good support during the birth was crucial. Kari made sure her husband and I (and her back-up doula) would be there to remind her she was safe.

Her line about being flexible was to remind herself not to be rigid, as she had been in the first mammoth birth plan. In the end Kari's labour was extremely short (three hours!). She went to hospital after only half an hour in labour at home as it was plain that things were progressing very fast. She delivered her son with the midwife, Allen and me in the room. She didn't use music or aromatherapy and the birth tub never made it out of the boot of the car. She said the pain was more intense than she'd imagined, but the birth was more amazing than she'd ever hoped it could be.

YOUR BLOOMING BIRTH PLAN – A TEMPLATE

This is just a suggestion for your final version. You certainly don't have to format your plan this way, there's no standard. The birth plan checklist, below, will jog your memory as you write.

Names (yours and partner) ....
Brief statement (sentence or two) about your general wishes, or greatest hope, for this birth

1 **Information** Practical information that will help you when you go into labour. Numbers to call when you go into labour (make sure you list the 24-hour maternity unit number here, not just the midwife's working hours number) and all the numbers (mobiles, pagers, work) for your support people (including babysitter's numbers if you have other kids).

2 **My main concerns** Your main worries about this birth. What prospect bothers you most? (Put it down and staff will hopefully be more sensitive should it crop up.) How will you cope if it happens?

3 **Pain relief preferences** What would you prefer to help you control pain? What would you like to avoid?

4 **Medical interventions** What is your attitude to them? Do you want to be consulted? What will you do if you're not in a position to make decisions? Are there any, particularly, that you would prefer to discuss or avoid?

5 **Second and third stage (pushing the baby and placenta out)** What pushing positions would you like to be in? Are there any interventions you do/don't want? Is there any specific help you'd like?

6 **Caesarean birth** See Chapter 6, page 198, on how to make caesarean feel more like a birth, when you're thinking this through. Do you feel strongly about this? When would you like to be told surgical birth might be a possibility (as soon as there's a worry? Or at the last minute?) Who should be with you? How do you want a caesarean birth to be?

7 **Baby care immediately after the birth** What do you want to happen to your baby as soon as she's out?

8 **Any other things you want your midwife to know about your wishes for the labour and delivery**

Blooming Birth Plan: checklist

Here is a list of 'issues'. Remember it's your plan – no one else's. Do NOT include everything in this list – that would be deranged – just look down it and pick out the points/issues that matter to YOU. Go back to Chapter 5: Your Options for a reminder if you're unclear about anything.

LABOUR

- **Your partner and other support**: who are your birth partners? Will your other children (if you have them) be there?
- **Induction**: your preferences, from natural methods to a syntocinon drip. If you know you're having an induction what issues bother you? (i.e. pain management? Feeling in control?)
- **Vaginal exams**: How often? Only if necessary? Don't mind? Not at all?
- **Dilation**: do you want to be told how dilated your cervix is? How often? Not at all?
- **Positions for labour**: freedom to move? Stand or walk? Remain in bed?
- **Fluids and food**: what you want to be able to consume when you're in labour?
- **Need to pee**: freedom to walk to loo; feelings about catheterisation?
- **Augmenting (speeding up) labour**: ways you want to try before medical methods? Artificial Rupture of Membranes: yes or no? In what circumstances would it be OK? Other ways to speed up labour e.g. syntocinon drip: your preferences/concerns?
- **Monitoring your baby's heart rate**: what kind of fetal monitoring do you prefer (see page 160).
- **Atmosphere**: privacy, respect, no strangers, medical reassurance, emotional reassurance?

PAIN RELIEF

- **Your general approach**: do you want to be offered/encouraged to have medications and/or anaesthesia? Do you want to try to avoid it? Have it ASAP? Only at your request? Only if you use your 'code word'?

- **Natural pain relief**: do you want to try bath or shower, relaxation, breathing, TENS, massage, aromatherapy, hypnosis, other kinds of assistance from your birth partners?
- **Medication** – what you want/want to avoid? (Injected analgesia, gas and air, epidural/spinal?)

PUSHING STAGE
- **Positions:** midwife's choice? Your choice? Freedom to squat etc.?
- **Where you'll give birth**: Bed? Water? Birth stool? Your free choice?
- **How to push**: negotiate on limits on pushing stage? Look at (i.e. have hand-held mirror) or touch the baby's head?
- **Instrumental birth**: how do you feel about ventouse? Forceps? How do you plan to cope should it be necessary? Anything they could do to help you through it?
- **Your perineum**: your feelings about episiotomy? Tearing? Stitches? Any means you'd like to try for intact perineum?

THIRD STAGE (DELIVERY OF PLACENTA)
- **'Managed'** i.e. made quicker with medication injection (reduces rate of haemorrhage)?
- **Made quicker** with massage of womb by midwife, encouraged with breast stimulation and breastfeeding?
- **Spontaneous** (i.e. let it come out on its own unless any danger)?

IMMEDIATE POSTPARTUM
- **Cutting the cord**: clamp and cut immediately? Partner will cut? Clamp and cut only after it stops pulsing?
- **Taking photos**: who? When?

IMMEDIATE BABY CARE
- **First to hold the baby**: do you want your baby put on you when he comes out? In your partner's arms? Straight to midwife for check?
- **Vitamin K**: not at all, orally or by injection?
- **Feedings**: breast or bottle?
- **Newborn exam**: who will witness your baby's first weigh-in, measuring, APGAR and physical check-up? (You're probably going to be pretty immobilised and you may want to request that your partner be with the baby rather than her being whisked into a corner of the room where you can't see her.
- **Circumcision**: rare for non-religious reasons in the UK. If your baby is to be circumcised what are your wishes for this?
- **If baby needs special care**: any particular issues you feel strongly about?

When things don't go to plan: some general tips for coping

Sometimes your baby just does need help to be born: anything from an episiotomy to a caesarean (see chapter 5, page 164 for information about possible interventions). Accepting this, wholeheartedly, is the biggest step you can take towards coping should it happen. **Get your birth partner to read the tips below: when an unwanted intervention happens, your birth partner is your lifeline.**

SIX WAYS TO DEAL WITH UNWANTED MEDICAL INTERVENTIONS

1 **Information:** make sure you know about common interventions – how common they are, what they involve and what the pros and cons are.
2 **Support:** your birth partner(s) should be right up close to you during the procedure, talking you through it, keeping you calm,
3 **Reinforcement:** your birth partner(s) should be helping you to focus on the reasons the intervention is needed.
4 **Reminders:** your birth partner(s) should remind you repeatedly that any minute now your baby will be out, you'll be holding her in your arms.
5 **Recovery:** your birth partner(s) can remind you, while the procedure is happening, of the ways they are going to help you recover when it's all over.
6 **Pain management:** basically, at this point, accept whatever it takes to get you through. There's no place for heroics in childbirth.

Tip: good support is the key to coping with interventions

Julia planned to have her first baby, Keaton, at home. She had a long and painful labour, transferred to hospital and finally had a forceps delivery. But Julia's midwife Kim gave her just this kind of support as each unexpected event cropped up: *'It was very powerful. Knowing I wasn't being left alone and that someone was acknowledging the change in plans got me through each unexpected thing that Keaton needed during his birth: the hospital transfer, my epidural, the syntocinon drip, forceps, episiotomy and antibiotics for Group B strep. Kim helped me feel that each intervention was what Keaton needed, and that I couldn't do anything more than I had done to change this. She gave me a lot of reassurance afterwards too. If a medical intervention is really necessary, and a woman has had all her questions answered, this kind of reinforcement can make an otherwise shocking experience entirely manageable.*

Communication with hospital staff

If your birth takes a turn for the unexpected, it's vital to be communicating well with the hospital staff. The last thing you want is people patronising you while your feet are in stirrups. And you don't want to be wasting valuable energy arguing or feeling affronted when you're moments away from another contraction.

You'll cope best in labour if you:
- feel you're being talked to like the intelligent adult you are
- feel like you have not suddenly lost all control
- feel respected, consulted and informed (see Chapter 5, Your Options, page 176)
- understand what is happening to your body and baby

You can't rely on the staff to make this happen. Many will bend over backwards to accommodate and respect you but some may not. No matter what you hear about 'informed consent' and 'patients' charters' and 'woman-led care' you're still going to be attended by real human beings who get tired, hungry, frustrated, grumpy, bossy and impatient. If it is a genuine emergency, there may be little time for niceties: you have to accept that these people are doing all they can for you and the baby and you must focus your energy on staying calm and getting through it. But if it's not a dire emergency, there are things you can do to change any dodgy dynamic. This way, you'll have a better chance of handling the unexpected, rather than becoming a victim of it.

As soon as you notice yourself feeling bullied/disregarded/bossed by staff, you and/or your birth partner can become (politely) more assertive.

FIVE TIPS FOR BETTER COMMUNICATION WITH HOSPITAL STAFF

1 **Be honest:** try and make everything you say, imply or insinuate, accurate. In labour, if you are telling your partner you want to die, but tell the midwife when she comes in that you're 'fine', you're not helping her to help you.

2 **Make communication a two-way thing:** after you clearly express your needs, really listen to your midwife/doctor's explanation. This can be harder than it sounds, especially when you're in labour. If you can't, get your birth partner to do this.

'I got the impression that there was a power struggle going on between the doctor and midwife. At one point they were literally arguing over my bed about what was best for me. I was so disempowered and never felt that I could make any decisions of my own despite a good degree, career and birth preparation.'
ADRIANNE (28) MOTHER OF HEATH (1)

3 **Eradicate the grey areas:** sometimes it's helpful to be clear about **why** something's being said. If the obstetrician starts referencing caesarean statistics stop her and ask her **why** she's saying this. Is this where you're headed? Does she think you need one?

4 **Keep communicating:** don't wait for the big moments during labour. Communicate from the beginning with your midwife, then if any big decisions need to be made you'll have a level of trust built up on both sides.

5   **Politely remind people who are talking over you/arguing about you/examining you thoughtlessly/patronising you** that you are a sentient, reasoned human being even if you appear somewhat undignified right now. Say (or get your birth partner to say) something like: 'This isn't helping. This is my body, and my baby. Please talk to me properly about what is happening.'

The unexpected in a homebirth

Homebirth expectations run high. You picture the romantic bits: giving birth to your baby on the bed in which he was conceived – a natural, pain-dimmed, aromatherapied dream. Homebirth can be a uniquely satisfying experience but to suggest that it's the 'best' way to give birth, puts considerable pressure on us all. Many women think that if they're going to have a homebirth they don't need a birth plan. This is a big mistake. Homebirths do – fairly frequently – end up becoming hospital births. If this happens and you've not considered it as a real possibility, it can feel like a traumatic disaster.

This is certainly Julia's experience with Keaton:

'I expected to give birth to Keaton in my bed and was so wedded to this that I was actually afraid to leave it in labour. I didn't: until I had to be transferred to the hospital. Family called to hear just as much about "where" he was born as how we were both doing. Those who knew we transferred to hospital were frantic with worry. A relative of mine actually said: "Ha! You thought you'd be able to birth at home! I told you couldn't! Bet you won't try that nonsense again!" With Larson, though I planned a homebirth, I also had a plan for how we'd transfer to hospital if that was necessary. I didn't get hung up on where he'd be born.'

It's vital, then, to plan how you will cope with pain (and anxiety) during any transfer, and how you'll deal with labour – and any medical interventions – once there, including how you'll cope with a caesarean.

My approach to Ted's birth was ambiguous. I was never obsessed with homebirth *per se*, but the idea appealed to me because my main fear was, again, unnecessary interventions. But I had to weigh my gut feelings against my desire for medical safety. In the end I decided to see how labour progressed. My community midwives were extremely encouraging and flexible about this. I got all the homebirth equipment, but also packed my hospital bag and planned how a hospital birth would be. In the event, labour went smoothly: I had a few contractions and called Penny, an experienced midwife, the head of the community team, who was fully aware of my neurotic debates. She came, I went into the living room with her and John, leaned on my birth ball and stayed there until Ted was born a couple of hours later. It didn't occur to me to go anywhere else and Penny monitored us both carefully throughout. If we'd have gone to the hospital, I know this would also have been fine – because it would have been the right thing to do.

A WORD ABOUT PAIN AT HOME | The other homebirth myth that's worth debunking here is that it'll somehow be pain free. It won't be. I actually found the pain of Ted's birth the most intense of all three of my babies. But if you are well prepared for it, feeling safe and having reduced your chances of needless intervention, you can certainly cope better with the pain, and will probably have a more positive attitude about it afterwards (women who give birth at home generally express high levels of satisfaction and certainly, if asked to repeat any of my three births, I'd choose Ted's).

Coping with an unexpected hospital transfer

THINGS TO CONSIDER IN ADVANCE | Talk to your midwife before you are in labour and ask:

- Why might I be transferred to hospital?
- To what hospital will we transfer?
- Will you (the midwife) stay at my side throughout the transfer and once we are in the hospital?
- Why would an ambulance transfer be necessary, and under what circumstances would we go in our car?
- How often have you transferred with your patients, and what is the procedure like?
- What things can we do so we're less overwhelmed by a transfer if it happens?

PREPARING FOR AN UNEXPECTED TRANSFER

1 **Ask your midwife to give you a 'heads up' (and put this in your birth plan)**: tell her you want to know as soon as any alarm bells start ringing for her during your labour. If she can give you even a few minutes warning, you'll cope much better with the trip to hospital when it's happening.

2 **Be prepared for an ambulance** even if it is not strictly an emergency. Most homebirth-to-hospital transfers are routinely done by ambulance. Your partner will usually follow the ambulance in his car.

3 **Have a 'just in case' bag packed** and take it with you, along with comfort things like a blanket/duvet/pillow.

4 **Don't give up on your birth if you have to go to hospital.** You may find there is more pressure to have interventions after a hospital transfer: make sure you've thought this through in advance and have mentioned your preferences in your birth plan.

5 **Let yourself off the hook:** if you want more medication than you'd thought possible, have it. Do what you have to do, to cope with your particular circumstance.

COPING WITH ANY TRIP TO HOSPITAL DURING LABOUR | It can be hard to get into a car and be driven to the hospital when you are having painful contractions even if this is something you were expecting to do. Here are some tips:

1 **Work out in advance who's going to drive you**. Your midwife (if she is with you) will not be allowed to drive you or go in your car. This means your partner (possibly tired and worried) will drive you. If you have a female birth partner she can be invaluable in your car (helping you cope while your partner drives).

2 **If you are in your car, get in the back seat, on all fours (this goes for any trip to hospital during labour)**. Use all your relaxation techniques to cope with the contractions. If you were listening to music at home, and have a portable CD player, put the headphones on (it'll blot out the car noise, and keep you in your 'labour world' as much as possible). Failing this, use the car stereo.

3 **Be prepared for a change in your labour pattern**. Be aware that the stress (physical and mental) of the move can either make you progress faster, or slow things down.

4 **Take your birth plan and all your comfort 'equipment' with you!**

When your newborn needs some help

It is worth taking just a moment to look this one in the eye (and note the details of BLISS, page 233 below). Although about one in ten babies born in the UK need some sort of special care in hospital, and around one in 50 of these need intensive care, few of us have thought about it in advance. *'Although none of us like to dwell on the possibility that anything might be wrong with our baby, there is a good chance that you – or someone within your circle of friends – will have a baby who requires some extra medical attention in the first few weeks of life,'* says Eleri Adams, consultant neonatologist at the John Radcliffe Hospital in Oxford.

A brief guide to the more common complications in newborn babies by consultant neonatologist Eleri Adams

Here are some common problems that could keep you in hospital longer than you expected.

PREMATURE BABY | This is one of the most common reasons why babies need special care. Babies who are born at 37 weeks gestation or more are considered to be 'term', i.e. they are fully cooked and ready for the outside world. Babies born before 37 weeks are considered premature. They may not suck properly, their temperature control may be poor and their lungs may not be quite mature enough. As a general guide, if your baby is born between 34 and 37 weeks then there is a reasonable chance that she might be able to stay with you on the postnatal wards (although this is not always the case) and not need special care.

If your baby is less than 34 weeks she will almost certainly need to go to special care. It can be very tough to be separated from your baby and it is likely to be a difficult and emotional time for you (to say the least).

BABY BORN A BIT TOO SMALL | Some babies who are born after 37 weeks are smaller than they should be ('growth restricted') and consequently have fewer fat stores. They may not be able to regulate their temperature well, and may have problems controlling the glucose supply in their blood. Your baby may be able to stay with you in the postnatal ward, but the doctors will probably need to do regular blood sugar checks to monitor her progress.

INFECTION | Infections in newborn babies have many, many causes and the symptoms of an infection can be very subtle. This is why paediatricians generally have a low threshold for prescribing antibiotics ('just in case'). Usually, they have to wait about 48 hours to get the test results that will show them what, if anything, is causing a possible infection. If the test is clear, and there is no infection after all, the antibiotics can stop and you'll simply go home as normal.

JAUNDICE | Jaundice may be caused by prematurity, the baby being bruised during birth, infection or exposure to certain drugs you were given in labour. The signs of jaundice are the whites of the eyes turning yellowish and the skin below the nipple line turning yellow. Most newborns will become a little bit jaundiced between day two and day seven of life, so if your baby looks yellowish then mention it to the midwife when she visits. She may take some blood from your baby's heel to check how jaundiced she is. Sometimes babies will need to be put under blue lights ('phototherapy') to reduce the jaundice level. If this is the case, you may have to stay in hospital with your baby for a few days. If your baby is less than 24 hours old and shows signs of jaundice you should call the midwife immediately, as this can be more serious.

A WORD ABOUT THE SPECIAL CARE BABY UNIT (SCBU) | You can't, of course, prepare yourself for every eventuality. But if your baby needs to go to the Special Care Baby Unit (SCBU) or even intensive care, support and information –for you and your partner – are vital. Detailed information about babies that need special care, whether they are unwell when they're born or are born prematurely, is of course beyond the scope of this book. However, BLISS, the largest UK premature baby charity, provides free support and information for all parents of babies who need special care: BLISS 68 South Lambeth Road, London SW8 1RL 0870 770 0337 email: information@bliss.org.uk Parent Support Helpline: Freephone 0500 618140 (Monday to Friday 10am–5pm) www.bliss.org.uk.

Many neonatal units also have their own home-grown information guides and there are usually local special-care charities (often run by parents whose babies have previously been in special care), that can give you a considerable amount of support. Ask for details at your antenatal visits if you think you might need to find out more (or afterwards, if it happens unexpectedly).

EIGHT TIPS FOR COPING WITH SCBU | Sarah Kilmartin, mother of Margaret, 18 months, who spent her first 3 weeks in intensive care after developing a lung infection at birth, has these tips:

1 **Ask for information about your baby**. It can be hard to get, so assert yourself and ask to see a doctor so that you understand any changes in treatment etc. You don't have to wait for the ward round or strain to overhear what the staff are saying to each other about your baby. **Doctor's eye view**: *'If the doctor doesn't come to find you, it means they are not overly worried about your baby,'* says neonatologist Eleri Adams.

2 **Take some breaks**. In SCBU they have a high ratio of staff to patients so they can look after your baby while you go out for a bit. Getting away with your partner to eat or walk for short periods is important because SCBU is quite a lonely experience. Your partner goes home each evening and you go back to the ward (full of new babies) or sit by the incubator on your own, then sleep on a ward full of new mothers and their healthy babies (which can be emotionally draining).

3 **Remember your baby belongs to you, not the medical staff.** You have a right to be involved in caring for your baby and you should always be kept informed about what is going on and how you can help to reduce stress for your baby (for instance, breastfeeding while a minor procedure is taking place).

4 **You can bond with a baby in an incubator**. Good staff can show you how it's possible to touch your baby even when she's in an incubator. Your baby will also recognise your voice, which can really calm her.

5 **Understand the monitors attached to your baby.** They are very sensitive, and understanding how they work saves you getting over-anxious as alarms tend to go off regularly and don't necessarily mean there is a problem. **Doctor's eye view**: *'If your baby has a setback in SCBU, ask your doctor to rate this on a scale of one to ten. This will give you a better idea of how things are going,'* says neonatologist Eleri Adams.

6 **SCBU can be quite an extreme environment**: babies arrive all the time and sometimes there are emergencies and several paediatricians appear. You need to be sensitive to other babies and their families when this kind of thing is happening; try to give other families privacy and train your visitors to observe the rules in SCBU.

7 **Don't give up on breastfeeding**. You can breastfeed even if you have a SCBU baby who isn't well enough to feed himself (by using a breastpump). Ask

to see the hospital's breastfeeding specialist and get her to show you exactly how – and how often – to use the pump.

8   **Finally...your amazing baby**. *'scbu is weird because on the one hand it's a nightmare, but at the same time it's also a magical experience because you have a new baby. We just couldn't believe how beautiful Margaret was and how much we loved her. Even now I sometimes use Milton fluid because the smell takes me straight back to scbu and the first precious days with Margaret...'*

· ·

FIND OUT MORE

Resources

Most of the resources you need to make up your birth plan are in Chapter 5: Your Options, where we discuss the nitty gritty of birth choices. You'll also need to prepare your BRAIN using Chapter 3: Fear and Pain, as coping with the unexpected is as much about mental preparation as it is practicalities.

Our website **www.bloomingbirth.net** has more on how to write your plan.

Grief and loss

It is very very rare for your baby to die but should this dreadful event happen you'll get immediate help and support from the nurses, midwives and doctors involved in your care. There are also a number of organisations which you might want to contact in time.

Stillbirth and Neonatal Death Society (SANDS) Support for parents and families whose baby is stillborn or dies soon after birth. 28 Portland Place, London W1N 4DE. Sands National Helpline: 020 7436 5881 (Monday to Friday 10 a.m.–3 p.m.) www.uk-sands.org

Foundation for the Study of Infant Deaths (FSID) Research into infant deaths, and provides a network of support to bereaved parents. Artillery House, 11–19 Artillery Row, London SW1P 1RT. Helpline: 0870 787 0554 General: 0870 787 0885 Fundraising: 0870 443 6814 www.sids.org.uk/fsid

Child Bereavement Trust Provides leaflets, books and videos for bereaved families. Aston House, West Wycombe,High Wycombe, Bucks HP14 3AG. 01494 446648 www.childbereavement.org.uk

Child Death Helpline A helpline for all those affected by the death of a child. Freephone: 0800 282986

Compassionate Friends Telephone support for bereaved families. 53 North Street, Bristol BS3 1EN. 0845 232304 www.tcf.org.uk

Group B Strep Support Helps families whose babies have been affected by GBS. PO Box 203, Haywards Heath, West Sussex RH16 1GF. 01444 416176 www.gbss.org.uk

Chapter Eight:
Blokes, birth and babies

'*What to Expect When You're Expecting,*
The Contented Little Baby Book, Raising
Happy Children, What Every Child Needs
Their Parents to Know: we had all the
books, and by the time Dora was born I
had read the first 19 pages of every one of
them.... Perhaps there are women who
feel that, come the big day, their partners
were just as prepared as they were. I
just don't happen to have met any of them.'

PETE PAPHIDES, JOURNALIST, IN AN ARTICLE ON
PREPARING FOR FATHERHOOD.[1]

1 **Produce regular presents,** flowers, chocolates or whatever your
   partner considers a treat both before and after the birth. During pregnancy she may quickly start feeling overwhelmed, unattractive or just
   plain mad. Remember, attack, so to speak, is the best form of defence.

2 **Make constant references** to how wonderful, beautiful etc. she is,
   how well she's coping and how much you love her.

3 **Put Mother's Day in your diary** and make a fuss of her on it, even if
   you think it's a naff and commercial marketing ruse.

4 **Negotiate realistically about domestic tasks** such as cleaning.
   Arguments about this will only get substantially worse over the next 18
   years if you don't sort things out now.

5 **Massage her in a nonsexual way** at any opportunity, and read our
   sex tips below.

6 **Make your 19 pages of preparatory reading** consist of this chapter
   and Chapter 9: The Love of a Good Woman. (OK, so that's more than 19
   pages, but what's a few extra pages between friends?) If you feel
   inspired by all this, add Chapter 10. Then read the rest of this book for
   good measure.

Until relatively recently, blokes had a pretty straightforward role when it came to
childbirth. You had to pace around a bit while all the messy yelling was going on,
smoking and intermittently trying to concentrate on *The Times*. You might have a
stiff whisky and soda to calm your nerves. Once the 'all clear' was given, you'd
light up your Havana then largely absent yourself until the little blighter was out
of nappies. Nowadays, it's all a bit more demanding. This is, of course, a
wonderful thing for you but at times it can seem that unless you have a PhD in
fetal development, midwifery and early infant care you're going to lack any
credibility as a father-to-be. Many men find the pressure to perform – as
prospective dad, birth partner or postpartum star of the show – somewhat
stressful. You may, in fact, find the whole notion of pregnancy and childbirth
entirely abstract. You may not have a clue what to do to prepare yourself for any
of it. As Pete Paphides writes *'I don't think I'm the first man in the history of the
universe to prepare for his child's birth by making her compilations of all his favourite
records...'*[2]

There are, of course, a few vital things you can do beyond burning a CD for the
baby. When you're in that delivery room, watching the love of your life attempt to
squeeze your progeny out of her vagina, childbirth will suddenly become
distinctly *real*. This is when it helps to know a bit about the process. A few hints
about what you can usefully do at this point may come in handy, to say the least.
This chapter will give you a sense of where you fit into the whole pregnancy, birth
and immediate postpartum. We can't tell you what the birth of your child will be
like for you or your partner. But we can show you how to make it decidedly **more**

manageable – whatever happens on the day. Before you know it you're going to be pacing round the kitchen at 2 a.m. with a yowling newborn on your shoulder. Read this chapter, and you'll be doing so with no regrets.

Fatherhood

There are many upsides to fatherhood. If this is your first time, all you need to know, really, is that the love, passion and protectiveness you'll feel towards that baby will be mind-blowing. It may also help to know that your role in your baby's life starts as it means to go on. Research has found that where fathers are involved, breastfeeding is more successful, postnatal depression reduced, children are more successful at exams at 16 and are less likely to have a criminal record at 21.[3]

If this is not your first stab at fatherhood, you may be wondering how you'll summon up the same degree of emotion for another child. The good news is that this time your love will be just as overwhelming as before. If it wasn't, Neanderthal man would have developed a far more sophisticated long-distance running capacity.

There are many other less profound reasons why fatherhood can be good. Behaving like a child can be immensely pleasurable. Indeed, one survey[4] found that more than 70 per cent of boys claimed their fathers spend more time playing with their toys than they do themselves, and 69 per cent of fathers were actually proud of this, admitting to buying toys for their children with their own interests in mind. Research has shown that fathers from a diversity of social and ethnic backgrounds usually say that fathering is the most important part of their lives.[5] You will, in short, experience the greatest highs of your life as a parent.

First time fathers: the wake up call

You may, when shown that plastic pregnancy tester thing, have initially felt a combination of shock, joy and general amazement that your sperm actually work. If the pregnancy was a 'surprise' you may also feel panicked. Once you've calmed down a bit, some other implications may also start to dawn. While most men are extraordinarily well adjusted when it comes to procreation, others hit the Rock Star Syndrome. If you have not yet become a rock star (billionaire/acclaimed novelist/astronaut etc.) this is the time when you have to face facts: it may not happen. *'I realised, when she told me she was pregnant, that I was never going to tour with Bono – that part of me was over,'* says Simon, 35, father of two. *'It sounds silly (I'm an accountant!) but it was actually rather depressing. I couldn't tell my wife about this – it would seem somehow disloyal given that we'd both decided it was time to have a baby.'* For some men, the Rock Star Syndrome may manifest itself in a freakish burst of self-improvement. Julia's husband got a personal trainer, started violin lessons and quit his job when she was pregnant with their first baby. Luckily, the frenzy was relatively short lived and he's now back working at Microsoft and eating doughnuts again.

The knowledge that in nine months time you're going to be responsible for another human being is enough to make even the best adjusted bloke reach for the Glenfiddich. But if you do pour yourself a snifter, beware: your partner can't join you. She's probably going to remind you of this, and of your lack of dietary restrictions, your continence and general freedom of bodily movement A LOT over the coming months, and she may not find it funny. Your best policy, now, and for the foreseeable future, is sympathy, understanding and the purchase of many gifts.

Performance anxiety – will I be a good Dad? – is another common fear for first timers, particularly those whose own father left much to be desired. But even the most unpromising fathers-to-be can turn out to be diamonds. Julia remembers one client who came into his own as a father:

'During the pregnancy Jose was pretty absent. We all worried that he would never be able to help his wife and, during the birth, this turned out to be true. He was completely unprepared, saying he did not want to read about birth in advance because he wanted to experience it without influence. On the day he found the whole experience traumatic. But he's turned into a fantastic dad. I recently bumped into him at a child's party: he was wearing a pink tu-tu and pirouetting while his 2-year-old shrieked with joy.'

'We're pregnant'

No you're not. Don't be tempted to say this. Ever. Yes, you are both going to have a baby. But **she** is pregnant, not you. The sooner you realise this, the better. You don't want to become one of those nauseating, obsessed fathers-to-be who strap bags of flour to their stomachs to 'share' her pain.

Whether or not you've witnessed your partner 'blooming' before, you may well feel a bit redundant while the baby's still inside her. This is fair enough: she's the one doing the gestating after all, and most men are fine with this. But it's worth knowing that feeling a bit left out or 'useless' is pretty common. Books about fatherhood bang on about this, particularly about how abstract it can feel in the early stages: *'Just about every study that's ever been done on the subject has shown that women generally "connect" with their pregnancies sooner than men do'* write the authors of *The Expectant Father*.[6] Now, you may have no desire to read books like this – the baby's in *her* belly after all, not yours. But there is a middle ground between sympathetic extremism, and absenting yourself entirely from the whole affair.

For a start, you do want, if possible, to preserve some sense of togetherness with your partner. And what's going on for her is pretty major. The best way to help is to stay involved in things like antenatal check-ups (at least make sure you know when they are, and what happens at them). Fetal development, if you get a good book (see Further reading, page 262) can be fascinating. Knowing a bit about what's *in there* might also help you connect with your baby when it comes out. As the authors of *The Expectant Father* put it: *'The general rule that women* connect with the pregnancy sooner than men has an exception: men who get involved early on and stay involved until the end have been shown to be as connected with the baby as their partners.' Most men go along to the ultrasound appointments (there are usually two, one early, one mid pregnancy). This can be very moving. In the first one (when your partner is around three months pregnant) the baby doesn't look much like a baby, but you'd be surprised at how choked up you can get over a grainy black and white shot of a king prawn. In the mid-pregnancy one, the baby looks more like a baby and this can be a big moment for fathers: *'I don't think I felt any connection to Sarah's pregnancy until I saw Jake's spine on the ultrasound. That was a wonderful, scary moment that made it all very real for me,'* says Tim, 33, father of Jake, 2.

A tip for second timers

If you are already a father, don't think this stuff doesn't apply to you. Getting involved during the pregnancy may in fact be **more** relevant this time than it was before. Your partner is going to be doubly exhausted, without the novelty factor and with a clear idea of what lies at the end of the nine months (labour). She's already got a belly full of stretch marks and she knows she's about to put on four-odd stone (yes, a big deal for most women). Your temptation will be to think 'she's done it before, she knows what she's doing, she doesn't need me'. This would be an error. No matter how delighted you both are to be expanding your brood, she'll need some bolstering.

Furthermore, if you have a small child or two you've probably already worked out that it's now your job to get up in the night to deal with them. Your pregnant partner needs REST (no matter how much of a trouper she is at 3 a.m.). She's growing a baby and that's a pretty major task even if she seems nonchalant. If your older children aren't already used to having things done for them by you (i.e. teeth cleaning/bedtime routine/park visits/dinner) now is the time to get into the swing of things. When their mother has a newborn attached to her breast round the clock, various routine tasks are going to fall to you. If she usually does most of the child-related tasks, they may demand their mummy. Press on, firmly, and you'll find they quickly accept that you are the one wielding the Barbie toothbrush, not mummy. You both have to be firm on this one, but establishing any new routines **before** your new baby arrives will significantly minimise the upheaval and psychological disruption for your older child (not to mention for you both). It may seem improbable that you could enjoy reading *Angelina Ballerina* every night, but many dads say that growing closer to their older child was an unexpected and profoundly satisfying side-effect of adding a newborn to the family.

Sympathetic pregnancy

There are, as you can imagine, different degrees of sympathy. If you find yourself developing morning sickness or sore nipples, do try pulling yourself together. If you can't, then it might help to know you're not alone. 'Sympathetic pregnancy' is a recognised psychological syndrome (the technical term is 'couvades syndrome'). Basically, some men get weird physical symptoms that may mirror their pregnant partner's. This is surprisingly common. Researchers say up to 70 per cent of fathers-to-be enjoy such delights as weight gain, nausea, mood swings or food cravings. Such 'symptoms' usually appear in about the third month of your partner's pregnancy, fade a bit, then re-emerge about a month or two before the baby is born. Psychologists say – and this is somewhat obvious – that these are down to sympathy or feelings of guilt for what your partner is going through, or (far less appealing) a touch of jealousy, but nobody really knows why this happens. None of it is new however: as far back as you'd like to go men have wanted to be involved in the gestation process. Indeed, the eighteenth-century Scots believed that during childbirth a nurse could use witchcraft to transfer the pain from the wife to the husband. If only.

As for weight gain, many men balloon during their partner's pregnancy simply because she, suddenly, has thrown dietary caution to the wind and is buying in crates of chocolate. Exercise a little restraint in the face of the pac man that was once your wife, and you'll be fine.

Personality changes

You may find your partner's ups and downs harder to handle than her physical transformation:

'Her moods became unpredictable in pregnancy,' says Darius, 40, father of three. *'Basically, she'd be incredibly emotional. She's a criminal barrister and I once caught her weeping in front of Pet Rescue on the TV. But also she'd get suddenly furious about things. In fact, it felt rather random, which way she'd go.'* She may also become weirdly domesticated. *'My wife has always been very focused and career-orientated. I naively thought that pregnancy wouldn't change her. But she stopped focusing on work. Instead, she would curl up with cookbooks and watch food programmes. We ate fantastically well for nine months, but it was strange to see her personality shift into domestic goddess overdrive,'* says Al, 30, father of Sarry, 1.

If this is your second baby, and your wife sailed through the first pregnancy being her usual sunny self, don't think she'll necessarily do it again. Every pregnancy is different. She may become Hannibal Lecter this time, so **make no assumptions**. While she's slavering over her filet mignon, you can be doing some useful tasks.

FIVE PRACTICAL THINGS TO DO DURING HER PREGNANCY

1 **Put all her antenatal and postpartum checks in your diary:**
   mention them in advance and ask about them afterwards if you don't go
   (and listen to her answers – she may test you on them later).

2 **Buy a present of some sort** to give to her when you bring your baby home. Make it a special one – she's just produced your infant, and as you probably noticed, it hurt.

3 **Take a bigger share of housework**/caring for your other children/cooking etc. even if this means performing *even more* tedious domestic tasks after work when you feel you've earned a rest.

4 **Update your will** to add your new child.

5 **Set up life insurance policies.**

TEN THINGS **NOT** TO SAY TO YOUR PREGNANT PARTNER – EVER

1 Do stop whining
2 Christ! your feet are enormous
3 This is the best martini I've ever had
4 You shouldn't have an epidural, it might harm the baby
5 You're eating again? Are you sure that's a good idea?
6 Labour isn't such a big deal
7 I've arranged for my mother to stay with us for three months after the baby's born
8 Why do I need to come to the birth class?
9 Blimey, are you sure there's only one in there?
10 So-and-so (naming non-pregnant female friend) looks gorgeous these days, doesn't she?

Common worries

MONEY | Having kids costs a fortune. Many men (and indeed women) worry about this – particularly when they're having more than one child. If this is something that's preoccupying you, why not look it in the eye now? Brace yourself – estimates vary but virtually all studies show childrearing is, indeed, ruinous. One 2004 study by a financial services company recently found that the total cost of raising a child in a typical two-parent working household from birth to age 21 is now an eye-watering £140,398. That's an average annual bill of £6,686 until your child is 21.

Of course, how much your children really cost you will depend on how much you're willing to lavish on them. Families manage on significantly less than six grand a year per child. Your wee one does not have to have the latest Nikes. But if you're feeling neurotic, do some sums – work out a budget, talk it over, even see a financial planner. Otherwise, assume you'll get by. We all do. Somehow.

CHANGING LIFESTYLE | If this is your first baby, you may enjoy frequent nights down the boozer, Saturday footie games and/or hours nerding in front of your computer. People will tell you this is all over once you have kids. To a certain extent, it is. But having kids doesn't mean you'll be confined to domestic duties alone after working hours. Men with children do still have social lives, play sport and all the rest. They may have to scale this down a bit – certainly initially – but life is not over. If this sort of thing is worrying you, try and talk to your partner about it. The worst thing you can do is bugger off to the pub leaving her with a screaming newborn every night. All of this may sound depressing, but the missing link, here, is the mind-altering love you'll feel for your small child.

THE CHILD IS NOT YOURS | This one's going to shock most women, but it's something many men worry about. One psychologist, Jerrold Lee Shapiro, interviewed more than two hundred men whose partners were pregnant, and found that 60 per cent of them 'acknowledged fleeting thoughts, fantasies or nagging doubts that they might not really be the biological father of the child'. Most, apparently, don't really believe their partners are having affairs. But on some level they feel they can't have possibly created another a human being: someone more potent must have done it for them.[7] One friend of mine forced her husband to come along to an NCT class with her. The task that day was for the men to write down the answer to various statements, so as to 'explore' their feelings about fatherhood. In response to the statement '*I would be most shocked if....*', her husband (who is Caucasian) wrote '*the baby is black.*' He wasn't entirely taking the exercise seriously, but as generations of psychologists, historians and literary critics have shown the 'anxiety of influence' is pretty pervasive.

Sex

You may find yourself vastly turned on by your partner's burgeoning form (those swelling breasts, at the very least, could get you going). Or you may become turned off by her morphing, unpredictable body. Enlargement – all over – is the name of the game. She'll put on fat as well as baby. This is normal. Her boobs, of course, are going to be temporarily pneumatic. But for many men this turns out to be the ultimate torment – they are often completely untouchable, as they'll become, at times, unbearably tender/rock hard/engorged with milk (during pregnancy, and afterwards). You may also find it hard, in a complex, confusing way, to separate her status as a mother, with her role as your lover. Which kind of Madonna *is* she these days? Sex with a pregnant woman can be a minefield for both of you. It's worth communicating about this if you can, because when you have a baby, the sexual distance, if it's there, is likely to increase rather than decrease.

'I had a huge problem seeing my wife as sexual when she was pregnant,' says Martin, 36, father of Aidan, 4. 'I was afraid I'd hurt her. We had sex a few times (on our sides), but I felt like I was in mourning for what I saw to be the end of our sex life. Then Aidan came and we were tired all the time. I think our marriage problems really started there. If we had just talked about it things would probably be better between us now.'

The ball, unfortunately, has to be in her court when it comes to how – and how often – you have sex. She really is in the grip of some serious chemicals and whatever she's feeling, sex-wise, just isn't her fault. Some women simply don't fancy it at all for nine months and you have to accept this – somehow. Others are raving balls of hormones, ripping your clothes off one minute, slapping you away in disgust another. Such a mixed bag can be hard to negotiate. The simple rule is: do not take it personally (after all, she loves you enough to have your baby). If you're feeling sexy, try and approach her sensitively. And, though this may go against your most basic nature, talk about it.

SAFETY CONCERNS | The baby is protected from your penis by:

- a kind of plug across the neck of the womb (cervix).
- the cervix itself, which is closed. (The opening of the cervix is what 'dilates' during labour. It has to get from closed to 10 cm open, to let the baby's head out.)
- a very resilient bag of waters (amniotic fluid).

Providing your partner has no medical complications in the pregnancy that have ruled out sex (ask the doctor/midwife for the go ahead if you are at all worried), your penis in her vagina will neither touch, disturb nor hurt the baby. The baby will have no idea what's going on and (I know, it's a mad concern, but it's in there for many of us) the baby is certainly **not watching**.

WHAT TO DO IF SHE DOESN'T WANT SEX | Above all, try to keep physical affection going. Make sure you continue to give her cuddles, kisses and to show her affection. Try to avoid simply giving up. Dr Petra Boynton, a psychologist specialising in sex and relationships at University College London says a dialogue is important: *'Try to talk to her about sex (but not when she's just rejected your moves – pick a stress free time). Explore why she doesn't feel like sex (for example, if she feels sick or tired she won't be interested, but if she feels she shouldn't do it, that's a different matter).'* Also, tell her how you are feeling about sex during her pregnancy (or the lack of it); let her know about your inhibitions, desires or fears. If your relationship is open, she may be happy for you to masturbate (she may even help you). But do avoid using masturbation as a bargaining tool (i.e. 'if you don't have sex with me then I'll have to masturbate/watch porn').

THREE WAYS TO MAINTAIN INTIMACY WITHOUT SEX

'Keeping the intimacy in the relationship is still necessary even if she doesn't want sex,' says Dr Petra Boynton.

1 **Keep the romance.** You don't have to be cooking elaborate meals or buying roses all the time. Just touching each other is good: cuddle her, hold hands, kiss her, hug her – whenever you can.

2 **Distinguish between sensual touching and sexual touching.**
This one is vital: you need to understand that if you give her a back rub
it will not necessarily lead to sex. She needs to know she can relax and
let you touch her without having to muster the energy to do anything
(or fear she's being 'unfair' to not want sex).

3 **Make the effort to communicate:** choose and watch a DVD together,
then talk about it afterwards instead of flopping in front of the telly;
have a telly free night a week – listen to music together, play music to
the baby, read to one another. These things sound contrived, but can
make a huge difference if you're feeling generally estranged by your
lack of sex.

BREASTS AND WHAT TO DO WITH THEM | Those girls are undoubtedly super-sensitive as well as, possibly, supersized. This may be a unique torment to you but you should know that even your most gentle nibbling might feel, to your partner, like you've taken a razor blade to her areola. The good news is that her breasts may also be extra-erogenous if you can work out how to touch them. Be more gentle than you'd think possible, and build up to the level, and technique she likes. If she can't have them handled, you can always just LOOK. One thing you may find freaky (and/or fantastic) is that sex with a pregnant or postpartum woman can bring milk out of her breasts (usually only a tiny amount in pregnancy).

HER CLITORIS | Masturbation and orgasms – yours or your partner's – will not hurt your baby. Her clitoris may feel more sensitive, because there is more blood in that area of the body during pregnancy, and more hormones floating around. But equally, it may feel totally unsensitive. And if she's got piles, constipation, is knackered and feels unattractive, no amount of clitoral technique is going to turn her into a sexual dynamo.

HER VAGINA | There is increased blood flow to the vagina during pregnancy, which can make it feel unfamiliar (it can feel either more, or less, lubricated) to some women. You can buy lubricant (such as KY Jelly) at any chemist. But if penetrative sex is no longer fun, oral sex (for both of you) can still be a good thing.

POSITIONS | Your partner – even if she tried to – is unlikely to be able to go through the whole pregnancy having sex in the missionary position. Lying on your back when pregnant can be unbelievably uncomfortable, especially in the later stages. There's a lot of weight in there, pressing on her spine and bladder when she lies down. Deep and thrusting penetration, too, can feel uncomfortable.
You're not going to squash or poke the baby (there's tons of fluid and flesh between you and it) but lying on her breasts will certainly cause her instant pain.

So, you have to experiment. This, for some couples, turns out to be fun.

A few good positions for pregnant sex:
- Lying side-by-side.
- Sitting (try using a chair too if you've got a big one).
- From behind.
- OK – any way she fancies (let her dictate what feels good). Try buying lots of pillows and using them in imaginative ways to prop up bits of her anatomy as you both try and manoeuvre into good positions.

The mechanics can get comical and it helps if you have a sense of humour and a flexibility that is not just physical. Sometimes – particularly later on – you may have to give up half way through a session if it all just 'feels wrong' to her. Be patient. Try thinking how sexy you'd feel with an 8lb baby lodged in your pelvis, and your balls wired up to the mains. Holding, stroking, reassuring and loving her, if penetrative sex won't work, is the only reasonable course of action (see sexual survival rule 1, below).

ORGASMS | Orgasms for her may feel different in pregnancy – more or less intense or satisfying. They can bring on mild, harmless contractions. And later in pregnancy, her orgasm might also make the baby wriggle around. This is absolutely normal and harmless, but it can feel a bit freaky if you're in porn land and suddenly you have a baby booting you (both!). The only advice here is to go with it and – as with childbirth – expect the unexpected.

How, when and with what degree of pleasure she orgasms can depend on anything from the state of her belly to the state of her mind (odd, usually).

FIVE RULES FOR SEXUAL SURVIVAL

1 **Make masturbation your friend.** You're probably going to need it over the next few months (and possibly years).

2 **Reassure your partner that she's beautiful.** If you find your partner's pregnant (or, even more dangerously, postpartum) form unattractive, telling her so, bluntly, is simply not an option. You really do just have to blame your lack of interest on Freud, or on your fears about hurting the baby.

3 **Inform yourself.** You will not hurt the baby by having penetrative sex, oral sex or any other reasonable kind of sexual contact. If she's on for it, and you are too, then enjoy it together. Once you have a wailing newborn in the room you may look back on these halcyon days with a touch of nostalgia.

4 **Avoid blame.** It's extremely rare for a couple with children (even if they're still inside the woman) NOT to have a disrupted sex life at some

point. You are not alone. Your partner is not frigid. You are not impotent and/or Priapic. How long your sex life will be disrupted for is anyone's guess but give it time, and if it becomes unbearable and you can't sort it out, do consider counselling even if the very notion makes you want to flee.

5   **Let your emotions in.** Childbirth may not signal the end of your sex life – far from it. Many couples find they reach new levels of intimacy after having gone through this unbelievable, intense, life-changing experience together.

A WORD ABOUT MEN AND MISCARRIAGE | When it comes to miscarriage, men's feelings are usually entirely sidelined. A miscarriage is, indeed, hardest on the woman (the physical event alone can be extremely distressing), but that doesn't mean you'll feel OK about it. Grief, disappointment, helplessness and depression are all common emotions in dads after their partner's miscarriage. It's important to remember, of course, that over 90 per cent of couples who experience a miscarriage will have a baby later, and that miscarriages are extremely common (see Chapter 1, page 34). Some books will also tell you that a miscarriage is a 'blessing in disguise' because it's 'natural selection' at work. But this kind of rational thinking often isn't terribly helpful when you're having a tough time coming to terms with what has happened. This is why counselling after a miscarriage can be immensely helpful for both of you – a way for you to talk through how you are feeling, and to get to grips with what has happened to you both. Your partner will certainly need you to listen to her, and to give her a lot of emotional support (sometimes for a very long time after the event, even when you think she should be 'over it' by now). But the key thing to remember is that it's perfectly valid for you to be upset and depressed about it too. As the authors of *The Expectant Father* put it: *'Until very recently, miscarriage, like the pregnancy it ends, has been considered the exclusive emotional domain of women. This is simply untrue. While men don't have to endure the physical pain or discomfort of a miscarriage, their emotional pain is just as severe as their partner's. They still have the same hopes and dreams about their unborn children, and they still feel a profound sense of grief when those hopes and dreams are dashed. And many men, just like their partners, feel tremendous guilt and inadequacy when a pregnancy ends prematurely.'*[8] (For more information about miscarriage, see Chapter 1, page 34.)

The birth

'Partners are terrific. But they often want to save the woman. That's what they're conditioned to do. But the women, in childbirth, don't want to be saved.' Kim Kelley, midwife

1 **Be there.**
2 **Keep her calm:** using talk, touch, distraction or humour – different things work for different women and you know her best.
3 **Fetch things:** give her ice to suck, mop her brow, bring her things she asks for, push the iv pole after her: then she can get on with her job.
4 **Massage her:** back, thighs, arms, hands, feet – whatever helps relax her.
5 **Keep her in gravity-friendly positions:** she should be sitting up, squatting, walking, leaning, standing, kneeling, rocking and should avoid lying on her back as much as possible. It's all about gravity.
6 **Guard her space:** keep the room quiet, the lights dim, the music on, and stop people from coming and going and talking unnecessarily (if this is what she wants).
7 **Ask questions about medical procedures** if she's not able to. Do your best to help her understand what's happening, and why, and that it's for the best.
8 **Encourage her through these medical interventions:** tell her she's done everything she can, that this is what the baby needs, that it'll soon be over and the baby will be out.
9 **Reassure her:** that she and the baby are safe, that she's in the right place, that the staff are looking out for her.
10 **Tell her you love her.** Repeatedly.

It's fair enough that you should feel discomfited at the prospect of a baby coming out of your loved one's holied vagina (or, indeed, abdomen). Even, or possibly especially, if this is not your first baby the idea of the birth can be daunting if you think about it. **And you should**. The last thing you – or more specifically your partner – want in the labour room is panic. Men are just as floored by the reality of childbirth as women are. One study of couples' fears about childbirth found that 'helplessness, powerlessness and the wife's death in childbirth were the most significant subjects of men's fears'.[9] It's not easy to stand by and watch the woman you love go through something as extreme and painful as childbirth. But it needn't be horrifying. It can be astonishingly moving. And – if you've prepared yourself – you almost certainly won't faint.

Should you be there?
Yes, really, this is a valid question. You may not feel this way when you're sitting on beanbags in some childbirth class, but if you seriously doubt whether you want to be there, open that dialogue **now**.

In 1965 only 5 per cent of fathers were at the birth of their baby. Today, according to the National Childbirth Trust, about 96 per cent of fathers are there.

The Royal College of Midwives does, however, acknowledge that some men might find giving support to their partners in childbirth hard. Often men worry about being at the birth simply because it's all so terrifyingly gynaecological and female. They can't imagine what they'll DO in the labour room (except faint, or be put off sex for life). But as any woman who's had a supportive husband by her side will attest, your role in labour really can be quite straightforward and crucial.

It may also help you to know that your presence can make a genuine difference to what happens during the birth. According to Jack O'Sullivan of Fathers Direct (the UK National Information Centre for Fatherhood) research has shown that when fathers are well informed about pregnancy and birth, mothers generally have shorter labours and need less pain relief, are more likely to breastfeed successfully and less likely to suffer from postnatal depression.

If you learn more about the mechanics of birth you may find it less daunting. Chapter 2: Birth for beginners, will give you all you need to know about what a straightforward birth can really be like – the real life version, not the text book one (read this even if you've seen birth before. Sometimes 'normal' things can floor you second time around too if you don't know about them). Men in general are woefully unprepared for witnessing childbirth, and are horrified or panicked by things that are basically normal and healthy.

It's worth recognising that there may be times, in labour, when you really won't be able to do much to help (except be there). *'When things got tough in Thomas's birth, I did feel helpless,'* says James, father of Margaret (18 months) and Thomas (4 months). *'The midwives were asking Sarah not to push, and she was screaming at them – in real pain. I found this very distressing. I just wanted it to be over.'* Hopefully, you'll only feel like this for short periods of time in labour, if at all. The trick, during the tough bits, is to stay calm – look at the medical staff for reassurance – and never underestimate the value of simply being with your partner, whispering loving, reassuring things to her. I know that during the births of all three of my babies, I needed John to be with me, regardless of whether he was 'doing' anything much. Whenever he left the room, I'd feel panicky.

Many men relish the births of their children, and for good reason. Andrew, a 39-year-old accountant, counts the births of his three children as the most outstanding events of his life: *'I'm normally your typically analytical Asperger's-type bloke – my hobby is physics – but the births of my children made me feel like a different person. I knew my wife really needed me. And when each of my children was born, I sobbed. I can't remember sobbing ever in my life. It really was an astonishing experience and any man who misses it is an arse.'*

HOW NOT TO BE AN ARSE IN LABOUR

Do not be tempted to:
- chat during contractions (to her or anyone else)
- run down to watch the baby coming out and forget about her, at the other end

- dominate proceedings in any way
- boss her around
- forget to eat – nobody needs a fainting dad
- get out your laptop
- become obsessed by machines, numbers and facts.

Practical help

Most childbirth books and classes give blokes a list of stuff to DO before and during the birth. The idea is basically that you won't feel 'at ease' unless you're hunter-gathering or performing some other function. You may, however, find the list of tasks you're given a wee bit manufactured. After all, there's only so much time you can spend plotting routes to the hospital and packing your sponge bag. If a list of things to do will make you feel comforted, here's one (below). But remember, the really important things you can do are all in the bullets on page 249. They sound woolly and touchy-feely, but they're what most women need in labour.

SIX HELPFUL FUNCTIONS FOR YOU TO PERFORM

Before birth:

1 Oh go on then – plot that route to the hospital, why don't you. No, seriously: it would actually be a bad idea to get lost with your wife hotting up in the back set. While route-planning, by the way, avoid bumpy roads/speed bumps/unnecessarily windy shortcuts if you possibly can. There's nothing like a jolting car plus contractions to enrage a distressed woman.
2 Remember to put the hospital bag and car seat in the car.
3 Take care of general practicalities: fill the birth pool, carry in stuff from the car when you get to hospital.
4 Don't forget to pack your mobile and camera (usually you can't use the mobile in the ward but it will still come in handy, for making odd calls, trips to the shop to get her the RIGHT kind of chocolate....etc).

During birth:

5 Mop her brow with a cool flannel and give her ice chips to chew if she wants them; fetch her things, press play when the CD stops, etc.
6 Don't forget to take pics if you've both decided you want them of the birth, or immediate post-birth.

Some common pitfalls

LABOUR IS NOT ABOUT YOU | One thing Julia has seen too many times is fathers who somehow contrive (possibly through anxiety) to make labour about them, not their partners. She had one client who she now thinks of as 'helmet dad' because he insisted on wearing his bike helmet throughout his wife's labour, in case he should faint. Understandably, this took much attention away from his wife. You are, I'm sure, not the sort of bloke to get his bike helmet on but do be clear that it's fine to feel nervous, scared or overwhelmed by birth. Above all else, your role is to focus on your partner, and make sure others do too.

EPIDURAL ABANDONMENT | Another no-no – again something Julia sees more and more of – is men who switch off when the epidural is switched on: *'I have seen this repeatedly: the man doesn't realise that it's not so great having a needle in your spine and being immobile. The woman will often be very anxious about how things are going to pan out over the next few hours. But the partner doesn't realise this, he feels liberated by the technology and trots off to get a sandwich, becomes obsessed with the sports page, (or worse still, switches on his laptop), leaving her very conscious and very alone.'*

Some women say their epidural was bliss. It can be a huge salvation. But others don't feel this way at all. So don't bugger off (physically or metaphorically), just because she's lying there looking calm with knock-out pain relief in her back. Even if you are just playing cards, or reading to her, or holding her hand as she sleeps, try to remember that you're still vital. That's not to say you *can't* nip out to get food, or pee or buy her a magazine. Just don't *assume* she's OK. And don't forget to tell her she's doing well and you love her.

NEVER GIVE UP | A survey of fathers, by the National Childbirth Trust,[10] found that more than two thirds felt frustrated during the birth that they were unable to help when their partner was in pain. One good tip for all fathers during childbirth is to **be flexible and don't give up**. You may have agreed, in advance, that you'll rub her back. But if she bats you off the minute you touch her, this doesn't mean your role in the birth has come to an end. You need to learn together – in advance and during labour – about the different things that help with pain. Sometimes nothing will seem to 'work'. This doesn't mean you aren't helping. If she doesn't let you 'do' anything, just be there, next to her, telling her you love her and she's doing well. It may even be that what she wants from you is for you to sit silently next to her for 18 hours. But do be sure this is, indeed, the case, before you oblige.

'My best advice for any father-to-be is to remember that the labour room isn't a theatre and you are not the audience,' says Rob, 30, father of Joe (3 months). *'In the end, I felt not like a viewer, but a participant. When Eliza started pushing, I had the instinct to go down there and watch the baby come out, but I couldn't let go of her hand. Beforehand, I had the vague notion that I should be with my wife on "her special day", but it really wasn't just her day, it was ours.'*

A WORD ABOUT THE BUSINESS END | My husband John is squeamish. Even the thought of blood makes him feel faint. Yet he was there (at the head end) for my daughter's birth (a caesarean) and he witnessed both his sons coming out of my vagina (for my first, he was holding my leg up and didn't look away; for the second, he was watching, excitedly, for the head). He says the blood just wasn't relevant. Indeed, he says there was surprisingly little of it (though there were apparently lots of 'fluids'). All of that stuff came second to the astounding fact that he was about to meet our baby. In cold blood birth does sound off-putting, but in the heat of the moment, seeing your baby enter the world can be miraculous.

You don't, of course, **have** to see anything gory. You can be at her head the whole time. But most men are very good at compartmentalising. Staying at your partner's head until the baby's head is just coming out is probably your best policy – but on the point of birth most men see the baby, not the vagina. Seeing our babies emerge, like this, certainly has not dented my husband's sex drive and this seems to be a common experience. *'To be honest, I'm just over the moon if she's feeling sexy at all,'* says Rowan (28), father of Oliver (2) and Fergus (9 months). *'The notion of being "put off" by some memory of witnessing childbirth when there's a prospect of a shag after many barren, baby filled weeks, is – to be honest – laughable.'*

Sticking around after the birth

You'll probably get sent home from the hospital once your partner and baby are 'settled'. Maternity units can be brutal (they also have to respect cultural differences: many women would be extremely uncomfortable with a man sleeping in a chair in the ward). A few modern NHS maternity units have overnight facilities for dads, and some even have private rooms, where you can sleep on a zed bed next to your partner and newborn. These rooms can cost anything from £50 a night to £200, depending on your hospital. Some hospitals let you book such rooms in advance (useful if you know the date your baby will be born on i.e. if it is by planned caesarean). Staying at the hospital, if you can mange it, can be a terrifically bonding experience for *all* of you, so do ask if you can somehow stay.

Babies

'I felt at first like the baby's real parents would be coming to get him soon. It took weeks for that feeling to go away. It took weeks for me to really understand that I wasn't babysitting – this is my kid.' Brian, 28, father of Alex (3)

FIVE FANTASTIC FATHER FEELINGS

1 Huge love for the baby
2 Amazement at what the female body can do

3   Amazement that you've made this new person
4   Pride at being a father
5   Protectiveness towards this defenceless baby/your partner

SIX SOURCES OF STRESS

1   Shock/upset after witnessing the birth
2   What happened to my old life? Guilt and hassle if you want to go for a beer with your mates
3   Shock (and or dismay) at how the baby changes relationship (including sex)
4   Weird feeling of detachment from the baby
5   Exclusion/redundancy (including possible sense that partner's body is out of bounds/her breasts now 'belong' to someone else!)
6   Stress about money/work/time

The first thing you're likely to feel, on meeting your baby (yes, even if it's not your first), is utter elation (and possibly relief). *'Most men say the birth of their child is the most profound thing that ever happened to them,'* says Jack O'Sullivan of Fathers Direct. However the early part of the postpartum period can take its toll.

'Postpartum is a time of great change, but also of great learning, for men too,' says Jack O'Sullivan. *'Nowadays most men take paternity leave or at least holiday when the baby is born, and are very keen to learn all there is to learn about being a dad. But there is not a lot of information out there aimed specifically at new fathers. You can learn from your partner, but most of all, you can learn from just being there.'*

If you think birth is the hard bit then read Chapter 10 of this book (Postpartum). In fact, reading Chapter 10 is the best thing you can do for yourself and your partner when it comes to the first few weeks of your baby's life. It will give you a flavour of some of the major things your partner may go through – physically and mentally – once the baby is out. It'll give you a sense of what life with your baby may be like, initially. And it will give you some ideas about how to make this easier, for all of you, whether or not this is your first child. Studies have shown that new fathers hold, touch, kiss, rock and coo at their babies as often as mothers do, and are just as emotionally involved with their babies as mothers are. So don't be afraid to let your inner Dad out.

Breastfeeding

No amount of inner Dad is going to get you far on this one. But you can still play a vital part in how your baby feeds. Breastfeeding really is by far the best way to grow a healthy baby (see Chapter 10, page 311, for 10 reasons why). Studies have shown that the dad's attitude to breastfeeding is one of the most important factors in breastfeeding success rates. You'd think breastfeeding was easy – it's nature after all. She just sticks the baby on when it's hungry. But often it's not this simple. Breastfeeding may – certainly initially – be hard to get the hang of. Some babies take a while to suck. Some boobs are agony at first. And getting a good 'supply and demand' thing sorted out can be hard. Many of us feel quite literally DRAINED by feeding in the first four to six weeks.

Breathing down her neck muttering 'no pain, no gain' or something equivalent, is probably the quickest way for you to find out what it's like to be bludgeoned to death with a rock hard breast. This is true even if this is not your first baby (breastfeeding can be a breeze with one baby, and difficult with another: same boobs, different infant). As with labour, your role is one of support and encouragement. Usually feeding settles down after about six weeks and initial problems, if there are any, should be ironed out.

Breastfeeding can make women feel:
- Blissful
- Invincible
- Beautiful
- Deeply maternal
- Miraculous

But also:
- Irritable
- Exhausted
- Sore
- Moody
- Tearful
- Despairing
- Bored

Possibly all at once.

Your partner may, then, become a wee bit challenging in those early days. She needs to eat properly, get rest and drink lots of water. It's your job to make sure, as best you can, that this happens.

TEN THINGS YOU CAN DO TO SUPPORT YOUR BREASTFEEDING PARTNER

1 Get the baby out of the cot at night to take him to your partner for feeds.
2 Change the baby's nappy, either before, after or during a break between breasts if he poos.
3 Walk around with the baby in a sling to stop her crying/distract her between feeds/give your partner a rest.
4 Stop your other small children from climbing on/demanding things of your partner while she is trying to breastfeed.
5 Tell your partner frequently that she's doing really well and that you know it must be tiring for her.

6 Bring her a drink of water, every time you notice she's feeding the baby.

7 Hand her a book, remote control or snack while she's feeding.

8 Take a big share of the shopping, cleaning and cooking or at least make sure that someone *other than her* is doing the bulk of this.

9 Collect a load of takeout menus, put them by the phone and use them liberally when Tip 8 has broken down (and it will).

10 Remind yourself of the ten good reasons (see page 311) why breastfeeding is best for your baby.

Breast tips (so to speak):

Prepare yourself: her breasts may be unrecognisable in the early stages of breastfeeding – huge, blue veined, bursting at the seams, with nipples the size of dinner plates. She may well sink her fangs into your hand if you try and touch them. This is normal but should not last more than a few days (if it does, she might need help from a breastfeeding specialist).

Some common postpartum dad concerns

Processing the birth

Many men feel that while there are many resources for women after the birth, few are aimed at them. Still reeling from witnessing the birth, you are thrown into parenting, often exhausted, and often without even talking about what happened. If the birth was difficult, men need to process it as much as women do. *'Go with your partner to see the midwife, and go through the birth together,'* advises midwife Jenny Smith. *'Labour, particularly a difficult one, can be fraught for men: they worry just as much about the baby's safety as the mother does, and then, they're worrying about the mother too.'*

'Provider Fever'

Of course, you probably won't get to 'be there' all day for long. Most men are forced to return to work soon after the baby is born. This brings a whole range of stresses. The main one is probably the headache of how to be successful at work without missing out on your children's lives. It can be hard to have to go back to work after only a week or so of unrestricted access to your baby. The law is gradually changing here (though some would say not enough), so there may be more ways than you'd think to get more time with your children. It's worth opening a discussion with your employer about this, no matter how unlikely it seems to you that they'll look favourably on your desire to be a hands-on dad (you may, however, be surprised: after all, your male bosses are probably fathers too).

The issue of work can also bring money worries to the fore. The balance really shifts when you have a baby. Your partner is suddenly at home, not earning (or earning little) while you're left as the sole breadwinner. *'This is the time of the greatest role segregation when it comes to breadwinning,'* says Jack O'Sullivan. Many men worry about money and feel a great responsibility on their shoulders: maternity pay often does not last – at least in full – for the whole period of maternity leave. This can be stressful in itself.

YOUR RIGHTS AT A GLANCE

Paternity leave

New fathers in the UK are now entitled to two weeks paternity leave. You get £100 per week, and you have to have been employed for 26 weeks before the 15th week before the due date to qualify.

Parental leave

You may be eligible for 13 weeks parental leave per child. This is designed to help you balance work and family responsibilities in the first five years of your child's life. You are eligible for parental leave if you have been with your employer for one year and have children born or adopted on or after 15 December 1999.

Where to go for help:

To get more information and make sure you are really up to date on any changes to these regulations, try the **Department of Trade and Industry** www.dti.gov.uk or www.fathersdirect.com.

Baby bonding

In the TV show *Cold Feet*, new dad Adam blurts out at his baby son's 'naming ceremony' that he feels absolutely nothing for his child. The episode shows him constantly pushed out by his partner Rachel who won't let him do anything. He's threatened by his son's closeness to Rachel, jealous, rejected, upset. Fundamentally when it comes to baby love, he just doesn't get it. It's only when circumstances force him into being an 'at home dad' that he realises he can do it. And, involved at last, he falls in love with his son. This is a lesson to us all: some women find it incredibly hard to relinquish control over their newborn, no matter how knackered and desperate we are. But if we want our partners to be great fathers, we have to let them. *'Get stuck in,'* advises Jack O'Sullivan, of Fathers Direct. *'Do all you can with your baby and instead of thinking "my wife just had a baby" think "we've become parents".'* You do not need to have your relationship with your child mediated by the mother (though be sensitive – many of us, particularly first time around, do find it genuinely, biologically hard to let the baby out of our sight). Spend time alone with your baby. Change her nappy. Rock her back to sleep at 2 a.m. Take her for a walk strapped to your chest in the baby sling. You are much more likely to enjoy the early weeks (not to mention fatherhood in general) if you are forming a strong relationship with your baby.

Fathering a newborn

'When I think back to those first few days and weeks, I don't think about the wailing and chaos,' says Julia's husband Buckley, 'I think of the early hours of the morning, sitting in the rocking chair, calming a little baby on my shoulder. I bonded with my babies by being alone with them, comforting them at 3 a.m. I was knackered most of the time, but I wouldn't give that up for anything.'

Fathers can actually be **better** at comforting crying babies than mothers. Many mothers work this out with subsequent children. Babies who just want comfort (not food, really) smell their daddies and know a boob simply isn't an option. Instead of screaming for a comfort suck, they crash out (possibly after a bit of a fight). Men are often less panicked by a crying baby (women are biologically hardwired to think it's an emergency). Put a mildly peckish baby near its mother and it'll be demanding a feed within seconds. Stick it on its daddy's chest and soon it'll be sleeping (unless it really *was* hungry). You could say that comforting fussy babies is a man's job.

As mentioned briefly already, one major problem, particularly with first-time parents, is that mothers can find it immensely difficult to relinquish control of the baby. As we hover over you, watching your big fingers fumble with our precious infant, few first-time mothers can resist barking orders. Or wrenching the baby back. You'll hold, touch, rock, move or dress your baby in a way her mother may find – at times – genuinely unsettling. (Men, incidentally, have been shown to hold babies differently from women.) If your wife is behaving oddly when you pick up the baby it's probably just because you don't do it her way.

You may also notice that many mothers become obsessed by the temperature of their infant. When my first baby was two weeks old, John took her round the supermarket in January wearing only a cotton babygro. Five years on I can barely write that sentence without a shudder. My baby did not develop pneumonia or turn blue or suffer any ill effects whatsoever but it took me weeks (OK, years) to forgive John. Both of you need to be aware that this mildly mad maternal syndrome is both genuine and in need of curbing. (The good news is that the more babies you have the less relevant this seems to become: mothers of small children are generally so **desperate** for any kind of respite that we don't quibble about technique half as much as we did first time around.)

The thing to remember, if she's criticising the way you're tilting the bottle, is that – unless you're genuinely incompetent, drunk or in some other way dangerous – the only reason she's unsettled is that **your way is different from hers**. There's nothing in the Y chromosome that means you can't be superlative at baby care. Indeed, around 155,000 men in the UK are 'Home Dads' and the number of men working part-time has rocketed, from only 300,000 in 1986 to 1 million in 2001[11]. If your partner has turned into a headmistress listen to her concerns and, if necessary, debate them, but try not to let her powerful maternal protectiveness undermine your confidence in your ability to pick up, change, jiggle and generally bond with your baby. No manual is going to tell you exactly how to handle your baby: it's up to you to work it out. You and your partner are in this together and both of you have to get to know that small, red, bawling bundle in your own ways. If you negotiate your territory now, your life is going to be much easier. And so is hers.

Equipment tip:
You no longer have to ponce around town with a teddy bear emblazoned nappy bag on your shoulder. 'Diaper Dude' has come up with some really quite acceptably blokeish nappy bags:
www.thebabycloset.co.uk/baby_blankets_diaperdude.asp

Mutual understanding

She thinks you have the easy life – getting to the office, meeting real people, going to the loo unaccompanied. You think she's swanning around all day drinking cups of tea with her girlfriends and watching daytime telly. The first few months can be tough for **both of you**, in very different ways. It really isn't reasonable for you to come home and express dismay that she has not tidied/cooked dinner/paid the bills. Looking after a new baby at home can be genuinely exhausting – the cumulative lack of sleep, the hormones, the physical rigours of feeding; the loneliness and lack of personal space can all be shattering. But then again, functioning on full throttle in the office on two hours' sleep, knowing you're going to go home to a newborn that needs jiggling and a wife that needs bolstering can also take its toll. This common misunderstanding can put vast strains on any relationship. You both need to talk about this **before** you get to boiling point. Aim to give each other support, not indulge in one-upmanship about who's the most knackered.

MUTUAL MISUNDERSTANDING | If you and your partner separate, and you are the one moving out, you will need to take proactive steps to be as involved in your child's life as you want to be. It is worth investigating your rights fully, and using them. The ins and outs of this are beyond the scope of this book, but a good first stop is Fathers Direct (see Find Out More, page 263).

Common domestic friction

For some couples, basic domestic tasks like cleaning become a minefield when a baby arrives. If your partner is the one who does the bulk of the cleaning (in most heterosexual relationships studies show that women do more domestic tasks than men, even if both partners work full time) **now** is the time to redress the balance. If you hear yourself uttering the words 'helping around the house' bite them back before she (or her best friend) comes at you with a blunt instrument. It is your house too, and your dirty sock on the floor, particularly after a new baby arrives, can become loaded with significance. The books all tell you not to care about mess when you have a new baby. Let the dishes pile up! This is all very well, but a filthy, messy house is, for many of us, fundamentally depressing. It's about keeping sane and calm amidst the obvious chaos of maternity. With a new baby you're both going to be around the house a lot more (even if it's just at weekends) and kids create nonstop filth. So, if cleaning's an issue between you both (whichever one of you is the 'clean freak'), something has to give: on both sides.

Isolation

If the stress of paternity is getting to you it can be hard to find a sympathetic ear in the first months after the baby is born. *'Many men are reliant on their partner for emotional support, but in the early days of parenthood, their partner is usually very busy,'* says Jack O'Sullivan. Some men find 'dad's groups' useful for a bit of moral support (see Find Out More, page 263). The NCT also run events specifically for dads.

Unmarried fathers

You need to inform yourself about Parental Responsibility if you are not married to your child's mother. Parental Responsibility is a legal status you can hold in relation to a child. It gives you all the 'rights and responsibilities' of a parent and it's vital to get PR if you want to have legal rights over anything from authorizing medical treatment to stopping someone adopting your child. Married parents have this automatically, and so do unmarried mothers, but unmarried fathers don't. To get PR you need to include your name on your child's birth certificate.

A WORD ABOUT POSTNATAL DEPRESSION | There is a possibility that your partner will develop postnatal depression. By the time she realises she's depressed, she may be unable to get help for herself. You are the best person to keep an eye out for this. Read the signs of postnatal depression in our list in Chapter 10 on page 304. If you think she is depressed you should contact your GP or health visitor straight away. It can be very serious, but is treatable.

Tip about depression:

Incidentally, you the father, could also get symptoms of depression after the baby is born. Many health professionals believe the causes, for men, are the same as for any other form of depression (while for women, there may be a hormonal cause for postnatal depression). Still, there's certainly nothing like the stress of new fatherhood to trigger any lurking depression, so if you're feelings are getting out of hand, try: Fathers' Matters, set up in 2003 by the South Essex Partnership Trust. Helpline 01268 556 328.

Sleep deprivation

Arguments about how to snap the poppers on a babygro may reach ludicrous proportions simply because you're both so knackered. The first few weeks can feel like crisis management, no matter how many babies you've had. *'Most of the time, during her labour and in those early days of parenting, I felt like a member of a*

Formula One pit crew: changing, moving, soaking, cleaning...' says Alan, 35, father of Oscar (2). The thing to remember, however, is that the real 'crisis' period is short lived.

'With our first baby, I felt like the first six weeks were the way life would be forever,' says Larry, 44, father of Grace (10) and Jack (8). *'I had no perspective on it, and it was hell: nonstop crying baby, my wife totally overwhelmed by feeds, nappies, nipples, piles or whatever. Second time around, I understood how fleeting that time is, really. Our second baby cried and pooed just as much, but I was so much more Zen about it. I wish I'd realised the first time that the panic doesn't last. Before you know it, your baby will be starting school.'*

Sex after birth

The official advice is to wait about six weeks after the birth before you have sex. This notion would make most women laugh were it not for the fact that we might burst our stitches. The reality is that – depending on what the delivery of the baby was like – it may be far, far longer than this before she's ready for sex. You don't need much imagination to work out why this is but reading Chapter 10 will give you a few concrete reasons. Many women take an awfully long time for the notion of having anything 'up there' to become even remotely appealing. Also, when breastfeeding, your body produces hormones that can suppress the sex drive, and make you less lubricated. So be patient. Some women find it takes as long as a couple of years (yes, really) after the birth until they're truly back on form. Touch, massage, cuddling and kissing are the best ways to keep a sense of intimacy. And some 'scene setting' might help – a glass of wine, a massage, a bit of romance. It can be hard for us to go from nappy changer to sex goddess with no steps in between. But equally, you may feel resentful that all her love is suddenly focused on the baby. Realistically, romance can be hard to achieve (certainly in the early days) when you're severely sleep deprived, somewhat on edge and one or other of you seems to be constantly jiggling, feeding or otherwise attending to a small, howling baby (not to mention appeasing any older kids you have). Again, be patient and do the best you can, when you can (see below).

FIVE IDEAS FOR INTIMACY

'You are, as a couple, role models for your child,' says psychologist Dr Petra Boynton. *'If your child grows up seeing you physical and loving, doing things for each other, and communicating well this can be incredibly positive. You don't have to be superheros, but you do have to negotiate and make the effort.'*

1   **Make an effort to hug/cuddle/kiss her on the lips** when you leave in the morning, and when you get home from work at night, even if it's just fleeting, before she thrusts the baby into your arms saying 'your turn'. You've made contact. This can be an achievement.

2 **Be physical.** You can hold her while she breastfeeds the baby; the three of you can even have a bath together. And no matter how sleep deprived you are, try and have even a short cuddle before you go to sleep.

3 **Make contact.** Try and phone her at least once during the day to tell her you love her and find out how she and the baby are doing. Your worlds are now very different and you need to make bridges between them.

4 **Be supportive.** Make an effort to tell her what a lovely mother she is – a lot.

5 **Talk.** Make a small amount of time, at the end of the day, where you just sit and listen to each other. You get ten minutes each to talk without interruption. In your ten minutes you tell each other how you are feeling. It's amazing how just this small, ten-minute slot, being listened to, can make you feel more connected.

FIND OUT MORE

Further reading

Two helpful books
The Birth Partner: Everything You Need to Know to Help a Woman Through Childbirth by Penny Simkin (Harvard Press, 2001) This is a good one for anyone attending a birth and will help you get to grips with what your role, among all that oestrogen, could – and should – be.

Becoming a Father: Men's Access to Information and Support about Pregnancy, Birth and Life with a New Baby, by D. Smith and M. Newburn (National Childbirth Trust and Fathers Direct, 2000) A good, no-nonsense general resource.

Some light reading
Fatherhood: The Truth by Marcus Berkmann (Vermilion, UK, 2005) An entertaining guide to sleep, breasts, baby blues and all the rest.

Parenting Made Difficult: Notes from the Alphabet Soup of Fatherhood by Phil Hogan (Piccadilly Press, UK, 2002) Jokey slices of life with four boys under ten, from his *Observer* column.

The Truth About Babies from A–Z by Ian Sansom (Granta, UK, 2003) Erudite and witty accounts of the 'secrets' about babies that nobody tells you, by the *Guardian* writer.

More on fatherhood

From Lad to Dad: How to Survive as a Pregnant Father by Stephen Giles (White Ladder Press, UK, 2005) Tackles pregnancy, from the father-to-be's perspective.

The Expectant Father: Facts, Tips and Advice for Dads-to-be by Armin Brott and Jennifer Ash (Abbeville Press, UK, 2001).

Becoming a Father: How to Nurture and Enjoy Your Family by William Sears, M.D. (La Leche League International, UK, 2003)

Fetal development

From Conception To Birth: A Life Unfolds by Alexander Tsiaras and Barry Werth (Doubleday, US, 2002)

What's Going on in There?: How the Brain and Mind Develop in the First Five Years of Life by Lise Eliot (Bantam, US, 2000)

Online

Fathers Direct Herald House Lambs Passage Bunhill Row London EC1Y 8TQ Tel: 0845 634 1328 www.fathersdirect.com This is the best place to start online – the UK's national information centre for fatherhood 'supports the welfare of children by the positive and active involvement of fathers and male carers in their lives'. Good source of information and even networking with other dads.

Good resource for single fathers Helpline: 07092 391489 or 07092 390210 www.dads-uk.co.uk

Helpful way to explore your employment rights
www.tiger.gov.uk/paternity/employee.

Chapter Nine:
The love of a good woman

'During labour my husband was wonderful,
but of course the things that worried me,
worried him too. The midwife was fantastic,
but she was also looking after other women.
There were times during the birth when
we felt very alone indeed, and scared, and
just didn't know what to do.'

CAT, 30, MOTHER OF DYLAN (1)

THE LOVE OF A GOOD WOMAN: FIVE REASONS TO HAVE
FEMALE SUPPORT IN LABOUR

1 It will reduce your chances of having medical intervention.
2 It will reduce your chances of having a caesarean section.
3 It will make you feel more positive about the birth, whatever happens.
4 It will be helpful for your partner, too.
5 It is now possible to hire labour support: a doula is specifically trained to support you in childbirth. She does not share your gene pool and will not take it personally if you hurl insults at her during labour.

Throughout this book we've banged on about the vital role of support – practical and emotional – during childbirth. In Chapter 5: Your Options we showed you how to choose and work well with your medical team. You're probably intending to rely on your baby's father for other support during labour. This is no bad thing. If he's well prepared he'll be indispensable. But it's worth thinking for a moment about his limitations. He's unlikely to be any more **experienced** than you are when it comes to childbirth. And even if he happens to be an obstetric genius, he's going to be watching you, the love of his life, in pain: he may not be as calm, collected and rational as you'd like to think. This is where a third person – preferably a woman who has given birth herself – can be a huge asset.

There is now good, solid, scientific evidence that having a non-medically trained woman supporting you during childbirth is beneficial. In 2003, a comprehensive review published by the Cochrane Library, the biggest source of evidence-based healthcare in the world, concluded that having a doula or other non-medically trained woman present at the birth significantly raises your chances of having a straightforward, manageable experience of childbirth.[1] The review examined 15 research trials involving almost 13,000 women giving birth and found that those who had continuous support from someone who was not a hospital staff member throughout labour needed less pain relief, had fewer caesareans and reported a far more positive experience than those who were cared for by hospital midwives alone.

None of this should diminish your partner's role. John could not have been more vital or supportive to me during all three of my labours. But, particularly first time around when the birth didn't go smoothly, I was acutely aware that he didn't know any more about getting babies out than I did. During a particularly tough period in Izzie's birth, I remember John muttering lovingly: 'It's all going really well,' and me thinking, quite clearly 'What the f*** do you know about it?'. I may have even said this. Possibly quite loudly. In short, the things that threaten to freak you out during the birth may well freak him out too (possibly even more). There may also be times when he's genuinely worried for your safety and this can be far from reassuring. When I got an epidural, during Izzie's birth, we were left with a trainee midwife. I began to shake uncontrollably. Neither John, nor I, nor the trainee midwife had any idea that such shaking can be a side-effect of an epidural. John's calm words, though I appreciated them, couldn't quite mask the look of panic in his eye. It would certainly have helped us at this point to have someone there whose job it was to reassure us and help us to cope.

Traditionally, of course, this is the midwife's job. A good midwife will **absolutely** give you a great deal of encouragement, reassurance and bolstering. But there's a huge national midwife shortage in the UK today. Continuous one-to-one care is just not the reality for most of us: your midwife (who you may never have met before you arrive at the hospital) is unlikely to be with you throughout your entire labour. There'll be shift changes, she'll probably be caring for one or more other women at the same time, and (particularly if there are complications) she may have to juggle your emotional needs with the demands of her medical role. She can't, for instance, be mopping your brow, whispering in your ear and keeping your husband hydrated if she's unhooking the umbilical cord from your baby's neck.

A doula or an experienced woman friend, on the other hand, has no medical role. She can be next to you whatever's going on 'down there'. When you and your partner are both wobbling, and the midwife is busy with the more technical side of things, it can be immeasurably beneficial to have a sane, calm, and most of all **credible** voice by your side going: 'This is normal, this is safe, you are doing well.' When you're exhausted and labour seems to be going nowhere, and the midwife is helping the woman in the next-door room, it can be incredibly helpful to have someone with you who knows lots of ways to get labour going; someone who knows about positions and techniques that will maximise the efficiency of your contractions, and minimise the pain. A good doula can also make an unexpected caesarean or an instrumental birth acceptable and manageable. It's no wonder many women say that hiring a doula was the best decision they made.

Of course, not all of us can hire one. Doulas are fast catching on in the UK (they've been around a while in the States) but it's early days, and in some parts of the country it can still be hard to find one. Doulas can also be expensive. But if you think you couldn't find or afford one **don't skip this chapter**. There are ways round the logistical difficulties and even if you don't end up hiring one, you may decide to have a female relative or friend with you and your partner at the birth (if you do, get her to read this chapter!). A female 'support person' even if she's not a trained doula can be an absolute godsend in labour. We'll explain here what your lovely lady – whoever she is – can learn from doulas about really helping you in labour.

What doulas do

The word 'doula' comes from the Greek word for 'woman's servant'. Doulas are women who are trained to give you emotional and practical support during pregnancy, birth, and sometimes after the birth. They are **not** medical professionals. Having a doula is hardly a new idea: for centuries women were attended in labour by a female relative – their mother, sister, cousin – as well as the midwives. In many cultures this still happens but in Britain (and indeed, much of Europe and the USA), the tradition has dwindled, probably because medicated hospital birth is now the norm. The recent rise in doula popularity in the UK shows we're not happy with this situation: we're starting to realise there are things we can do to get a better birth – if we take the initiative.

You may encounter two different kinds of doula: a 'birth doula', specially trained to give you support during childbirth, and a 'postnatal doula', trained to support you after the birth (she'll know about mother and newborn care, be able to give breastfeeding support and advice and help with cooking, childcare, errands and light cleaning). Many doulas (Julia is one) are trained in both birth and postnatal care.

Most birth doulas will meet with you two or three times before the birth and will be there consistently for telephone/email support in the run up to it. When you go into labour your birth doula will usually come to your house. Then, when you're ready, she'll go to the hospital with you, and will stay with you until you're settled with your baby after the birth. Once you come home, she'll probably see you once or twice in the first few weeks but if you want to discuss the birth at any time in the future, she'll usually be there for you.

A BIRTH DOULA (OR A GOOD FRIEND):

- Gives **you and your partner** continuous emotional support during the pregnancy and birth.
- Helps you to inform yourself properly about childbirth, and any pregnancy issues you encounter.
- Provides non-medicated pain relief during labour (e.g. positions for pain relief, acupressure, counter-pressure, massage).
- Suggests non-medical ways to try and slow or speed up labour if wanted.
- Gives comfort – in many forms – to you and your partner during labour.
- Protects your birth environment: keeps it quiet and calm with no bystanders or unnecessary strangers.
- Makes sure you feel consulted and informed during labour, not bullied or patronised.
- Respects you and your partner's intimacy during the birth.
- Helps you to connect with your baby during the birth.
- Works alongside the midwife, respecting her role.

She should NEVER:
- Give medical advice (though she should help you find it).
- Come between you and the medical staff who are caring for you.

- Leave when the birth goes in a direction she does not approve of.
- Say any unsupportive things or suggest any negative scenarios to you or your partner.
- Persuade you to give birth in a certain way.

Why do doulas do it?

'Attending a birth is amazing,' says Shona, a doula for five years. 'You're so exhausted you could weep, you haven't gone to the loo for nine hours even though your bladder's bursting, and there is still no place in the world you'd rather be.' Most doulas are motivated by a passion for childbirth. They usually have a strong belief that women who are supported properly can have a far more positive experience than they otherwise might. They are really interested in the emotional side of childbirth, and how it can affect your overall experience. Jennifer Nunn, former president of DONA International (the biggest US-based doula organisation) has been in maternity care since 1989. She used to be a midwife but felt that while 'the physical factors of labour are supposedly understood, the emotional aspect has been understated. As a midwife I saw doulas as being the one thing that could change maternity care; whispering to the mother, not telling her what to do, but empowering her.....[this is why] I opted for the subtle empowerment of being a doula'.

Tip: some doula synonyms:

Labour support professional, labour companion, birth partner, birth companion are all synonyms of 'birth doula'.

Why hire one?

The short answer is simple: because researchers have found the birth is more likely to be straightforward if you do. One seminal study[2] looked at the effectiveness of doulas by comparing three groups of first time mothers: those who received active doula support, those who did not, and those who were only observed by a doula. The women who received doula support had fewer epidurals, used fewer drugs to speed up labour, had fewer admissions to neonatal intensive care, shorter labours and fewer surgical deliveries (indeed, the women who were simply observed, also had reduced rates of intervention, pain, epidurals and complications).

Beyond all this data, the main reason to hire a doula is that by doing so your birth should be a **significantly** more positive experience, whatever happens.

This testimonial sums up the advantages brilliantly[3]:

'Ava was finally born about 22 hrs after the doula had arrived at our home...... she must have been exhausted but it didn't show. Having the doula there as added support really was the best decision my husband and I made during pregnancy... despite ending up in hospital with an epidural and eventually ventouse, I feel very positive about the decisions we made and the overall experience. I felt completely

*supported and my husband felt supported too..... I would recommend anyone to
consider having a doula – it may feel like an extravagance to some but it really does
make a difference to what is one of the most scary, amazing experiences of our lives.'*

How are doulas organised?

The best place to start is with **Doula UK** (DUK), a non-profit organisation for
doulas and those who want to find them. Most doulas are currently hired by
middle class, professional working women, generally in the London and
surrounding areas. **But this does not have to be the case**. Doulas are
springing up all over the country. And doulas in training will take on clients for
little or no fee. Many doulas also have a sliding scale of fees, depending on what
you can pay. **Always ask, if money is a problem.** Don't think a doula is just an
indulgence for posh Islington types.

In the US, the 'doula movement' is far more substantial and structured than it
is here (though we're getting there). There are two major organisations: DONA
International and Association of Labor Assistants and Childbirth Educators
(ALACE). DONA has recently set up training in Britain.

A few misconceptions about doulas

Many people have funny ideas about what a doula is for. Here are some of them.

1   **DOULAS ARE GLORIFIED DOMESTICS** | Many people bracket all doulas
    somewhere along with maternity nurses or housekeepers. The idea is that
    they are rather bossy ladies hired by posh girls to come in, clean the house,
    give foot rubs, do the shopping and help pop a baby out. Postnatal doulas
    may, indeed, perform some domestic tasks that will allow you to rest so you
    can bond fully with your baby, and establish breastfeeding successfully. But I
    have to say that Julia, as my birth doula, was never once moved to change my
    bedlinen or clean my loo (if only!). Domestic relief is not the core of a birth
    doula's role. Her primary role is to support you during childbirth.

2   **DOULAS WANT TO BE MIDWIVES** | Doulas are not medically trained. Yours
    will **not** be instructing your medical team to hold that caesarean (though she
    may be helping you to ask key questions so you feel informed and consulted
    about procedures). She will not be sewing you up, assessing your baby's heart
    rate or bickering with the midwife about what to do next. Her job is to give
    you comfort and NEVER to interfere in the medical side of birth.

    As Julia explains:

*'A doula is not a barrier between you and the medical staff. At times she might be
a buffer certainly – helping you finish a contraction before you have to speak to a
new doctor, for instance – but not a barrier from medical counsel.'*

3 DOULAS ARE A POINTLESS LUXURY | *'Why would you fork out three hundred quid for someone just to stand and hold your hand?'* This is a common question. Particularly from men. And yes, it's another misconception. Doulas don't just mop your brow (unless this is what you've asked them to do). You hire a doula because she has a huge array of skills to help you in labour (as well as before and afterwards). Her techniques and strategies can help you with anything from pain relief and relaxation, to slowing a fast labour or speeding up a slow one. *'I knew I was a real doula,'* says Claire, a doula for 11 years, *'when my nine-year-old son was watching a woman give birth on the Discovery Channel. She'd been pushing for a while and HE shouted at the TV "Get her to squat!!"'* If you've read the rest of this book, you'll understand this anecdote by now. (We explain more specifics below.)

4 DOULAS ARE ALL HAIRY HIPPIES | Many women assume that doulas are a hairy-legged, natural birth troupe who'll insist you have to have a homebirth with no pain relief. Julia's sister Susan says, *'I'd heard about the benefits of labour support – ad nauseum – for years and when I became pregnant I had a competitive reaction – I didn't even consider hiring a doula. I had an idea that my sister attended births of hippies and commune women. My labour was really hard, but the hardest thing for me is how alone I felt. The staff were swamped, my husband was in at the deep end, and I felt hopeless. I had the caesarean I ended up demanding – and I will never again make light of the importance of labour support. It's not a luxury or a natural birth thing. I regret not having support tremendously.'* You will be glad to know, incidentally, that Julia (like the vast majority of her colleagues) is neither hairy nor smelly; she reads *Hello* magazine with the best of us, drives an SUV, drinks lattes and no one could mistake her house, husband and two kids for a commune. Some doulas may indeed be earthy types but all good doulas have to be highly organised, committed and reliable.

5 DOULAS ARE ONLY FOR WOMEN WHO WANT A NATURAL BIRTH | Doulas are there to help you whoever you are, and however you want to give birth. They're passionate about making childbirth better for ALL women. As Julia points out: *'You have to be. To want to get up at 3 a.m., work for anything from two to 120 hours, sometimes with no or little pay and without a break; to risk missing your own child's birthday or recital, to smile reassuringly in the face of bodily fluids and abhorrent cursing and to explain your job to hospital staff again and again.'* Julia set up the 'New Hope' project in the US – a group of volunteer doulas who work with women who are relinquishing their babies for adoption. Renowned childbirth expert Sheila Kitzinger set up Holloway Birth Companions here in the UK, providing doulas to mothers in prison (it marked the birth of the doula movement in this country). Doulas do all this because, as Jennifer Nunn, former DONA International President puts it: *'Being a doula is a privilege.'*

6   **A DOULA WON'T LET YOU HAVE AN EPIDURAL** | Doulas and epidurals are in no way mutually exclusive. *'I am still stunned when I hear of a doula that leaves when the mother gets an epidural,'* says Jennifer Nunn. *'A doula is there for the mother – wherever the mother is and whatever her needs are. I have certainly attended many births that were medicated. In the end, we are there to comfort the labouring woman, NOT to have opinions about what she should do. It's her birth after all.'*

7   **DOULAS ARE AGAINST CAESAREANS** | Again, a doula wants you to have a good experience whatever happens to you. A doula can be a huge asset if you end up with a caesarean (and even if you plan one). Peggy Fitzgerald is a certified doula and mother of triplets. Her story illustrates how a doula can help WHATEVER your birth scenario turns out to be:

   'My birth was very high tech, very high risk, with many complications. I don't remember it....[but] my doula was wonderful. She attended my emergency C-section. She was the only one who was there, out of 25 people, solely to recognise that it was a birth of three people and simply witness it. I was practically unconscious and Charles was trying to keep track of three babies, one obviously very sick indeed. My doula wrote my birth story and it's the only thing I have. She also took a few pictures and they are such a gift. Don't underestimate what a doula can do, even if it's not about labour.'

8   **HOSPITALS DON'T LIKE DOULAS** | Hospital staff who have worked face-to-face with a doula are generally very supportive. Penny, the midwife I had for Ted's birth here in Oxford, was relaxed with Lucy, my doula, and even asked her opinion at one point. However, the majority of health professionals in Britain may still be unaware of what a doula really does (and therefore possibly suspicious). Some midwives may be defensive about their 'territory' and worry that a doula will meddle in medical matters. This should change as more and more doulas show up – and show their mettle – in delivery rooms across the country.

9   **DOULAS EXCLUDE DADS** | You might think a doula will muscle in on your partner's territory. What will his job be while the doula is rubbing your back? Many men, quite understandably, feel suspicious (if not outright threatened). This is groundless. *'The partner is emotionally connected,'* says Jennifer Nunn, *'making objectivity difficult or impossible at the birth. The doula relieves that anxiety, letting the partner do what he does best, without the added pressure of having to be the expert on birth.'*

   Your doula, then, rather than getting between you, your man and your baby, or 'robbing' him of his role in the birth, will actually **help** him to stay useful, calm and genuinely supportive. She'll make sure he pees, eats, drinks and stays on top of the great emotional wave that is the birth of his child.

She'll make sure he won't pass out, fall asleep or panic when you need him most. She'll show him how to give you comfort if he's uncertain about what to do. She'll make sure he understands what's going on so he's not scared. She'll reassure him, so he can reassure you. She'll prevent him from feeling, as many men do, that he is redundant, or helpless or unable to comfort you. In short, a birth doula can transform a man's experience of his baby's arrival.

My husband John initially felt hostile at the idea of a doula. His first reaction was 'so what will my job be then?' However, once we hired Julia, he quickly realised that she was an asset:

'Having doulas at the births of our second and third babies was a totally different experience for me. With Izzie, our first, we didn't have a doula. The childbirth classes all made me feel that the main way I could be helpful during the birth would be to become knowledgeable and somehow advocate for Lucy. In the event I realised I wasn't knowledgeable at all - that whole idea felt like a complete con - I felt intimidated, panicked, nervous and useless most of the time. With our second baby, Julia worked with us a lot during the pregnancy to unpick Lucy's fears. This helped me realise that what Lucy needed most of all was for me to be reassuring, solid, calm and loving. This felt like a huge release: all that other stuff was not my job - I didn't need to be second-guessing doctors or asking pertinent questions. Julia also made sure that we were both at all the meetings with her during the pregnancy - had she not done this I'd have felt like a spare part.'

10 DOULAS ARE POLITICAL | Most doulas believe that the maternity system could change for the better. But they don't all agree on how. And they don't all spend their time thinking about this. Their job is much more immeditate (you!). Having said all this, there are still a few rogue doulas floating around. These women have a fixed idea of the 'right' way to give birth and are not afraid of foisting their opinions on any client that comes their way.

As Julia puts it:

'I have had women come to me saying they've called other doulas who 'wouldn't DO' hospital births. We are hired to comfort the labouring mother and her partner, and to stick to her birth plan. A good doula should attend your birth whether it's at home or in the hospital. Her job is to help you have the birth you want - as simple as that. She may tactfully open your eyes to certain scenarios and options you had not previously considered. But ultimately, the choice about where and how you give birth must be yours. Women can find satisfaction from any scenario. We know that we're useful to any woman who wants to hire us, regardless of her birth plan.'

A doula should not interfere with the medical side of things, but at times she can be a great a buffer between you and a difficult situation with hospital staff. Valerie, a doula from Kent says:

'I remember one dad – Richard, expecting his first child – who was not pleased with the fact that the midwife kept coming in the room unable to remember anything, as if she hadn't read the notes. He would have shouted at her but he said to me "I am leaving – Valerie please deal with her and call me in a little while".… He needed some fresh air!'

If you don't have a doula… how to choose and prepare your support person

'Women through the centuries have had other women with them while they are giving birth. Not specially trained women, just women who have had babies and can be there with them during labour,' says Sheila Kitzinger, author and social anthropologist of birth, who founded Holloway Birth Companions. It may not be possible – for financial or geographical reasons – for you to hire a trained and experienced doula. You may decide, having weighed it up and even spoken to a few doulas, that you'd rather not hire one. This does not mean you should abandon the idea of having another woman with you in labour. Having a carefully chosen and well-prepared female friend or relative at the birth is also very likely to increase your chances of coping. But you **do** have to choose her carefully. And prepare her well. Here are some important issues you should explore before you invite your mother, sister or best friend to show up at the hospital with her camcorder.

Who will she be?

Your mother may have been a paragon of good sense when calming your wedding jitters but seeing her baby *having* a baby could do her head in. Your best friend may have three kids, but the fact that she wants to leave her husband and marry her anaesthetist might inhibit her ability to support your waterbirth plans. Here are a few things to consider when choosing your support.

SPECTATOR SPORTS AND WHY BIRTH ISN'T ONE | The last thing you need, in the labour room, is a spectator. Some childbirth experts argue that we give birth more smoothly if we have as much privacy as possible (see Chapter 3 Fear and Pain). Obstetrician Michel Odent is the best-known proponent of this (indeed, he believes we need to 'mammalianise' childbirth: in other words, get back to our animal roots and give birth in relative privacy). Odent argues that anything which stimulates the neocortex of a labouring woman can slow or impede their ability to give birth. Even a video camera, he claims, can be detrimental to a labouring woman. *'A feeling of being observed,'* he writes, *'is another type of neocortical stimulation. The physiological response to the presence of an observer has been scientifically studied. In fact, it is common knowledge that we all feel different when we know we are being observed.'*[4]

Of course, your birth may not progress smoothly and you may need or choose to have medical interventions. If this happens, you may not have privacy and calm: unfamiliar faces can quickly start appearing, lights may go on. Having a trusted, reassuring person by your side at this point can allow you to block out the hubbub. If your friend is making you nervous or self-conscious, this won't work. You may think you can't possibly be inhibited by the presence of someone you know well and this may be true – particularly if they are helping you to feel safe, unbothered, secure, reassured. But if you feel that person is watching you anxiously or worst still judgmentally, if they're interfering or making unhelpful comments then their presence could well nudge you in the opposite direction.

YOUR SUPPORT PERSON SHOULD BE:

- There for the right reasons (yours, basically)
- Aware of her role to support you in any way you need her to
- Able to cope with the reality of childbirth
- Able to put aside any childbirth 'baggage' of her own
- Able to support you to have the birth you want, not one she thinks you should have

Here are a few questions to help you decide whether she can do this:

1 **'CAN I BE NAKED IN FRONT OF THIS PERSON?'** | And it might not just be nudity – you may fart, poo, throw up and/or utter abysmal profanities in front of this woman. The last thing you want is to feel self-conscious or inhibited.

2 **'WHY DOES SHE WANT TO COME?'** | If you suspect that she wants to come just so she'll have a cracking dinner party story afterwards, she may not be your best bet. If she wants to come because she wants to be the first to see the baby, think again. Obligation, duty, guilt or even love, are not good reasons in themselves to ask someone along. The only good reason to do so is if you think her presence will be beneficial.

3 **'WHAT BIRTH BAGGAGE DOES SHE HAVE?'** | A woman who has given birth herself may have insight and compassion that will be uniquely helpful to you when you are in labour. Alternatively, she may be a total psycho about the whole business. Having an experienced mother with you in labour can be fantastically reassuring as long as she's **well-adjusted** about birth. It's worth asking yourself (and her) what her preconceptions are about childbirth: how was childbirth for her? Does she think there's a 'right' way to do it? Does she believe it's basically normal and healthy?
   'I once attended a birth that was going well,' says Jennifer Nunn. *'The woman was in late active labour, concentrating beautifully and it was all smooth sailing ahead: until her best friend barged in and said, during a contraction in a*

loud voice, 'Why don't you have an epidural now?' That friend had had a very difficult birth, resulting in a very difficult caesarean. Now she was passing her birth issues on to a well-progressing labour.'

Exploring her birth baggage is, then, a vital part of working out if she'll be a positive addition to your labour.

4 **'CAN SHE FIND THE TIME?'** | She needs to be there when you want her there. This means she has to be willing – and able – to get up at 4 a.m. when you call and to stay with you for as long as it takes. If she has three kids under four and a husband who works nights, she's unlikely to be much use if your waters break at an inconvenient moment. Can she find the childcare? Get someone to feed the cat? Take the time off work? Finally, do you know she'll come?

If you're happy with the answers to these questions then the next step is to give her an idea of the things she can do for you.

What your friend can learn from doulas
A GOOD LABOUR SUPPORT PERSON WILL
- Respect your birth plan and leave her plan for your birth at the door
- Ask questions on your behalf if needed during the birth
- Make sure you understand what is happening during the birth
- Help keep you calm, coping and as comfortable as possible during the birth
- Stay realistically positive and encouraging: she'll agree with you in advance to give you an honest sense of how you're doing.

FIVE WAYS TO HELP HER TO HELP YOU

1 Get her to read this book (this chapter, and Chapter 5: Your Options).
2 Get her to buy and read *The Birth Partner* by Penny Simkin (see Further reading, page 282). This book has everything a really good doula should know, and is small enough to go to the hospital with you.
3 Get her to come to a birth class with you, even if she has been to them for her own pregnancies. Going with you will give her a new perspective on the whole business.
4 Ask her to watch a good birth video. Again, even if she's done it herself, she'll get to see things from a very different angle.
5 Go over your birth plan with her in detail.

Helping you to feel in control

One of the most crucial aspects of a doula's role is to help you to feel relatively in control of anything that needs to be 'done' to you during the birth. During labour you might be faced with choices about medical interventions or procedures. If you're being bombarded with contractions, haven't slept for 24 hours and are at the end of your tether, it can be hard to weigh things up and make rational choices. This is where an experienced doula can be helpful. She can help you to understand what's going on and to feel as if you are being properly consulted. You don't have to be a medical expert to do this. You just have to be rational and calm enough to ask why something needs doing, what the pros and cons are, and what the alternatives are. Your baby's father may well be (on some level) too frazzled and anxious to do this effectively. A doula, on the other hand, is less emotionally involved. This is part of her job. Studies have shown that feeling consulted and respected, and understanding the reasons for any procedure can make your experience of childbirth more positive, regardless of the circumstances.

Ten more things good doulas do

1 **ENCOURAGE YOUR RITUALS** | Women in labour get great comfort from ritual: moaning, swaying, dim lighting, music or sounds. A doula will keep this consistent for you: she'll try and keep the room undisturbed by passers-by and will tactfully remind any noisy staff that you want the room to stay quiet. She'll help you find your own way to give birth, then support you to do it.

2 **KEEP YOU WALKING** | A doula will map out a walking route for any hospital, hallway by hallway so you don't have to think about the way back to your room. Walking is an excellent way to keep early labour progressing.

3 **USE MASSAGE** | Most women in labour love hand and foot massages. A hand massage can help release the hormones that keep labour going. Doulas know lots of massage moves.

4 **USE COUNTER PRESSURE** | Counter pressure is also a great doula trick for pain relief: she simply presses firmly on the lower small of your back during a contraction, to counter the pressure of the baby inside. *'I have attended labours where I sat for hours on the sistern of a toilet, bending to give counter pressure during each contraction,'* says Julia. *'The combo of sitting on the toilet (her release) and counter pressure (comfort) can really help her to move the baby down.'*

5 **KEEP YOU BREATHING** | Your childbirth class should teach you how to breathe deeply and for maximum relaxation during contractions. A doula will remind you of this, but most of all will remind you simply to breathe at all (rather than to hold your breath and tense up during contractions, thereby heightening the pain).

6 **KNOW THE GOLDEN RULES OF BIRTH BREATHING** | She will help and encourage you...

- not to hold your breath at any time during a contraction
- to breathe slowly and deeply during each contraction, releasing tension on each exhalation
- to take a deep breath and let it out as you think to yourself 'goodbye' when a contraction is done. (This will lower your shoulders, relax your stomach and refresh you for the next one.)

7 **KEEP YOU RELAXED** | Mostly this means just keeping the room quiet, with only your trusted 'team' in it (or, however you want it). A doula will remind you of any methods of relaxation that you've practised.

8 **KEEP YOUR MUSIC PLAYING** | A doula will keep your music playing even when you're not consciously aware that you need it. Your partner may be too distracted to press 'play'. A doula will know music can be comforting to you, even if you're not consciously 'hearing' it.

9 **BE INVALUABLE AT THE PUSHING STAGE** | A doula during the pushing stage may be the only one who's really focused on YOU – encouraging you, up there, at your end, when every one else is locked down there, peering at the baby's emerging head. Melanie, a doula for seven years, says *'You are often the only one in the room whispering in the woman's ear: "Listen to your body, you are doing such a great job, look down, push your baby out, just like that, you are fantastic".'*

A doula can also help you if the midwife asks you not to push (this sounds bizarre, but it does happen if, for instance, you are having the urge to push but your cervix is not fully dilated yet). She'll probably get you to pretend to have a feather in front of you and ask you to blow the feather with soft little breaths.

10 **KEEP YOU POSITIVE** | All doulas know that the labouring woman's attitude is KEY. If she's negative, depressed and gloomy, the birth tends to mirror this. If she's upbeat she may be surprised by labour, but will generally cope well. A doula's general reassurance, ideas and comfort can help to keep you from despair or negativity during the tough times of birth.

A DOULA'S BOX OF TRICKS

Your female friend can bring some of these things to the labour room, too:

Rice sock

An ordinary man's sock, filled with normal white rice (jasmine rice has a nice smell) with maybe a drop of essential oil such as lavender, tied with string at the top, or sewn tightly, so it won't open no matter how roughly you treat it. You can put it in the freezer then use it as a lasting cold pack. But more often doulas put it in the microwave for about three minutes and use it for pain relief on your lower back (or indeed anywhere that helps). You want it hot (but not burning). Unlike a hot water bottle it smells soothing, will mold to fit nooks and crannies of your body and is weighty enough for gentle counter pressure.

Tip: After it's been in the microwave, rest it on your forearm. If it's too hot there, it will burn the woman in labour, so wait for it to cool a bit.

Hot water bottle/ Ice pack

Either can be soothing on her lower back.

Soft drink can/Water bottle

Freeze a regular water bottle or take a soft drink can just out of the fridge. Roll this on the woman's back to cool her down and relieve pain (also, when the iced bottles melt the woman can drink the cold water).

Comb on pressure points

Get the woman to press a couple of small plastic combs into the palms of her hands for instant (and controllable) pressure-point pain relief.

Lemon

The scent of a lemon helps with nausea. In a hospital, the smell of real lemon or other essential oils (you can put some drops on a flannel and hold it near her face) can also help mask the unfamiliar chemical aromas.

Small fan

A tiny hand-held fan (small enough to not tire out the woman who is holding it) can be good for soothing and cooling in labour.

Spray bottle

Fill this with cold water and use it along with the fan to cool down a woman during a hot summer birth.

Scents: lotions, candles and lights

Candles may be banned from hospitals for obvious reasons, but at home they can be relaxing. Plain massage oil, some drops of essential oil on a flannel or lotion with drops of essential oils in it can do the same thing in a hospital. Massage the woman with these, and keep replenishing the drops of oil on a flannel.

Hand mirror

Some women want to see their baby's head when it starts to emerge. Often midwives suggest this as a fantastic incentive to push in the final moments.

Mints

Doulas might bring mints to the birth to offer anyone with stinky breath. A whiff of someone's lunch, or smoke on a midwife's breath, can seriously turn a labouring woman's stomach.

Tip: It's all in the details

A doula will also encourage you not to wear your contact lenses in labour and to take off any body (particularly clitoral/labial) jewellery.

Finally: the perfect friend

Your ideal labour support person has to be pretty committed to her role. She should be prepared to:

- listen to you and abandon her own agenda
- support your preferences and understand that plans change.
- keep you informed and fully aware of any choices that are being made on your behalf
- wipe your brow, fetch you snacks and possibly even clean up after you, quietly and respectfully
- understand that the normal relationship rules don't count when you're in labour. She can't take things personally: if you want her to leave at any point, she has to go, then come back when you're ready, preferably with flowers and coos for your new baby and definitely with **no hard feelings**
- do or say nothing disturbing or controversial

In short, she has to understand that seeing you give birth is a real privilege as well as something that you'll both treasure forever.

. . . .

FIND OUT MORE

Doula details

How do I find one?

No one organisation fits all doulas just as no one doula fits all women. Finding a doula in Britain today is getting easier. Your best starting point is to make sure you fully understand what you want, and what doulas in general, are for. Currently, in Britain, the best place to find a doula is through Doula UK (DUK) – a non-profit organisation run by women who feel passionately about birth. DUK doulas have private clients but also work in a variety of venues such as prisons, projects for teenage women or refuges. DUK has a map on its website through which you can find a doula free of charge.

There are currently about 150 doula members. About a 30 per cent of these are birth doulas only. Seventeen per cent are postnatal doulas only and the remaining third (that's over 50 per cent) do both.

Doula UK (DUK) P.O. Box 26678, London N14 4WB. 0871 433 3103 www.doula.org.uk

DONA International This is a US based non-profit organisation run by and for doulas. Right now they are just setting up doula training in the UK. DONA International is the largest organised body of certified birth and postpartum doulas worldwide. In 2002 they had 4,550 doulas worldwide, with 2,432 of those certified. For more information: www.dona.org

Tip:
Many doulas in training programmes will either not charge or charge very little, and can be extremely dedicated and useful.

OTHER WAYS TO FIND A DOULA | There are other organisations in the UK which claim to be THE way to find a doula. Some charge hefty placement fees and some run training courses for doulas which are frankly inadequate (and even misleading). **Avoid any organisation that charges you a placement fee.**

If you can't find a doula in your area do not give up. Some doulas, particularly those in training, will travel from neighbouring counties for you. My doula, Lucy, came from Berkshire (I was giving birth in Oxford).

HOW MUCH DOES A DOULA COST? | A birth doula found via DUK can cost anything from £200 to £500 depending on the area and the doula. Most offer a sliding scale of fees depending on what you can afford. Birth doulas should charge a flat fee (**not** by the hour). **If you can't afford to pay anything at all, don't give up.** Doulas do sometimes work free of charge (at their own discretion). Some, when they are starting out, will work free of charge just to get the experience (even a less experienced doula can be an asset). DUK also have a small hardship fund (paid to the doula) to cover costs in some circumstances.

A postnatal doula usually charges between £12 and £15 an hour. On average, she works a few times a week (three to four hours) for up to six weeks.

Again, other agencies in the UK may charge fairly large fees for getting you a doula. **Avoid these.**

CERTIFICATION AND TRAINING | DUK have a code of practice and several accredited trainers. To become recognised by DUK as a doula, you have to have completed one of these trainer's courses and have attended a minimum of four births.

Further reading

The Birth Partner: Everything You Need to Know to Help a Woman Through Childbirth by Penny Simkin (Harvard Press, US, 2001)

Mothering the Mother: How a Doula Can Help You Have a Shorter, Easier, and Healthier Birth by Marshall H. Klaus, John H. Kennell and Phyllis H. Klaus (Da Capo, US, 1993)

The New Experience of Childbirth by Sheila Kitzinger (Orion, UK, 2004)

Ina May's Guide to Childbirth by Ina May Gaskin (Random House, US, 2003)

A comprehensive article on doulas
Doulas: The Future Guardians of Normal Birth? (MIDIRS Midwifery Digest 13:3) 2003 Contact: **Midwives Information and Resource Service (MIDIRS),** 9 Elmdale Rd, Clifton, Bristol, BS8 1SL 0800 581 009. Or get this online at www.doula.org.uk/books/stockton.pdf (they have great links to other articles on doulas, from the national press and other sources: worth a browse).

Online

DUK: www.doula.org.uk

DONA International www.dona.org

Association of Labour Assistants and Childbirth Educators www.alace.org

The National Childbirth Trust's information about 'Birth Partners' www.nctpregnancyandbabycare.com

Chapter Ten: Frozen peas and pyjamas – postpartum and how to prepare for it

'The first two months were more amazing, but also harder than I'd expected them to be. I'd spent all my time preparing for – obsessing on – the birth that I almost forgot there'd be a real baby at the end of it. With my next baby I'm giving it an awful lot more thought.'

KEIRA, 32, MOTHER OF MARK (2), PREGNANT WITH HER SECOND CHILD

1 **Immediate postpartum help.** Make a list of friends/family who have offered to help when the baby comes and organise them accordingly.

2 **Your relationship.** If you have relationship troubles try and work through them now: the demands of a new baby can turn a fixable relationship into a crisis.

3 **Acquiring basic baby equipment.** You don't need much, really, but it's worth getting what you do need before the baby is born, as shopping with a newborn can be fraught (see Find Out More, page 323).

4 **Getting supplies to help you recover postpartum.** There are some simple things that can make a big difference to your comfort in the hours, days and weeks after the birth. See page 322.

5 **Childcare.** Good childcare facilities can be booked up a year or more in advance so, if you'll need one, start to investigate nurseries when you're pregnant. You can always change your mind when you get to know your baby. Also consider whether you need childcare for your other child/children, both for the birth itself, and for the weeks afterwards. If you have a first child under school age, you'll almost certainly need more help than you think you will.

6 **Your camera.** Yes, really: if it doesn't work, get it fixed or buy one (digital can be good for emailing pics to friends/family) or you'll regret it. And if you think you're not the camcorder type, you're about to be wrong. Get one now if you can possibly afford it.

Why bother planning?

Nowadays we are encouraged to leap up the moment we've given birth, slap on our lippy and pretend nothing has happened. We're congratulated if we leave hospital early, manage to squeeze into our jeans and not complain about our sore bits. Consequently, many of us have unrealistic expectations of ourselves postpartum. We're supposed to be 'successful', to 'bounce back', to get our lives back. But our lives, not to mention bodies – have changed. The world shifts when you have a baby: it now contains someone you love more than you love yourself; someone you'd die for without hesitation; someone whose smile is awe-inspiring, who fills you with emotions deeper and more mind-blowing than any you'd imagine possible. This someone also keeps you up all night, poos, wees and throws up on you, eats endlessly, and can be funny, shocking, adorable and alarming. Sometimes all at once. Like birth, you can't control what sort of baby you have. But you can prepare yourself to cope brilliantly with this transition period: those first few fraught and magnificent weeks.

Birth takes recovery – in the old days this was known as a 'lying-in period'. Childbirth educator Sheila Kitzinger has dubbed the period after your baby's birth, when you two (or three, or more) should be simply reveling in your new found love, the 'babymoon'. It's a time for bonding and you'll never get it back. But unfortunately nowadays most of us seem to ignore this notion. And this is just not sensible. It's quite simple: if you prepare properly for the immediate postpartum period, and look on it (at least for the first couple of weeks) as a time to rest and recuperate, you'll really be able to enjoy your baby. Leave it all to chance, and you may find yourself – at times – drowning rather than waving.

A cautionary tale from Julia:

*When I was pregnant with my first baby, Keaton, I covered all the birth eventualities but I never prepared for my postpartum. The books focused on childbirth and that seemed overwhelming enough. I just thought I'd come home, change nappies, be a tad tired... no big deal. When I got home from the hospital with Keaton, my fever rose but I was so focused on the baby that I ignored it. Eventually I was hospitalised with an infection. Meanwhile Keaton developed jaundice. I wanted Buckley to be at home with him, so I was completely alone in hospital during these heartbreaking days. ALL of this nightmare was **avoidable** and it took a long time to bond with my son: I remember telling my midwife he was nice, but I didn't feel connected to him. With my second baby, Larson, I was so anxious about my postpartum that I actually paid a chef to make months' worth of meals and load them in our freezer. We asked our fortnightly house cleaner to come every week for a bit. We organised a new laundry system. We lined up friends and neighbours to come and play with Keaton. We prepared like lunatics and had a great postpartum.*

Julia's first postpartum was unusually dire. There are, however, countless milder variations on such stressful times that really could be mitigated with a bit of planning. And – as Julia's second postpartum showed – if you plan for the worst, you'll get the best.

FIVE COMMON MISCONCEPTIONS ABOUT POSTPARTUM

These five came up repeatedly when we asked women with more than one child what their biggest misconceptions were first time around:

1 **I've run a business, I can manage a small baby.** You're used to managing teams and running complex projects so how hard could dealing with a newborn be? The challenges aren't comparable: motherhood strikes at the very heart of who you are, constantly. It can be bliss or hell. Or both at once. Business skills may get you a fantastic weaning schedule, but they won't help you sing 'baa, baa black sheep' in exactly the right, sleep-inducing key.

2 **You're either a stay-at-home mum or you work.** For many of us, working life changes dramatically after we have children (most

commonly, after we have a second child). Some of us find ways to become freelance. Some go back to the office part-time. Some set up our own projects with more flexible hours. Many of us simply work harder and longer at odd times of the day, to compensate for time spent with our children. It is rarely simple. I've lost count of the amount of telephone interviews I've done while jiggling a baby/breastfeeding/ trying to ignore the howls of my children beating each other up in the other room.

3 **I won't need postpartum help.** You will (see below, page 287).

4 **I will fall in love with my baby the minute I see him.** Many of us feel alarm, indignation, surprise, indifference, shock or confusion in place of instant maternal love. It can take weeks, months and in some cases more, to fall in love with your baby. None of this will mean you're not cut out for motherhood.

5 **Being pregnant was so difficult, being a parent has got to be easier.** When pregnant, your child, crucially, is inside you, and therefore its sphere of influence is somewhat limited (though it can seem significant enough). Inside you, your child is unable to fully exert the power of her personality. Other peoples' babies may have seemed featureless and blob-like to you but your own will be infinitely complex and permanently life-altering.

How long does postpartum last?

Everyone has a different answer to this one and you may experience postpartum differently with each child you have. Julia says hers, with Keaton, lasted three months – one month of which was 'intense'. With Larson, who is now over two and has never been a good sleeper, she wonders 'am I still postpartum?' Most women say that dealing with a newborn gets distinctly easier when you all pass the three-month mark, hence the notion of the first three months with your newborn being 'the fourth trimester'. There is a medical term – 'puerperium' – the period usually described as six to eight weeks after childbirth, where your womb and other organs and structures which have been affected by the pregnancy are returning to their non-pregnant state. At the very least, take this period seriously: you have a genuine physiological (not to mention psychological) need to recover.

It can take a while for your baby to start feeding and sleeping more predictably (colicky or fussy babies tend to get mercifully better when they're about 12 weeks old). In this chapter we're concentrating on the immediate postpartum: the first three months of your baby's life. This time – when you're establishing yourself as a mother (or a mother of two, or more) and getting to know your beautiful baby – can be bliss. **If you prepare for them**.

Getting help postpartum

Rest and how to achieve it

The number one rule for a productive postpartum is simple: take rest very, very seriously. Stress and tiredness are implicated in anything from mastitis to postnatal depression. But in order to rest you'll need plenty of help (even – indeed possibly especially – if this is not your first baby). Whether it's a team of highly-paid nannies, or merely regular packages of your mother-in-law's baked goods, you should plan – in advance – how you'll get the help you need.

TIPS FOR EVERY POSTPARTUM WOMAN

- **Put your pyjamas on** and stay in them for at least three days (and preferably more) after you get home from hospital. You can't dash around town in your jimmies. Take no pride in being up and about: it's not going to do you or your baby any good.

- **Avoid walking up stairs** for three days if you can. *'You have a wound inside you where your placenta was so help yourself heal it,'* says midwife Kim Kelly. Let others bring your food to you, and keep your baby with you for the whole three days. It's a cliché, but this is time you'll never get back.

- **Cook and freeze lots of healthy meals** that you actually like (borrow a friend's freezer space if you don't have a freezer, or consider buying one if you can possibly do so – they are invaluable for feeding babies and children in a remotely healthy way).

- **Create a six-week support plan** so you can rest, and not become overwhelmed by your new situation (see The Skeeter Effect below).

- **Include your other children in your postpartum** – get them to hold the baby, touch her, count her toes, change her nappy. And get help with them, so that you are not left feeling guilty/overstretched/overwhelmed.

Options for postpartum support

POSTNATAL MATERNITY NURSE | The idea is that they satisfy the worries and concerns of the new mother. They can cost a fortune (about £600 a week, via an agency). You hire one for the first week or two following the birth to help you establish breastfeeding schedules, and to give you confidence and tips for dealing with your newborn, and to let you rest. People normally book one for at least two weeks. They can be lovely, or bossy, or both. But most will have their own very fixed, and sometimes rigid, system for dealing with a new baby that can, for some mothers, feel overpowering. They'll expect to live in.

NIGHT NANNY | Again, a posh option for those who are really obsessed by sleep. Can also be a lifesaver if you have twins (or more) or a sick baby. Night nannies will normally look after the baby in your house from 9 p.m. to 7 a.m. They cost around £70 per night. If you are breastfeeding, they will bring the baby to your room for feeds and take her away afterwards, doing all the jiggling and nappy changing while you crash out.

POSTNATAL DOULA | Trained to help you cope brilliantly with the early days, her main agenda is to help you bond with your baby, and not feel over-stressed. She'll do anything from advise you about feeding, nappies or newborn sleep patterns, to nipping round the supermarket for supplies. They usually charge between £10 to £15 per hour and probably ask for a deposit. They're not just for first time mothers. A friend of mine, who has three children, hired one when she had her fourth and fifth babies: twins.

'MOTHER'S HELPS' | Terrible term, but a catch-all for teenage girls to whom you and your partner can ruthlessly pay a pittance in exchange for basic help around the house – washing up, laundry, hoovering, jiggling baby's pram, changing the odd nappy, answering the front door. Remember, though, that teenage girls can be fickle (i.e. they may not show up). And they should not be expected to behave like nannies (i.e. look after your baby for long periods unattended).

FAMILY/FRIENDS | Consider getting a family member to come and stay after the birth with the explicit purpose of helping. But be clear about what you may need them to do: cook dinner? Clean the kitchen floor? Look after your other child/children? Just hold the baby while you sleep? Some people say tension with family members became significantly better with the arrival of a nappy-clad mutual distraction. Others say it all exacerbated an already inflammatory situation. Only you can judge how your particular family psychodrama might play out but the golden rule is: if they're not helping, tell them (tactfully if you can) to go away. And have a back up plan.

Some common family pitfalls

Close family members are ideal postpartum helpers. But think hard before you commit. Many women think the baby will heal rifts, help them bond with estranged parents or siblings, even 'change' people. Maybe it will, in the long run, but the first few weeks postpartum are not the time for family therapy. So:

1 **BEWARE THEIR EXPECTATIONS** | *'My mum came expecting fun and joy,'* says Len, 34, mother of Liam (1), *'and got stress – I was ill and her grandson was*

colicky. It was a BIG mistake having her come so soon – she was anxious, and it made us even more stressed. Next time I would have her there, but I'd talk to her about exactly the kind of help we'll need, before she comes.'

2 **BEWARE CHANGES IN PARENTING** | It's been years since your parents had a newborn on their hands. Ideas may have changed. It's your turn to make your own mistakes, and if they can't recognise this, it's probably worth a conversation early on, as things will only get worse.

3 **BEWARE THE BAGGAGE** | Julia has seen many idealistic clients: *'One client, when I asked her about her postpartum plan, said her mother would be flying in to help. I asked if they got on well and there was a pause before she said, "Well, she's a practising alcoholic and that's been really hard on our relationship, but I think this will really bring us together." Eventually, after much discussion, she invited her mother to come out when the baby was a bit bigger.'* Use your judgment about how helpful your family will actually be: it's a bit like when you chose your birth partner – loving that person isn't a good enough reason in itself to invite them to stay during the precious early days of your baby's life.

Tip for organising postpartum help:
The *'Skeeter Effect'* is a system Julia suggests her clients use to organise a support network of friends in the first few weeks (Skeeter was her baby son's nickname). You just get several of your friends to agree to take one or two days of each week to check on you. In the first week after your baby's birth they bring you a meal on their day (they just make two dinners in that first week – one for their own family and one for you). After that first week, they agree to phone you on their chosen day for at least six weeks more. This way, you won't feel isolated or alone (at least you'll get a phone call a day). This can also be a good way to spot symptoms of postnatal depression. Julia has had clients' friends calling her weeks after a birth to tell her they've noticed symptoms of postnatal depression in the new mother.

A WORD ABOUT VISITS | These can be overwhelming in the immediate postpartum, especially if they all expect you to make them tea and feed them cake (or worse, real food). Do not try and pretend you're normal. Get them to make their own tea and bring cake with them. Set particular times for their visits and tell them how long to stay. If they offer to help, or bring food, say yes without hesitation or guilt.

Releasing your helpers
Once you have accepted help it's important to find a reasonable time to let go of it. Julia has seen some clients over-use their poor friends and relatives. *'For most of us, who are healthy and have healthy babies, the 'crisis' period postpartum, where*

we really need urgent help, lasts two or three weeks (this is not to say we don't need help after this, just not so much, or so intensely). Eventually, you've got to work out how to cook and get laundry done. That's not postpartum. That's life with kids.'

When to venture out

In some parts of India, twenty-two days of rest after birth is the common practice. Women are served and pampered, able to recover and adjust to motherhood in their own time. Until relatively recently, even British women had a long 'lying-in' period (sometimes months). These days, however, you're meant to be scooting round Sainsbury's within days of popping that baby out. For first time parents, just leaving the house with a newborn can be daunting, and if you've got other children, going out in the early days can become a major (and majorly stressful) event. You might feel, first time around, like everyone is watching you to see whether you're incompetent. You might be terrified in case your baby cries at the checkout or poos on her babygro (she probably will). You might wonder how you'll carry a tantrumming toddler and a baby in a car seat, while wheeling a trolley across a busy car park (answer: a trolley with infant seat AND toddler seat, grim determination, thick skin and lots of patience).

TAKE OUTINGS ONE STEP AT A TIME

- Don't feel you have to go out if you feel you want to stay in and rest. There is no right time.
- A walk, with your baby in the sling or buggy, is a good first outing.
- Make your outing – whatever it is – short.
- Get your partner or friend to come too.
- Be aware that your baby is not used to noise, bright lights, odd smells. The outside world, the first few times, can be pretty alarming for them too. Crying is pretty normal for a first buggy trip.
- Be aware that if you have other children, particularly if they are small, they may play up simply because they're not used to your attention being divided.

Your body postpartum

'Try not to worry at this stage, that you feel a bit as though someone has implanted a bunch of miniature bananas into your vagina: a bruised vulva is part and parcel of a normal delivery, and no-one gets away without some discomfort.' Journalist Joanna Moorhead in an article in *Junior Pregnancy and Baby* magazine[1].

What's the fuss about?

Nobody tells you what postpartum can feel like. But one of the most common things women we spoke to for this book said about postpartum was: *'no one told me it'd be like this*'. This is a diary I wrote, for a newspaper, when my second postpartum was fresh in my mind. Look at it as a cautionary tale: I had been totally focused on having a good birth and had NOT prepared for the after-effects of a vaginal birth. I therefore had no idea what to do about them. I was living far from home and family, in Seattle, and had very little help or support. You, of course, will manage your postpartum MUCH better than I did. This diary isn't meant to scare you, but here you go: I'm telling you how it *can* be if you are not prepared for it.

DIARY OF A POSTPARTUM WOMAN

Zero hour

Having heard many friends liken childbirth to melon-pooing, I beg to differ. It is more like completing a triathlon while simultaneously attempting to turn oneself inside out, labia first. Improbably my beautiful baby is finally born. A flood of utter relief, helped massively by a rush of endorphins.

20 minutes

Euphoria. I am distracted by sight, feel, smell of beautiful, salty, messy baby. I need stitches and the midwife calls for an obstetrician who, she claims, is a 'devil with a needle'. Having endured childbirth you'd think a few little stitches with an anaesthetic would be a piece of cake but they're quite sore. I focus on my astonishing baby boy who is now snuggled against my chest. Everyone is congratulating me. I feel like I've achieved a miracle. And so I have.

45 minutes

The midwife wants to tell me all about my 'tear' and is slightly taken aback that I don't want the details. She takes my husband outside to debrief him. When she comes back (John with a 'bright smile'), she says she should put a catheter in as it might be a 'bit sore' to pee. I consume handfuls of painkillers in anticipation of the local anaesthetic wearing off. **Tip:** *'Your right to know everything includes your right to NOT know everything,'* says Julia. *'You can always ask your midwife later if you decide that you want to know the nitty-gritty after all.'* (Also, with a straightforward vaginal birth like this one, a catheter is uncommon in the UK, and definitely optional – it's usually better for you to go to the loo on your own. You can ask to have your first pee in a bed pan if you don't want to get up.)

One hour

Warm, flooding feeling in the bed. I ring the bell in a panic, but it's just the catheter bag, 'malfunctioning'. My stomach is still vast, as if another baby is lurking in there. The midwife explains that it takes six weeks for my womb to shrink back to normal size. She prods it regularly over the next two days to see that it is doing this and to check that there are no signs that I have retained any of the placenta or have any infection.

Six hours
Still haven't dared get up as I'm feeling distinctly bruised. Fortunately, my baby is a great distraction: he is alert, and beautiful, and gazes up at me with huge eyes and I spend a lot more time gazing joyfully back at him than I do worrying about the state of my vagina. Even though this is my second child, it still seems genuinely astounding that I've given birth to this fantastic baby boy.

Seven hours
Catheter is removed and I am guided to the bathroom to 'get cleaned up'. My legs shake and ache. My head is light. I have the distinct impression that my intestines and colon are going to fall out of my vagina. But, I am still euphoric at having produced an actual, healthy baby so – astoundingly – none of this matters. Afterwards, I put on a pad and a pair of paper knickers. They have small pink sprigs on them, a nice touch. **Tip:** Bleeding is painless and normal after childbirth. Peeing in the shower or the birth tub in those first hours after the birth may not be ladylike, but will make that first pee much less of an ordeal. Alternatively, ask the midwife to bring you a jug of warm water and when you sit on the loo, pour it over your parts as you have your first pee.

Day one
I have to recline since sitting is painful. I refuse to look down there and also refuse to let my husband look as I don't want him to retain any negative image. He thinks I'm mad, as he saw Sam come out. My stomach is still inflated. My shoulders, oddly, ache as if I've carried a piano around for several days. My breasts are producing pale liquid called colostrum that Sam laps up round the clock but other than this they don't feel any different. I have been given 'stool softener' pills but apparently may not be able to 'go' for quite some time. **Tip for inevitable constipation:** soak 1–2 teaspoons of linseeds or psyllium seeds in a cup of warm water, leave to swell into a gel for 15 minutes, drink at night. Or soak same amount of linseeds overnight and add to breakfast cereal. Take any stool softeners you are offered.

Day two
I am still having painful 'contractions'. This is my womb shrinking and shouldn't persist. Walking out of the hospital is a challenge. I have to stick my bum out and take tiny steps like ancient tribal dancer. I look pregnant still. I am unable to sit down in the car and have to perch, one

cheek on the side of the seat, swearing. But I feel triumphant: bringing my family home. **Tip:** Afterpains are worse with your second, and subsequent babies. Take plenty of paracetamol and try lying on your tummy. If it's painful to sit on your bruised perineum, you can hire a 'valley cushion' from the National Childbirth Trust (see Find Out More, page 326) designed specially for comfort after birth.

Day three

I now see the need for stool softener and can confirm it has failed. I am genuinely alarmed by my piles. My perineum still aches when I move, and it hurts to sit down. My boobs have inflated to the size and texture of medicine balls, my nipples are bright red and I keep crying. ('Baby Blues', I am told by a sympathetic midwife; a normal hormonal day-three thing – my oestrogen and progesterone levels have 'dropped precipitously'.) **Tip:** Keep up with the linseeds for constipation and drink plenty of fluids. Baby blues are normal and should pass within a day or two. Bathe your piles in cotton wool soaked in witchhazel, which you keep in the fridge. You can also use over-the-counter haemorrhoid cream. Use sore vagina/perineum/stitches methods we've outlined on page 295. For ways to cope with engorged breasts, see page 298.

Day four

My husband insists on taking a look at my parts. I am sure he'll never desire me again, but right now couldn't care less. He claims – to my astonishment – that they look almost normal. I know he is lying because when I move I can feel the wind whistling up there and things flapping. Also, the midwife told me she put in purple stitches. Love is a wonderful thing. Sam is feeding constantly, and my milk supply feels good. His two-year-old sister holds him on her lap, and John and I look at them both and feel, suddenly, like a 'real family'.

Week two

Still incontinent, still huge. Sam eats round the clock (what happened to 'four hourly schedules?'). My boobs feel variously engorged and completely drained. And I now have a suspicious red, painful lump on one breast. A day later, the whole side of it is red and inflamed. I have a fever. Midwife diagnoses mastitis – an infection of the milk ducts – and prescribes rest (ha), steaming them over a pan of hot water, massage and antibiotics. **Tip:** There are many ways to treat sore nipples, lumps and other breastfeeding difficulties (see page 298). In the vast majority of cases these things happen because your baby is not latched on properly. Get advice straight away from a breastfeeding specialist (ask your midwife for details of the hospital breastfeeding clinic) if any problem emerges. **N.B.** Many women at two weeks postpartum feel fantastic: their stitches have healed, breastfeeding is established, their help and support are really working for them and they begin to feel human again!

Week three

The mastitis has gone, I can still feel the bruising on my perineum if I'm up and about too much, but am now much more mobile than before. Sam is sleeping more, and my mother has arrived, so for the first time I am able to just sit and marvel over him (while my mum takes my two-year-old out for treats). **Tip:** Gentle postpartum yoga moves and stretches will help to increase your energy, manage stress and heal faster.

Week six

My book talks about 'easing back into sex'. Ha, ha. One of the tips is 'don't be discouraged by pain' **Tip:** Some women feel sexy surprisingly early (sort out your contraception!), others find that, with the recovery from the birth, and with hormones released from breastfeeding (not to mention interrupted sleep) it's months – and often up to a couple of years even – until they feel sexy again. The general advice is: take sex at your own pace, don't feel pressure to be sexy and – if you do – go gently at first.

Week seven

Fretful baby and very little sleep. I have been told that Sam's elephantine wind problem could be a result of dairy produce in my diet and so have cut it out, which is not helping my stress levels. He is still farting and writhing. My health visitor gives me a questionnaire to check whether I have postnatal depression. Apparently not. My mood is, she says, 'normal'. **Tip:** Tiredness often catches up on you surprisingly late, and can make you feel down. This is usually also when you are alone with the baby more. Join local groups, even if you're not a 'joiner', as being with other new mothers can be your salvation. If you're worried about postnatal depression talk to your midwife or health visitor (who should be checking you for this anyway). Many babies have settled well by seven or eight weeks, and are sleeping more and feeding more regularly. If yours is very 'windy' see a breastfeeding specialist to check that you are latching him onto your breast properly, before you start to alter your diet. I took Ted, my third (equally windy and fretful) baby to the breastfeeding clinic at my hospital when he was six weeks old. They explained that I was latching him onto my breast in an inefficient way when feeding him. Doing it correctly turned him into a different baby overnight: peaceful, non-windy, content. This might not work with a genuinely colicky baby, who can be extremely exhausting (see page 307). Most fretful (and even colicky) babies have settled down by 12 weeks postpartum so remind yourself this will pass and GET SUPPORT.

Week eight

Life is looking up. The piles have almost gone. I can now walk for half an hour without discomfort. I slept for three consecutive hours two nights in a row and I managed faintly to twitch my pelvic floor yesterday. I'm still exhausted and feel fat. But my baby smiles now as well as farts and his sister claims she loves him, even though she's cross with me, and wants to hold him all the time. I think they're the most beautiful human beings in the world. Which makes it all worthwhile.

Immediate postpartum

Your vagina

If you gave birth vaginally then let's face it your faithful friend has been through the mill (particularly if it is your first time). It needs tender loving care to recover properly, not stoic, gritted teeth. **One rule**: put nothing in your vagina for three weeks after the birth – no tampons or (god forbid) penises or vibrators. If and when you do begin to have sex, you might want to use a lubricant at first (e.g. KY gel from any chemist) as your hormones may make your vagina less lubricated for a while (and it may still be tender).

TRICKS FOR SOOTHING SORE BITS

Try the following until you find something that works for you

1 **Frozen peas:** put them in a ziplock plastic bag, wrap in a thin towel or pillowcase and put them on the sore area. They mould well to the shape of your body and can feel hugely comforting. You can also buy slightly pricey 'gel pads' from Boots that are specifically for postpartum use on your perineum – same effect (though quadruple the cost) as the peas.

2 **Squirty bottles:** many women have several days of perineal/labial pain while peeing after giving birth. Ordinary little plastic bottles with squirty tops (a bit like small washing up liquid bottles) are commonly handed out to new mothers in American hospitals. You can buy their equivalent plastic bottles with squirty tips in Boots, marketed to store your cosmetics in when you are on holiday. Alternatively, on your first trips to the loo after birth, go armed with a jug of warm (not hot) water and pour it on your labia/perineum as you pee. The water will dilute the acidity of your urine and massively reduce the stinging feeling.

3 **Cold maxi pads (get cottony feel ones):** sprinkle your sanitary pad with cool witchhazel from the fridge. Witchhazel is soothing and antiseptic. Change your pads very frequently. Keep pads in the freezer and use them cold to soothe and reduce swelling.

4 **Gentle drying techniques:** never rub your vulva dry: always just pat it very, very gently.

5 **A 'sitzbath':** this is a small tub that you fill with warm water and put on the loo, or sides of the bath, so you can bathe your parts in it (a washing up basin will do at a pinch). It can be immensely soothing – and quick to do – after a vaginal birth. (Ordinary baths work too, but are more time-consuming and harder to get regularly when you have a newborn.) Some midwives suggest adding a few drops of lavender essential oil (dilute it in a couple of tablespoons of milk so it does not just sit on top of the water). Herbalists say some herbs are good for soaking your bum. Buy all of this before the baby is born. If you have a bidet, this will do as well.

6 **A 'valley cushion':** A special cushion designed to help you sit more comfortably while your perineum is bruised or stitches are healing. You can hire these from the NCT (see Find Out More, page 326). They are now recommended by midwives instead of the old 'ring' shaped cushions.

Bleeding

Expect to bleed for a few days as if you're having an excessively heavy period – you might pass some large clots – then as if you have a normal period, for a month or so after the birth, getting gradually lighter as the days pass. This is normal. It also happens after a caesarean. It's called 'lochia' and it's your womb shedding its lining. It's why you initially might want disposable knickers (available from Mothercare, Boots and large supermarkets like Tesco and Sainsbury's – in the baby aisle usually) and to buy in crate loads of sanitary pads before the birth (see Appendix). An alternative to disposable knickers is to wear old or cheapo knickers you can bin. You'll need to buy a lot of the thickest sanitary pads for wearing at first; later on, they can be reduced down as the bleeding slows.

Tip: Put an old towel under your sheet to protect your mattress.

Afterpains

These are period-like cramps you get after the birth (for about a week) as your womb begins to shrink back to its normal size. They'll be stronger if this is not your first baby – your womb has to work even harder this time to regain its pre-pregnancy shape and size. They can be more intense while you breastfeed, because of our old friend, the hormone oxytocin: this is responsible for the letdown of your milk and also causes your womb to contract. **How to cope:** try massaging your lower abdomen, lying on your stomach with a firm pillow under it, putting a hot water bottle on it. Take the maximum dose of paracetamol in the first few days. **Tip:** If you have a TENS machine (see Chapter 5, page 167), you might want to keep hold of it for a few days after the birth as it can be good for afterpains.

Incontinence

I know. But it happens to the best of us. I remember peeing myself as I walked upstairs to the loo about a week after giving birth – totally unable to control the flow. I felt like a distraught old lady. No one had told me incontinence could be a temporary side-effect of giving birth. Do your pelvic floor exercises as soon as you can bear it (or sooner). At first you may feel absolutely nothing. Again, no one ever tells you this and it can be immensely frustrating. But keep doing it and gradually you'll regain some control. It's essential to do pelvic floor exercises regularly (see Chapter One, page 30, for instructions) to minimise future incontinence, improve your sex life and avoid other problems with your nethers as you get older. If your incontinence remains problematic, discuss it with your midwife. It's incredibly common after childbirth and so many of us don't mention it. She can help you sort it out with special exercises and refer you to a physiotherapist if this does not work (in some cases it won't, and you will need extra help but in the long run, you should be fine). It's normal to leak a little bit of pee when you cough or sneeze, for up to a year after the birth.

Experienced mother's pelvic floor tip:

If you're mentally prepared for dodgy bladder control, and know it won't last (if you do pelvic floor exercises), it's perfectly manageable: use sanitary pads, even when you stop bleeding as this takes the anxiety away a bit.

Your bottom

Yes, just as your progeny's poo can be a source of concern, so can your own. At least in the first few days postpartum. **Constipation** is common, can be eye-wateringly painful and is caused by your changing hormones. **Ways to cope:** try linseed as in the tip on page 292. Drink eight glasses of water a day and make sure you are eating fibre rich food (wholegrains, fruit and veg – hard to do in the first few days, but try or you'll be trying harder on the loo). Take any remedy or 'stool softener' your midwife suggests (usually lactulose or fibrogel). Another glamorous after-effect is **piles** (haemorrhoids). These can be shockingly pronounced after birth. **Ways to cope:** bathe your bottom with cotton wool soaked in witchhazel, apply over-the-counter medications and use wet wipes to wipe for a bit. And talk to your midwife: some suggest raising your bottom above heart level with cushions at night (helps the piles go back in!). Your midwife will not be in the least surprised by the conversation. Indeed, she may be wondering why you haven't already raised the issue.

Experienced mother's bottom tip:

'My birth ball, after I'd delivered, turned into the most comfortable chair in my house for a while.' Jo, 38, mother of Lucinda (4 months)

Your belly

The first thing you may notice is that you **still look six months pregnant**. This is because your womb has only just started shrinking. The next thing you'll notice is that your stomach has metamorphosed into a large squishy sponge (in texture and appearance). Stay calm. It will (particularly if you exercise later) firm up again. The sponge effect, even if you do no exercise, is short lived (how short lived will depend on anything from your genes to your pregnant size).

Your breastfeeding boobs

The other day I looked down at Ted – now a big, chubby, healthy four-month-old baby – and it occurred to me that he has been fed on **nothing but me** since he was a small bundle of multiplying cells. This is quite an achievement, when you think about it. Breastfeeding is a miraculous extension of pregnancy: your boobs, which have spent their whole life propping up your wonderbra (or whatever) finally get to show what they're made of: they'll produce milk that will feed a real baby. But like all achievements, this can involve some effort and determination. The best preparation for breastfeeding is mental: get information. There's tons of research to show that breastfeeding is incredibly beneficial for your baby and for you, but it isn't always easy. If you are prepared for this, and informed, you can tackle any problems that arise and go on to feed your baby for as long as you want. The best thing a midwife ever said to me was: *'Breastfeeding may be natural, but it isn't instinctive.'* **You have to learn**. Start by reading our Breastfeeding basics on page 311.

YOUR BOOBS IF YOU ARE NOT BREASTFEEDING | If for some very rare reason you are physically unable to breastfeed, then your boobs may feel normal after the birth. However, if you are choosing not to breastfeed, they can become engorged with milk for up to a week or so. **How to cope**: do not stimulate your breasts at all, take paracetamol regularly, use breast pads for leakage. A warm flannel or hot water bottle may also help soothe non-breastfeeding boobs.

Your skin

You may sweat a lot in the first few days after giving birth, especially at night. This is your body getting rid of the extra fluid it has amassed during pregnancy. The look of your skin might change too: in pregnancy you may have noticed increased pigmentation ('cholasma', sometimes called the 'mask of pregnancy') and maybe even hair growth on your face. These, you'll be relieved to learn, should go away postpartum.

But when it comes to postpartum skin, most of us are more worried about stretch-marks than sweating. If your smooth tummy has turned into a crumpled page of red scribbles it's easy to feel dismayed. The books will tell you they're feminine badges of motherhood – great in theory but not enough if you're shocked by yours. The good news is that almost all stretch marks will fade and become *far* less noticeable over time (though this can take months). You can't get rid of them, but you can buy sexy one-piece swimsuits to replace your outdated bikinis, know that you are most definitely not alone and – yes – cultivate a 'don't care' attitude.

Sweaty nights tip:
Sleep on a towel so you don't make endless laundry for yourself.

Your hair

Hair becomes thicker in pregnancy then falls out, sometimes alarmingly, afterwards. This is normal. Your hair actually falls out all the time when you are not pregnant: you just don't notice it. During pregnancy, your hormones simply slow this natural falling out routine. This makes your hair seem really luxuriant. Many of us rush to the hairdresser as soon as possible after the baby is born, desperate to feel more glamorous (unlike the rest of your body, hair is something you can control, at least superficially). It can, therefore, be a bit of a downer when your hair starts falling out. But fall out is normal. You are not going bald – merely returning to your usual follicular state.

Your smell

It is fine to have a bath any time after you've delivered your baby (the view that you should only have showers until your blood flow has dried up is very outdated). Watch out for hot baths in the hours after the birth though, says midwife Jenny Smith: *'Most women are usually exhausted after labour and there's a danger of fainting if you have a hot bath.'* Not getting time to bath or shower once you've left the hospital, on the other hand, is one of the things many women find hard in the early weeks. Particularly first time around, we're terrified to leave our baby unattended for even ten minutes. But if your baby is sleeping in his cot/Moses basket somewhere safe (and you know where your cat/other children are) you can just take the baby monitor to the shower with you. Don't panic if your baby wakes up and howls for a few minutes while you're rushing to dry your tender bottom. He is safe (you'd hear on the monitor if some predator appeared in his bedroom). He may be cross. But he's fine. You are not a neglectful parent. Another tip is to make an agreement with your partner (or pay a teenager to come for an hour) for a set time each day when he'll watch the baby while you shower or soak in the bath. It can be nice to know that you are, just for that short period, not going to be interrupted. **Tip:** wear earplugs while you bathe, or earphones. Yes really. This way, you won't leap out guiltily at the first wail.

Experienced mother's tip:
'I just let mine cry, if necessary, safely in the bouncy chair next to the shower,' says, Manju, 38, mother of three. *'It's stressful, but effective. I was determined to start my day with a shower. I got clean and I knew the baby was not being tortured by the other*

children. I look back on my first baby – when I virtually never had a proper shower –
and wonder why I didn't just let him yell for a minute or two.'

Your teeth

Pregnancy can affect your teeth so try and get to the dentist reasonably soon postpartum. If you are lucky enough to have an NHS dentist, you get free dentistry throughout pregnancy and for a year after the birth. But take your partner. You don't want to be wrestling with your howling newborn while gagging on a tamp. If you're breastfeeding **tell the dentist** before they start any work on you (anaesthesia and drugs can pass through the breast milk).

Your body image

Julia believes that it's important for women's psychological health not to turn into unwashed, uncared for beasts postpartum. Obviously, if you were such a beast in the first place, then motherhood doesn't mean you have to slip into heels, lippy and a bright Stepfordian smile. The real issue, of course, is more complex than a bit of lippy might suggest. Your body has been through something extreme and somehow not entirely reasonable. You may feel like a huge, spongy, mildly psychotic milch cow for a while and this is fine. I remember walking up a very steep hill in Seattle with John (who had our tiny son in a sling and was pushing our two-year-old in the buggy). We were both out of breath (me more than him) but unlike him, my thighs were wobbling, my perineum was aching, my boobs were throbbing, my waistband pinching. And I suddenly felt wildly jealous that he was so unencumbered. It's not easy, at times, to adjust to your postpartum body. But it **will** change. *'I remember the glee I felt when out for a country walk some time after my second baby was born,'* says Linda, 48, mother of two teenagers. *'I realised I could just hop over a fence. It was a profoundly liberating moment.'* The postpartum rebound effect: it **will** happen.

Your weight

Childbirth educator Sheila Kitzinger once wrote that many women love pregnancy because it's the first time it's socially acceptable not to be skinny. But when the pregnancy is done, the 'too fat' pressure descends once more. You will, unless you've been starving yourself in a stupid way during pregnancy, be somewhat over your ideal weight after you have had a baby. Some women don't mind this one bit, others find it depressing. You'll lose weight rapidly in the first few days after delivery because you will pee out the extra two to eight litres of water your body carried in late pregnancy. But after this things may slow down somewhat.

'I tell women not to expect to be back to normal for at least a year,' says midwife Jenny Smith, 'this way, you are off the hook. I see some women who become so thin so fast after the birth it just isn't healthy. You should be enjoying your baby, not worrying about what you eat.'

WEIGHT ADVICE FOR SENSIBLE WOMEN

- **Do not diet if you are breastfeeding:** weight loss after pregnancy will be gradual (remember the old adage: 'nine months on/nine months off').

- **Eat well:** good nutrition is essential postpartum to stop your body's natural resources, such as your calcium supply, from becoming depleted in the long term. Plan frequent, healthy snacks if you are breastfeeding, to keep your energy levels up.

- **Do gentle postnatal exercises:** as advised by your midwife or health visitor in the weeks after the birth. They will help you get back in shape.

- **Breastfeed:** it can help you lose weight (it burns calories).

This is all technically correct. But many of us are not so well-balanced. We worry that we'll never lose the baby weight. We feel depressed when we catch sight of our bellies and bottoms in a shop window, or when we can't fit into clothes three times our normal size. We get grumpy when our partners tell us we look lovely when we feel fat. We try to restrict our eating even though we know we shouldn't. And because we're knackered from dealing with, not to mention feeding, a small infant, we then crack and eat all the wrong things at the wrong times. We don't cook curly kale because we're too tired and haven't got to the shops anyway. Instead, we eat frozen pizza and hobnobs, then worry that our bums will forever reach the backs of our knees.

WEIGHT ADVICE FOR THE REST OF US

- **Let yourself of the hook,** for God's sake. You've just produced a baby. Prepare yourself for weight loss being slow, and for this being OK and totally normal.

- **Do not go on a fad diet when breastfeeding.** Really. Just don't. Your breastfeeding body needs balanced nutrients for long-term health, not a carb-free, food combining, cabbage soup extravaganza.

- **Don't weigh yourself for three months** – at least – after the birth. It won't help and it will probably just depress you. Put away the scales.

- **Don't exist solely on Marks and Sparks ready meals** if you can possibly help it. Freeze batches of healthy food, like vegetable soup, in individual portions, before your baby is born. Defrost them for three minute lunches. Boring, perhaps, but effective.

- **Make it easy to lay your hands on a healthy snack.** Planning snacks probably isn't going to be your top priority but there are easier ways to cut back on cake than willpower alone. Buy more fruit and fewer hobnobs. If fruit isn't enough, eat toast and marmite with low fat spread; a (preferably wholemeal) hot crossed bun, a granary roll with cheese or a handful of nuts. Put dried fruit on your shopping list, and remove crisps.

- **Have the odd treat.** For crying out loud, you deserve it.

- **While breastfeeding uses up calories** (about 500 a day) many of us don't lose any weight while doing it, because we stuff ourselves with cake (see above) and don't get enough exercise (or we're simply more hungry all the time: who can blame us?). Even if you are not an exercise person, try walking with the baby in a buggy for 30 minutes a day, five days a week, once your midwife or health visitor says it is ok to do this.

- **Dress like a non-pregnant person.** If you can afford it, take a trip to some super cheap clothing shop like Matalan, or a Hennes or TopShop sale. Buy a couple of pairs of trousers and some tops or dresses that you can give away as you shrink out of them. Many of us feel significantly more human in something without stretchy panels. A stretchy black dress can also be a versatile godsend.

- **Hide your jeans.** Store away your old jeans in a distant cupboard and do not touch them (or even look at them) for at least six months, if not a year. I remember, about three months after Izzie was born, attempting to get into my 'fat' jeans. I couldn't even get them over my knees. I whipped them off, assuming I'd mistakenly picked out my 'skinny' pair instead, and had to sit down when I saw they were, indeed, my most capacious denims. Expect a few instances like this and **keep a sense of humour.**

PHYSICAL WARNING SIGNS POSTPARTUM

Call the doctor/midwife if you experience any of these symptoms postpartum:

- Passage of a blood clot larger than a lemon. Heavy bleeding that soaks a maxi sanitary pad in an hour
- Fever of 100.4F/38C or higher on two occasions
- Problems when you pee: burning, or blood in pee, inability to pee
- Very foul fish-like smell to vaginal discharge (this can signal infection)
- Pain at site of episiotomy or tear or redness and pain on your caesarean scar
- Swollen, red, hot painful area on the leg, especially the calf (can signal blood clot – a huge emergency – so call immediately).
- Sore, reddened, hot, painful area on breast, along with fever or flu-like symptoms (this could be mastitis, see page 316).

Your mind postpartum

Your body is oddly shaped and surging with hormones, you've had less sleep than you thought physically possible and you've fallen in love. These things can affect your mental state. Here are a few common worries and what to do about them.

Anxiety taking the baby home
It's surprisingly easy to become institutionalised in hospital, comforted by those lovely midwives with their understanding smiles, advice and sympathy, their safe medications and the doctors on hand; the regular (if revolting) feeds you get, the routine, the noise, the smell. It's like being a small child again – everyone else is in charge.

Putting on clothes, strapping your defenceless infant into a car seat that suddenly seems the size of the Titanic, and walking out of the door can feel terrifying. The whole world swells dangerously around you: how will you keep this small creature alive? Safe?

Going home – particularly with your first baby – can be a tremendously vulnerable time. Most of us feel like this – it's normal, and says nothing about your ability to cope, but don't underestimate its power to freak you out. Remember, the midwife is coming tomorrow. And there is always one at the end of a phone.

Tiredness
The physical act of giving birth would be enough to send most of us to bed for a month. When you factor in a wakeful newborn, the tiredness can feel catastrophic. Don't think that if you're the kind of person used to working lunatic hours in the office you'll breeze through sleep deprivation as you've always done. Baby tiredness – the hormonal, physical, emotional blend – is a different kind entirely. The only thing you can do about it is REST. For this, given that a small creature is waking you up night and day, you will need help.

Sleep deprivation: mental preparation tip:
Julia knows how acute sleep deprivation can be hard to handle: *'Don't assume that you'll be tired for a little while then all will be normal. Just as you planned for a long labour and hoped for a short one, plan for a baby who doesn't sleep (and hope for one who does). I treated Larson's bad sleeping as a temporary thing: I just kept going like it would end soon. We had 18 months of not more than four hours sleep a night and it was so hard: on us, on our work, on our four-year-old and hardest on our marriage. If I had to do it again, we would have taken naps, hired childcare for our eldest and made a point of getting out regularly without the kids, instead of ignoring the effects of this sleep deprivation, and hoping it would end soon.'*

Baby blues

On or around days three to five after the birth, it is normal to start feeling weepy, depressed, desperate or helpless (about 50 to 80 per cent of new mothers experience this). Midwives spend a lot of time reassuring new mothers who've hit the day three blues. It is, however, a normal mood response to a rapid drop in your hormone levels after birth, and the hormonal changes as your milk supply begins. What you need most is support and reassurance. Baby blues should fade away after a couple of days.

WHEN IT'S WORSE THAN THIS:
HOW TO SPOT POSTNATAL DEPRESSION (PND)

Ten to 15 per cent of new mothers develop PND at some point in the year after their baby is born. This is a treatable illness, but it's called the 'silent epidemic' because it's so often left unspoken, sometimes with catastrophic consequences (one to two per cent of new mothers develop a severe illness called 'postpartum psychosis'). No one really knows why such illness affects some women more than others (there is some evidence that it can run in families) but if it happens to you **get help**.

PND *warning signs*

You may have symptoms of the baby blues AND
you may have any combination of these symptoms:

- despondency and hopelessness
- feeling exhausted all the time
- being unable to concentrate
- feeling guilt/inadequacy
- anxiety, feeling unable to cope
- feeling uninterested in the baby
- feeling hyper-concerned about the baby
- obsessive thoughts
- panic
- fear of harming yourself or your baby
- headaches/chest pains
- not caring about your appearance
- sleeplessness (even when the baby is not waking you)

Severe PND (or postpartum psychosis) warning signs

The above symptoms plus you may also:

- not want to eat
- seem confused
- have severe mood swings
- feel hopeless or ashamed
- talk about suicide/hurting the baby
- seem hyperactive or manic

- talk quickly or incoherently
- act suspiciously or fearful of everything
- have delusions of hallucinations

Spotting PND tip:

PND can happen late in postpartum (up to a year after your baby is born). This means it might not be recognised as a postpartum illness. The medication used may be different for women with PND than for women with general kinds of depression. If your depression isn't acknowledged as PND, you can go on suffering for years on the wrong treatment. If you think you (or someone you know) may have PND, treatment from a specialist is essential.

Where to go for help:
Write down your symptoms. Talk to your health visitor and your GP (if possible, take your partner with you). And try:
Association for Post-Natal Illness (APNI) 145 Dawes Road London sw6 7EB
Helpline: 0207386 0868 www.apni.org

Further reading:
Coping with Postnatal Depression by Fiona Marshall (Sheldon Press, UK, 1993)
Antenatal and Postnatal Depression by Siobhan Curham (Vermilion, UK, 1999)

Online:
What is PND? www.rcpsych.ac.uk/public/help/pndep/postnatd.htm
BBC PND page www.bbc.co.uk/education/health/parenting/yoblues.shtml

Piecing together the birth

Postpartum is a good time to sort through what happened at the birth. If your birth was difficult, and you feel upset, now is the time to get help. Many women find it's best start piecing together what happened by writing it down (do this even if your birth went well – it might help you plan your next birth, if there is one). Who did what? Who said what? How long did various stages take? How did it feel? Emotionally and physically? What shocked you? What didn't? What was amazing? Then sit down with your midwife and birth partner(s) to fill in the gaps and get explanations.

Your baby

Your baby may seem like a frighteningly complex (if stunningly beautiful) being comprised of strange noises, smells, emissions and moods. In your addled state there are a few key things worth knowing about. Detailed baby care is beyond the scope of this book so find out the rest from trial and error, your baby, your midwife, your health visitor, friends, family and the legion of child-rearing books and websites out there.

FOUR THINGS TO DO BEFORE YOUR BABY IS BORN

1 **Get excited:** birth is just the beginning. Parenting is the biggie.
2 **Arrange help and support:** you're going to need some.
3 **Decide how you'll feed your baby:** if you are to breastfeed, make sure you have read about it first (see page 311) and know where to go for help as you are learning.
4 **Buy a good medical 'new baby' book:** so you can look up things that worry you as they crop up. Understand what professional support (i.e. health visitor/midwife/GP) is available to you.

Real mother's tip:
'Buy a few photo albums before the baby is born. If you have them handy then early photos won't go missing or get drooled on. You'll be glad you did this later on!' Kate, 50, mother of 3 teenage boys

A WORD ABOUT YOUR HEALTH VISITOR | I certainly didn't understand, with my first baby, what the health visitor was for. I've now discovered, with my third, that they can be a good source of ideas, support and information. Health visitors are nurses or midwives who have been specially trained (in child health and health promotion) to help you adjust to being a parent, and to cope with the hiccups and worries you experience: medical or not. You'll bring your baby to see your health visitor for regular weigh-ins, checkups and immunisations (often at a weekly 'baby clinic' attached to the GP's surgery). Your health visitor should visit you when your baby is about 11 days old (they will ring you – your midwife will have told them about your new baby. If you don't hear from a health visitor in the first ten days, ask your midwife why not). Don't hesitate to phone your health visitor for advice if anything is worrying you, or go to the baby clinic, even if your baby isn't 'due' a check-up. That is what they're there for. (But remember they may not have the detailed expertise of a breastfeeding specialist, so if your problem is breastfeeding related, get specialist help.)

Baby basics: a few things new babies do that can be worrying

1 **CRYING** | Newborn babies may be very peaceful and sleepy for the first few days. It's like they lull you into a false sense of security and then let loose the guns of war around days three to five. Often this coincides helpfully with your partner's return to work. There are many supposedly 'logical' approaches to decoding a baby's cries: indeed some bright spark – a Spanish engineer – has actually invented a machine that diagnoses the reason for a baby's cry, which says something for our faith in maternal/paternal instinct. You'll be advised to go through a little checklist: Wet? Stinky? Hungry? Hot? Cold? In pain? Uncomfortable? Just needs a cuddle? But sometimes the baby just seems to *want* to cry (old ladies will tell you 'he's exercising his lungs, dear'). Baby

books or online baby guides can be helpful, as can other mothers for tips on things like baby massage, but largely it'll be up to you to get to know what your baby wants. Most parents will tell you that the most helpful thing of all, when it comes to a crying baby, is to remember that the baby WILL STOP. Eventually. He will not cry forever (even if he tried to he'd be scuppered by **growing up**).

How to cope with your baby's wailing: This doesn't mean you should grin and bear it if your baby's crying is upsetting you badly. If she seems uncomfortable a lot after feeding (tucking her legs up, yelling, writhing), get advice from a breastfeeding specialist about your feeding technique (see Breastfeeding basics, page 311). If your baby is not unwell, but just keeps crying all the time, this may be colic. Colic can be genuinely traumatic – for all of you.

A WORD ABOUT COLIC | Colic is a term used to describe the inconsolable crying/screaming and apparent tummy pain of an otherwise healthy young baby (up to about six months). The reasons for this are unclear, but in some infants painful gut contractions might be at least partly to blame. Many babies are fussy, but a colicky baby is one who cries like this for long periods (hours, even), most days of the week. The symptoms usually start when the baby is around three weeks old (though can start later). It is worst at about six weeks and usually ends when the baby is around three months old.

> **Where to go for help:**
> Talk to your midwife and health visitor who should give you advice and tips for coping.
> **Serene** incorporating **The Cry-Sis Helpline** Serene provides support and non-medical advice to parents/carers of excessively crying, sleepless and demanding babies and young children. BM CRY-SIS, London WC1N 3XX. 020 7404 5011 (this is the national switchboard, they match you up with a local contact who can talk to you). www.cry-sis.org.uk
> **National Society for the Prevention of Cruelty to Children (NSPCC)** www.nspcc.org.uk/html/home/needadvice/copingwithcryingbabies.htm NSPCC Publications Unit, 42 Curtain Rd, EC2A 3NH. 020 7386 0868 has free information about dealing with crying babies, stress, and general coping with parenting issues. And if you've reached the end of your tether or just want someone to talk to about this, call the NSPCC **Child Protection Helpline:** 0808 800 5000 (you won't be judged!)
>
> **Further reading:**
> *The Happiest Baby on the Block: The New Way to Calm Crying and Help Your Newborn Baby Sleep Longer* by Harvey Karp (Bantam, US, 2003)
> *365 Ways To Calm Your Crying Baby* by Julian Orenstein (Adams Media Corporation, US, 1998) Written by an American paediatrician, this has lots of ideas, particularly relevant to the first three months.

2   **SLEEPING (NOT)** | Expect little sleep. Your baby will feed about every two hours in the first few weeks, even possibly this much at night. Again, remember that this period WILL PASS. The books all tell you that new babies sleep 16 to 19 hours a day, but what they don't tell you is that most of the time they'll want to sleep on – or right next to – you. Even if your baby will sleep in her bed, allowing you to achieve more than one-handed tasks, resist the temptation to get things done the minute she nods off. You, too, need to nap as much as you can because if you don't, you will go nuts in those first few weeks.

A WORD ABOUT COT DEATH | **What is it?** Cot death is the sudden and unexpected death of a baby for no obvious reason and it's what many of us worry about a lot in those early months. You'll hear about it because it is the leading cause of death in babies over one month old. According to the Foundation for the Study of Infant Deaths (FSID) *'Cot death can happen to any family, though it is more frequent in families who live in difficult circumstances or who smoke a lot. It is uncommon in Asian families, for reasons that are not yet understood.'* According to the latest statistics from FSID, 89 per cent of all sudden infant deaths in England and Wales occurred among babies aged under six months. But mercifully, these days cot death is rare: it has fallen in the UK by 75 per cent since the introduction of the government's *Reduce the Risk of Cot Death* campaign in 1991. So take this advice seriously:

What can you do to prevent it? FSID's new advice to parents on reducing the risk of cot death is:

- Cut smoking in pregnancy – fathers too!
- Do not let anyone smoke in the same room as your baby
- Place your baby on the back to sleep
- Do not let your baby get too hot
- Keep baby's head uncovered – place your baby with their feet to the foot of the cot, to prevent wriggling down under the covers

It's safest to sleep your baby in a cot in your bedroom for the first six months (see UNICEF below).

It's dangerous to share a bed with your baby if you or your partner:

- are smokers (no matter where or when you smoke)
- have been drinking alcohol
- take medication or drugs that make you drowsy
- feel very tired
- if the baby is less than eight weeks old
- It's very dangerous to sleep together on a sofa, armchair or settee.
- If your baby is unwell, seek medical advice promptly.

Where to go for help:
UNICEF advice on bed-sharing There is on-going debate about the risks and
benefits of sharing a bed with your baby. Where your baby should sleep is certainly
something you should research for yourself. Start here.
www.babyfriendly.org.uk/press.asp#160104
Foundation for the Study of Infant Deaths, Artillery House, 11–19 Artillery Row,
London SW1P 1RT. 020 7233 2090. 24 hour helpline: 0870 7870554.
www.sids.org.uk/fsid

Further reading:
*Healthy Sleep Habits, Happy Child: A Step-by-step Programme for a Good
Night's Sleep* Marc Weissbluth (Vermilion, UK, 2005)

Newborn breathing tip:

Most babies don't have a very steady breathing pattern, and may gasp a bit from
time to time. Lots of new parents think their baby has asthma or some other
breathing problem, when she's actually perfectly healthy. Talk to your midwife or
health visitor if your baby's breathing is worrying you. *'Try not to obsess on your
baby's breathing, it can sound really odd at times. I did a lot of panicking and now
realise he was fine – healthy colour, no sign of pain or distress. I just got myself into a
cycle of worry.'* Angela, 35, mother to Eric (8) and Jack (3)

3   **POOING** | It's no idle cliché: mothers do, indeed, care deeply about their
     child's poos – from day one. Poo will be a large part of your life for the next
     two years at the very least. The good news is that you'll be broken in gently to
     the world of nappies and bottom wiping – newborn poos are surprisingly
     manageable, and always **far less** revolting than you'd think.

A WORD ABOUT YOUR BABY'S POO | Your new baby will, in the first day or two,
do a meconium poo that looks like tar (it's a very sticky black/brown maybe
greenish tablespoon or so – though it might be more – and is totally normal).
Breastfed babies may then start doing non-stinky mustard-coloured, liquidy
poos. How much and how regularly your baby poos is one way to see if she is
getting enough food but it can vary massively from baby to baby. My first emitted
an almost constant stream, my second and third could go for three or four days or
more without a single one. Formula-fed baby poo can be more stinky, browner
and heavier and your baby might be more windy and more likely to be
constipated. Sometimes a baby's poo will be greenish and stinky. This can be a
sign of slight illness or a reaction to something you ate, if you are breastfeeding.
Diarrhoea is when the frequency of poos increases suddenly and they are more
watery: more than eight very watery and copious poos in 24 hours counts as
severe diarrhoea. Again, if you are worried at all about what's normal, do phone
your health visitor.

Bottom wiping tip:

It is probably best to use only cotton wool and warm water to wipe your baby's bottom in the early weeks. You might want to use unperfumed baby wipes later as they make things easier, but you can of course keep using cotton wool. Baby wipes – and indeed other baby bath products/lotions – can contain some quite harsh ingredients that can irritate a baby's skin. Always wipe your girl from front to back (i.e. vagina to bottom) to reduce the risk of a urine infection.

4   **CHANGING COLOUR** | Most babies are a greyish blue colour at birth (even black babies, which can be unsettling if you aren't prepared for this) but within just a few breaths they turn a more normal colour. New babies can still look oddly coloured for a while – very red, blotchy, lighter or darker than you'd think. They can also turn very bright colours when cross (red, puce, purple). In the first 24 to 48 hours, sticky secretions that your baby has swallowed during the birth can occasionally get stuck in his throat, making him choke and sometimes turn blue. If this happens, advises neonatologist Eleri Adams, put him over your knee, face down and give him a firm slap between the shoulders. You might need to repeat this to clear his airway, but if this doesn't work, call for help immediately.

A new baby's skin can peel or seem very dry. It can also be spotty: you might see small white spots (noticeably on the face). These are hormonal, healthy and may take several weeks to clear. **What's not healthy:** If you see your new baby's skin turning yellowish, it could be jaundice. See Chapter 7, page 233, for more details.

A WORD ON THE UMBILICAL CORD STUMP | You'll get instructions on this from the midwife. It will look black and crusty, and you'll probably think 'that can't be right' – ask if you're worried. Usually the advice is just keep it clean but basically leave it alone and be careful when bathing/dressing your baby. It normally just drops off within about ten days.

NEWBORN WARNING SIGNS

Paediatrician's tip: *'Doctors tend to worry more about a very quiet baby who doesn't seem quite right than they do about a noisy one,'* says consultant neonatologist Eleri Adams. **If you see any of these signs in your newborn you should get medical help.**

Call the doctor urgently/call ambulance:

- Problems breathing: blue lips, struggling to breathe, flaring nostrils, deep indentations of the chest when breathing, unable to finish feeds because breathless or sweating when feeding.
- Excessively or uncharacteristically fussy or irritable; unusually lethargic or sleepy; feeding poorly/differently; crying in a high-pitched way.

Call the doctor to see soon:

- Fever higher than 100.4 F/38 C rectally or above 99.50F/37.0C under the arm
- Vomiting: forcefully or more frequently than usual (not just spitting-up)
- Repeatedly refuses feeds for more than six to eight hours
- Diarrhoea: unusually frequent and very watery poos; blood or mucus in poos

Talk to the midwife:

- Dry nappy for six to eight hours, or fewer than five wet nappies in 24 hours (after your milk has come in); dry mouth; dark yellow urine; sunken fontanel – the soft part on the top of your baby's skull, where the bones have not yet joined together. (Call the doctor to see soon if this is combined with significant diarrhoea or vomiting: see above.)
- Shows signs of jaundice (unless under 24 hours old, or is very sleepy and not feeding, in which case, call urgently).
- Doesn't pass a greenish-black poo (meconium) within 24 hours of the birth. Most babies (94 per cent) will pass meconium within 24 hours of being born. But two to four per cent of normal babies don't pass meconium by 48 hours. If your baby has not passed meconium after about 24 hours, then do mention this to the midwife. If, however, your baby is vomiting, or has a very distended tummy and has not passed meconium, then talk to the doctor/midwife immediately.
- Problems with the umbilical cord: redness around the cord, foul odour or pus, bright red bleeding

Breastfeeding basics

TEN GOOD REASONS TO BREASTFEED

1 Breast milk is the healthiest food for your baby: it provides everything your baby needs for the first six months.
2 Breastfeeding reduces your baby's risk of developing gastroenteritis, respiratory, urinary tract and ear infections, eczema and childhood diabetes. There is some evidence to associate breastfeeding with a lower risk of developing childhood leukemia.
3 Breastfeeding is healthier for you too: you will have a lower risk of pre-menopausal breast cancer and ovarian cancer and, later in life, of hip fractures.
4 Breast milk is always available, requires no equipment and is instantly at the right temperature.
5 It's free (breastfeeding rather than formula feeding saves you an estimated £450 a year).

6   Breastfeeding is good for your baby's neurological development. Studies have found that breastfed infants test higher on IQ tests than bottle fed infants.

7   Breastfed babies are less likely to be obese as adults, and to suffer from cardiovascular disease.

8   Breast milk burns up to 500 calories a day, so it can help you lose weight.

9   Breastfeeding saves the NHS money: the NHS spends an estimated £35 million a year treating gastroenteritis in bottle-fed babies in England alone.

10   Breast milk is ecofriendly: it's organic, and comes without unnecessary packaging or waste.

How does it work?

It's a great system. When the baby is born your breasts produce their first food: colostrum. This is usually thick and yellowish and there is not much of it, but it's packed with nutrients and will protect your baby from all sorts of infections, so feed your baby as often as he wants in the first day or two (you may feel like he's permanently attached to your breast in those first couple of days). The hormone that is responsible for producing milk is called prolactin. Prolactin can't work until the hormones from the placenta have gone from your bloodstream – usually one to four days after the birth. The prolactin then tells the cells in your breasts to start making milk: this is when they can feel full, tight or 'engorged'.

Your baby's sucking then sends messages to the pituitary gland, in your brain, which triggers the release of another hormone, oxytocin. Oxytocin (which your body produced when you had contractions in labour) makes the muscular walls of the milk-producing cells contract. This contraction ejects the milk down the duct and out through your nipple into your baby's delighted mouth. This is what they call 'supply and demand'.

A WORD ABOUT EXPECTATIONS | As with birth, the textbook version may not be the reality for you. A huge part of breastfeeding success is trusting that your body **will** do it, even if your breasts do not seem to be doing what 'most' breasts are supposed to do. When I had Izzie, I was told that on day three after the birth my boobs would swell and gush 'real' milk to feed her. I was in the hospital for five days after my caesarean. The patient midwives showed me various positions for feeding and gave me a breast pump to try and 'get things going'. I waited with a growing sense of hysteria and inadequacy for the 'engorgement' to happen but it never did. This didn't mean I couldn't breastfeed but it caused me unnecessary angst (my confidence in my body, after the birth, was at an all time low anyway). My milk 'came in' slowly of its own accord and not very noticeably. This happened with all my babies. The lesson here is that if your breasts don't follow the textbook pattern at any point there is **no reason to assume they are not**

doing perfectly well. (There is, incidentally, some evidence to show that having a caesarean can delay your milk coming in, so this experience is actually quite common among caesarean mothers.)

Is breastfeeding easy?

Breastfeeding can certainly be marvellously simple: no sterilising bottles, no fuss, no expense. For many women, it's a happy, healthy, unproblematic experience. It can also be deeply fulfilling: breastfeeding your baby really does create a unique bond. But when you are a learner it can be a painful, frustrating and very tiring. *'Breastfeeding doesn't come naturally in our bottle-feeding culture: it is a learnt social skill,'* says midwife and breastfeeding specialist Sally Inch. *'The reason many women have problems breastfeeding is that they are not given the opportunity to learn that skill.'* If you get support from breastfeeding professionals, you should be able to sort out any problems and go on to feed your baby for as long as you want (the current advice is to breastfeed for a minimum of six months if possible).

Many of us – perhaps because we're not expecting it to be a challenge, or don't know how to get support (or get the wrong advice when we do ask for help) – give up breastfeeding way sooner than we want to. Although 69 per cent of mothers in the UK initially breastfeed, a fifth (21 per cent) of these give up within the first two weeks and over a third (36 per cent) give up within the first six weeks of their baby's life. By four months only 28 per cent of all mothers in the UK are breastfeeding and by six months this has gone down to 21 per cent. Ninety per cent of mothers who gave up breastfeeding within six weeks of birth say they would have liked to have breastfed for longer.[2] The key thing to do, then, if you are having any problem with breastfeeding – no matter how seemingly insignificant – is GET HELP from a breastfeeding specialist. By far the best place to start is by asking your midwife **before your baby is born** if there is a breastfeeding clinic or an infant feeding specialist at your hospital.

Breastfeeding basics

It's hard to overstate this: **latching the baby onto your breast properly is crucial to breastfeeding success**. A poor latch-on is responsible for the vast bulk of problems you might encounter. The reality for many of us is that the first few days of breastfeeding can be painful (usually because of sore nipples). But as you learn to latch your baby on right, any pain will stop and your baby will have satisfying feeds that contain both foremilk (the watery first part of the feed) and hindmilk (the richer second part of a feed). If you get the latch-on right, don't restrict the time he can stay on your breast, and offer a second breast when he comes off the first (he may refuse), then your baby should automatically get the right amount of food and it should NOT hurt.

If you are in pain or discomfort, if you develop any of the problems below, if your baby is not gaining enough weight, or is colicky or windy then a dodgy latch-on could well be the cause. You need to get an infant feeding specialist to sit and watch you latch your baby on. Sometimes what you are doing wrong is incredibly subtle and no matter how much you've scrutinised the diagrams, you might not be able to work out what the missing link is. An infant feeding specialist will. (Not all midwives or health visitors are as up to date on breastfeeding as they'd like to be. This is why it's the **specialist** you need to see.)

A WORD ABOUT YOUR PARTNER'S SUPPORT | You'd think a bloke's role on this one would be curtailed by his anatomy. But studies show that the attitude of the baby's father is one of the most important factors in whether or not a mother begins and continues to breastfeed. So talk to your partner about breastfeeding, both in advance, and postpartum. Show him the list of ten reasons above, and make sure that he is aware that it can take practice to get right, and that you may need moral support.

Why might breastfeeding be harder than expected (and what to do if it is)

1   **WORRIES ABOUT YOUR MILK SUPPLY** | Studies have shown that nearly half of us give up in those early months because we are under the impression that we have 'insufficient milk supply'. It can be hard to have faith in your breasts when you can't actually **see** the amount of milk glugging into your baby, like you can with a bottle. In reality it's extremely rare for women to be physiologically unable to produce enough milk (reasons for this may include breast surgery or a retained placenta in the first week or so post-partum). If your baby is latching on well, it should take about a week for the supply and demand to balance out (after this, your baby will probably have one or two growth spurts, where she is sucking away to get your milk supply to increase). If your baby is latched on properly and you are feeding her when she wants to be fed (and not when some very persuasive book tells you she should be fed!) you have to have faith: your milk supply will be enough for her. Sometimes women lose faith in their milk supply because they stop being engorged and their breasts feel 'normal'. Your breasts do not need to be engorged or Dolly Partonesque to produce adequate milk for your baby.

2   **UNPREDICTABILITY OF FEEDS** | Hardly any breastfed babies stick to a fixed schedule for feeds. For the first 24 hours your baby will probably hardly eat at all. Then he'll unleash his appetite on his unsuspecting mother: for a couple of days, feeds can be unbelievably frequent, day and night (he may even feed every hour). This will gradually slow down as your milk supply sorts itself out and you learn to get him latched on well.

3   **ENGORGEMENT** | Starting a few days or more after the birth and lasting until you've learned the best way to feed, your boobs might become intermittently 'engorged' (flushed, rock hard, full of milk and very painful to the touch). This

is usually because they are producing more milk than is being removed. Engorgement should quickly subside when your baby starts to remove milk efficiently from your breasts, as long as you are not withholding feeds.

How to cope: You need to work on increasing the amount of milk that is removed from your breast. There is a common misconception among health professionals that if you remove milk with a breast pump, you will make the problem worse (because your breast will then produce even more). This is not the case: gently using a breast pump after a feed may make the problem better. So will improving the way the baby is latched on. Again, get an infant feeding specialist to check how your baby is latching on.

Tip: You might be told that putting Savoy cabbage leaves over your breast will reduce swelling, but trials have shown that they actually have no effect on engorgement beyond being quite cold, and therefore soothing. By all means stick a couple on if it's going to make you feel better, but a flannel will do just as well. Expressing a small bit of milk before your baby latches on (during a warm bath or shower is easiest) can also release some pressure.

4   **PAINFUL NIPPLES** | In the first few days most women's nipples feel sore – sometimes acutely so – when the baby feeds (and sometimes in between). If this carries on, it is almost always because – yes, you guessed it – the baby is not latching on in the right way. He should have your nipple at the back in his mouth as he 'milks' the areola, rather than having his tongue press painfully against it. Again, get help from a specialist. You should NOT have nipple pain, except fleetingly. As the NCT put it: *'It's breastfeeding, not nipple feeding.'*

What to do about your sore nipples: Obviously, sort out your latch-on. But while you're doing this put Vaseline or a lanolin-based cream on them (such as Lanisoh, which is available in Waitrose, Mothercare, Moss pharmacy, NCT and online from www.lanisoh.co.uk) and make sure you keep feeding (you want to prevent drying and scabbing over). Don't put soaps, creams or lotions on your nipples. If it's too sore to feed, use a pump or hand express, then feed your baby with this expressed milk from a bottle, while you're sorting out a visit to a specialist. Remember you **will** sort this out with help: your boobs are not defective in any way. Breastfeeding isn't 'sensation-free' (i.e. it can feel odd if you've never done it before), but it should not hurt like this.

Thrush: sometimes very sore nipples can be a sign of thrush – a treatable yeast infection of your nipple and the baby's mouth. Your nipples may be bright pink and tender, you may get shooting pains while breastfeeding, and between feeds. Your baby may have white patches in her mouth (these look like milk curds) that won't wipe off. Get treatment from your GP (for you and the baby) but avoid antibiotics unless really needed (they increase the likelihood of yeast infections). Some nutritionists advise lowering the sugar in your diet to avoid thrush outbreaks.

5 **BREASTFED BABIES MAY NOT GAIN WEIGHT EXACTLY ACCORDING TO THE CHART** | *'My doctor kept pressurising me to switch to formula, saying my baby wasn't gaining enough, against the chart,'* says Regine, mother of Kimberley (5). *'Eventually, I switched to a black doctor who told me she was a perfectly healthy size for an Afro-Caribbean baby.'* The weight charts currently used are based on data from largely Caucasian and formula-fed babies. Most breast-fed babies gain weight, perfectly healthily, at a different rate. Usually, breastfed babies gain weight quicker than the average on the chart in the first couple of months, then, around two to three months, they'll start to look like they're not gaining enough according to the chart. The Child Growth Foundation recently produced 'Breast from Birth' charts which your health visitor may have.

6 **OTHER PEOPLE CAN MAKE YOU FEEL UNCOMFORTABLE** | This is a can of worms. Breastfeeding in public is not against the law. What you are doing is normal and natural. Cultural mores, of course, dictate that flashing your naked boobs around with abandon may make people uncomfortable but if you're relatively discreet, you should not be made to feel uncomfortable about breastfeeding in cafes, pubs, trains or wherever and whenever your baby needs to eat.

What do to: Remind yourself that there is nothing wrong, or embarrassing, about feeding your baby. On a practical level, before you whip out your boob use your judgment about how you're going to feel feeding her where you are (you may not feel like a confrontation with your baby actually latched on). A good place to start, if you're initially nervous about feeding when out and about, is bigger branches of Boots, which have mother and baby rooms. Some supermarkets (Tesco and Sainsbury's for instance) also have a national policy of providing a place for baby feeding. Your County Council may produce a guide to smoke-free places to eat, and many include details on whether a place 'welcomes breast-feeding mothers'.

7 **MASTITIS AND 'BLOCKED DUCTS'** | Mastitis is an inflammation of the breast tissue. It is almost always caused by 'milk stasis'; in other words, the breast not being emptied thoroughly by your baby when she feeds (yes, that pesky latch-on again, though sometimes it can be caused if you suddenly drop a feed). It can start with lumpy, painful areas in the breast (the size, roughly of a coin) but not much pain or inflammation (usually people call this a 'blocked duct'). If the milk stays there, the pressure then rises even more and forces the milk through the lining of the milk ducts and into the surrounding breast tissue. You then get acute inflammation inside the breast, redness and pain. If the milk then enters your bloodstream, you start to feel fluey, with a fever. Your body's immune system is treating the milk like it was a foreign protein. This is mastitis.

How to cope: Don't linger if you feel a blocked duct: get help. If you improve how the baby is latching on, she'll remove the milk properly during a feed. Most GPs mistakenly think of mastitis as an 'infection' and prescribe antibiotics, but mastitis is actually **very rarely** an infection (it's an inflammation, which is different). Antibiotics can help because they are anti-inflammatory, but they will only treat the symptoms not the cause. I learned this the hard way, having had mastitis a ludicrous and very grim nine times before I finally saw the breastfeeding specialists at my hospital, one of whom (Sally Inch) wrote the World Health Organization briefing on mastitis[3]. Ibuprofen (which reduces inflammation) can also help the symptoms, as can using a breast pump after a feed (to ensure that the milk is moving through your breast even if the baby isn't latched on well). All the advice people give you about hot flannels, hot showers and massaging your boobs are missing the point with mastitis (and may on occasions make it worse). Whatever you do, don't stop breastfeeding as this will make things worse (there'll be even more milk hanging around in there).

The Breastfeeding Network has an excellent information leaflet on mastitis (see page 318).

8 BABY NOT CONTENT | If your baby is:
- Not coming off the breast spontaneously after he's fed
- Restless or writhing as he feeds
- Not satisfied after a long feed
- Very windy/uncomfortable after feeding
- Taking a long time (30-40 minutes per breast after the first few days)
- Feeding tons (more than ten feeds in 24 hours, after the first few days)
- Hardly feeding at all (fewer than three feeds in the first 24 hours; fewer than six feeds in 24 hours when 24-48 hours old)
- Still doing black poos when he's 36-48 hours old

Then you should get some specialist breastfeeding help.

How to latch your baby on correctly
Your baby needs to take a big mouthful of breast. To do this, his chin should be close to your breast and his bottom lip curled back. Before the feed begins, make sure his shoulders and chest are turned towards your breast and his nose/top lip is opposite your nipple. Before you bring him to your breast, let his head tilt back slightly so that his chin, not his nose, touches your breast first. When he opens his mouth wide, anticipating the feed he's about to get, his bottom lip should be as far from the base of your nipple as possible.

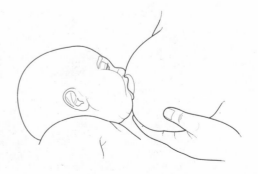

Where to go for information, help and support with breastfeeding

- **A trained breastfeeding specialist** is essential if you are having any of the problems above (or indeed, any others!). Ask your midwife or health visitor, when you are pregnant, if there is a breastfeeding clinic or an infant feeding specialist at your hospital (or one nearby). Midwives may not be up to scratch on breastfeeding, and many of us are bombarded by conflicting advice.

- **Other support organisations:** counsellors who'll speak to you on the phone and even visit are easy to find (see below). These can be a fantastic source of reassurance and emotional support while you're learning (but do be aware that advice can sometimes be conflicting).

> **Helplines:**
> **National Childbirth Trust (NCT) Breastfeeding helpline:** 0870 444 8708
> www.nct-online.org.uk
> **La Leche League,** Great Britain Helpline: 020 7242 1278 www.laleche.org.uk
> **The Breastfeeding Network Helpline:** 0870 900 8787
> www.breastfeeding.co.uk/bfn
>
> **Further reading:**
> *The National Childbirth Trust Book of Breastfeeding* by Mary Smale (Vermilion, UK, 1999)
> *Breastfeeding: Getting Breastfeeding Right for You: An Illustrated Guide* by Mary Renfrew, Chloe Fisher, Suzanne Arms (Ten Speed Press, UK, 1990)
>
> **Online:**
> Find out more about breastfeeding from **The Unicef UK Babyfriendly Initiative** at www.babyfriendly.org.uk

Postpartum second time around

If you have had one baby already, you probably think you'll know what you are doing this time. In some respects you do. In others, you could be in for a shock – particularly if your children are close together in age. I thought I'd breeze through postpartum with my second baby. The delight at having what seemed suddenly like a 'brood' was incomparable, but I had no idea what life could be like dealing simultaneously with a newly 'assertive' two-year-old and a wailing, hungry baby. I felt guilty, exhausted, stressed, inadequate and largely panicky for about six months (come to think of it, at times, I still do). Again, my stress was intensified by my total lack of preparation for postpartum. But even if you're lucky enough to have good friends and family around, do take all our 'getting help' recommendations **seriously**. You'll look back on having just one baby and think 'what was I fussing about?'

Some of the problems can be practical

Books and advice columns can be wildly unrealistic, particularly if your other child is very young. The silliest advice I ever read was 'lay out nice toys for your toddler to play with in a safe place while you and the baby nap next to him'. This would be a delightful idea were it possible to nap with small fingers poking in your eyes, a little voice going 'Wake up! Mumeeeee!' or little (surprisingly strong) arms deciding now is the time to 'cuddle' (i.e. wake up) the tiny sibling. Yes, how, exactly, do you simultaneously breastfeed a baby and read to a wriggling toddler – by growing extra hands? How, exactly, do you make your hungry toddler's dinner/get him down for a nap/play lego with him while your baby is wailing for attention/milk/cuddles (which will, if answered, upset your toddler)? How, exactly, do you 'nap while the baby naps' if your toddler has his hand in the toaster?

The only way, really, is to compromise, muddle through, survive, savour the good moments and try to laugh about it all if you can. You should also get help, network like a maniac with other mums and at truly stressful moments (and you'll have them) remind yourself that it won't always be like this. One day they'll be sneaking off down the pub with their underage friends and refusing to acknowledge you in public and you'll get all misty eyed about their toddler days.

Three ideas for dealing with small children and a newborn

1   **DEFUSE THE ARSENIC HOUR** | It's easy to understand why, in the Seventies, valium was called 'mother's little helper'. A friend of mine, who has two children, calls 5ish to 6.30pm (the time before your partner gets in and your children are demonic) the Arsenic Hour. Getting strategic help at key times of the day can work wonders. Many people hire a teenage girl to come during the Arsenic Hour (or hours) to help with tea/bath/bedtimes: an extra pair of hands can be all you need. **If you can't afford to pay anyone**, draft in friends and family as much as you can, again at key times of day. The second best thing for the Arsenic Hour is to have a friend with her kids round. Adult company really eases the pain, and releases your tension.

   How to meet other parents: The National Childbirth Trust has 40,000 UK members in 400 branches around the country helping 300,000 new parents locally. It's a great place to start. MAMA (meet-a-mum association) provides friendship and support to mothers and mothers-to-be who are lonely or isolated after the birth of a baby or a move to a new area. Try one of these even if you're not a 'joiner' (see Find Out More, page 326).

2   **BANISH GUILT** | Guilt can be major, when adjusting to having a second baby: you never feel like you're paying either child enough attention. One friend of mine summed it up when she said: *'It was like having an affair. As soon as my son was out of the room, I'd be cooing over the baby. Then when he came in, I'd leap up and pretend I wasn't doing anything.'* You may be shocked to find that you no

longer think your first child is quite as cute or small as you did before the baby came along: this can feel like a betrayal. Remind yourself that you are giving your first child an amazing gift – a sibling – even though they may not quite see it like this at this stage. You are teaching them to share, to be tolerant, patient and loving. You may also feel guilty for taking out your sleep deprivation on your first child. We've all been there. The best approach, when you realise you've yelled unreasonably at your poor child is to apologise. Explain why you yelled. Admit your mistakes. Small children can be very forgiving.

3   **HELP YOUR FIRST CHILD TO ADJUST** | Plan regular time to spend *just* with your first child, who may be feeling ousted. This may even mean booking someone to look after your new baby for short periods – just so you and number one can go to the park for 20 minutes.

Talk, before the birth, to your first child about what having a new baby will be like (read books about new siblings, discuss what babies sound like, what they do, how tiring they are). Then they'll know not to expect a smiling ball of cuddles (all the time).

Reassure your first child – constantly – that you love them as much, if not more, than you did before their little brother/sister was born, and that they're very special to you.

Involve your first child from the start with the baby: nappy changes, baths, dressing, even if they're so young as to be no *real* help whatsoever. And praise them for it.

Postpartum play tip:

Keep a stock of cheap new 'emergency' toys: pick up incredibly cheap bits and pieces in the school fetes, jumble sales, NCT 'nearly new' sales or whenever you spot them. Then stuff them away to be pulled out on rough postpartum days. Toy Libraries are also good for novelty value. **National Association of Toy and Leisure Libraries** has more information: 020 7255 4600. www.natll.org.uk

More than one baby

It can be a whole different ballgame with twins, or more

The logistics of feeding, burping, dressing and cuddling two or more babies can be initially mind-boggling. Your map of the local area will metamorphose into double-buggy friendly routes. And you may feel both immensely proud (if not superhuman) for producing more than one baby, and flattened by the effort of caring for them. Support, reading and preparation for coming home with more than one baby are vital. Sadly, this is beyond the scope of this book. Take the following as a starting point then go forth and inform yourself.

MULTIPLE BIRTH AND POSTPARTUM TIPS

- **Get help, and make sure it is reliable.** There's nothing worse than counting down the minutes for someone to arrive at 3 p.m. so you can finally sleep after two days of no sleep, only to have them cancel on you.

- **Make sure you have significant breast-feeding help/feeding advice** before you get the babies home and know where to go for feeding help once you are home with them.

- **Consider finding peer support.** There are countless issues with multiples that you will run into that are not addressed by many singleton pregnancy/birth books (including this one!). Finding support and advice from parents who know is really useful.

- **Do not underestimate how much work it will be in the beginning.** It is very tiring in those first few months, especially if you are breastfeeding or pumping.

'The only thing I can tell you about postpartum for me was that I was ABSOLUTELY CRAZY for about two weeks. I didn't know who I was, didn't recognise people, didn't remember phone conversations, don't remember most of the first time I had with my three girls, didn't know my milk would come in, didn't care that I had children, didn't know how old they were.... Yet I looked "fine" on the outside. I just never realised exactly how nuts you can go postpartum.'

PEGGY, MOTHER TO ONE-YEAR-OLD TRIPLETS

Where to go for help:
The Twins and Multiple Births Association (TAMBA) 2 The Willows Gardner Road, Guildford, Surrey GU1 4PG. 0870 770 3305 Fax: 0870 770 3303 www.tamba.org.uk A nationwide UK charity providing information and mutual support networks for families of twins, triplets and more.
The Multiple Births Foundation Hammersmith House Level 4, Queen Charlotte's & Chelsea Hospital, Du Cane Road, London W12 0HS. 0208 383 3519 Fax: 0208 383 3041 Email: info@multiplebirths.org.uk www.multiplebirths.org.uk Great, informative website including link to 'twins clubs' around the country.

Tell us about it

We want to hear what happens! Send your blooming birth story to us at: www.bloomingbirth.net.

Postpartum shopping list

* = BASICS (if nothing else, get these)

FOR YOUR PARTS:
- *Several small packets of frozen peas (to soothe sore perineum)
- *Squeezy bottles for every loo in the house or a big plastic jug by each bathroom sink to pour on yourself while you pee (reduces stinging)
- * Large sanitary pads (make them 'cotton feel', not plasticky cheap ones)
- * Disposable knickers (buy 10 to 15 pairs), or same number of pairs of old or cheap knickers you can chuck out
- Couple of pairs of comfy pyjamas (that fit you when pregnant!)
- Bottle of Witch Hazel
- A sitzbath (or plastic basin you can use just as well!)
- Pure lavender essential oil or herbs to use in your sitzbath/bath **Herbalists at Neals Yard Remedies recommend**: a few drops of hypericum & calendula tincture in a bath or diluted in small amount of water to make a wash that will help heal a sore perineum. Your midwife may have other herbal recommendations worth trying.

FOR YOUR BREASTFEEDING BOOBS:
- * A good breastfeeding book (see page 318)
- * 2–3 soft breastfeeding bras
- *The telephone number of your hospital's infant feeding specialist
- Breast pads (again, avoid plastic) – these stop your breasts leaking onto your shirt (but not all breasts leak)
- Extra pillows: good for propping up the baby while breastfeeding
- A footstool – can help with a good breastfeeding position, and ease your tired feet (old phone directories taped together with masking tape work as well)
- 2 big water sippy bottles – one for by your bed and one to put by your other main resting place to keep you hydrated as you feed the baby

GENERALLY:
- *Large pack of paracetamol (for afterpains, etc.)
- * Hot water bottle (ditto)
- * Lots of healthy meals for your freezer (e.g. portions of homemade soup, casseroles, pasta sauces)
- Soft stretchy clothes like sweatpants
- Any midwife-recommended postpartum vitamins and iron tablets

Basic baby shopping list

Don't get hung up on buying nappy disposal units and other frankly nonsensical pieces of equipment (unless you're rich, and this sort of thing makes you happy). In the early days babies really have very simple requirements (somewhere to sleep, a buggy or sling for outings, some clothes and nappies). You don't have to buy everything new, either. Try NCT nearly new sales, EBay (online auction www.ebay.com) or even your local newspaper. This kid is going to cost you thousands over the next 18 years (plus) so you might want to reign yourself in while he's small enough not to want the latest Nikes.

ESSENTIALS:

- **Nappies and cotton wool:** you'll need TONS of newborn nappies (you'll change a newborn's nappy about 60 times a week at the start) and big rolls of cotton wool for wiping. Re-usable nappies are far more environmentally sound and nappy laundering/delivery services are springing up all over the place. Ask your midwife for recommendations. You might want a pack of unperfumed baby wipes for outings.

- **Car seat suitable from birth**: According to the Department of Transport, 35 children aged 0–11 were killed and 480 seriously injured in cars in 2002. In 2003, a survey conducted by TRL showed that 6 per cent of 0–4-year-olds were not restrained in any way in the rear of cars. For a free leaflet on choosing the right car seat and fitting it correctly: call 0870 1226 236, product code T/INF/697. www.thinkroadsafety.gov.uk/advice/childcarseats.htm. A car seat should have a British Standard Kitemark or European Regulations Mark (EUR 44.03). Never buy a second-hand car seat unless you know its history (i.e. no accidents) and have the instructions, so that you can fit and use it correctly. Fit it in the car before you have the baby as they can be baffling.

- **Stroller/pram**: just make sure it's 'suitable from birth' – all the other extra features are your choice.

- **Crib, cot or Moses basket** with mattress that's British Safety standard certified.

- **Baby clothes minimum**: 6 cotton vests, 6 cotton babygros, 6 pairs socks, 2–3 cellular blankets (duvets are dangerous for babies), 3 cardigans (easier than jumpers), couple of cotton hats. A winter baby needs an all in one padded warm suit.

OTHER RECOMMENDED EQUIPMENT:

- **1 baby monitor** – so you can hear your baby wherever you are in the house/garden.

- **1 nappy bag** (consider your partner's feelings here: he may not want to parade around town with pink teddies slung over his shoulder. Indeed, nor may you once the hormones have worn off.) This is to put those essentials into each time you leave the house: nappies, wipes or whatever you use on her bottom, small pot of nappy rash cream, complete change of clothing (for the baby), extra socks (they always get lost), toys, books (for both of you) and a water bottle and snack for you. (For subsequent babies you'll probably just use your usual shoulder bag because you'll be sick to death of nappy bags).

- **About 10 muslin squares (get them in packs from Mothercare or Boots)**: very handy for wiping up baby sick, protecting your shoulder from dribble, lying the baby on in a park...any number of things, really.

- **1 baby 'gro-bag' with shoulder straps**. Good for babies that kick off their covers, then get cold and wake you up.

- **1 sling baby carrier** – good for fussy or colicky baby, or for just getting around when she's small enough to be easily portable.

- **Basic childproofing stuff** for your house. Newborns don't get into much mischief, but it's easier to do childproofing when the baby's still inside you. Also, the new friends you'll make with this baby may have other kids who can easily burn down your house or seriously injure themselves in it if it's not childproofed. It's not rocket science, and starter kits are available at Mothercare shops (www.mothercare.co.uk).

- **Bottles, infant formula and sterilising equipment** if you don't plan to breastfeed. Ask your midwife for advice on which kinds and how much.

Baby clothes tips:
Expect your baby to get through up to six outfit changes a day. Buy only babygros that have poppers from neck to crotch and down legs as buttons and poppers on the back are a pain in the neck when changing a baby's nappy. Buy soft stretchy cotton clothes as babies often yell when you are getting them dressed and you want it to be as quick and soft an experience as possible. Borrow stuff where possible! Your baby grows out of it so quickly some clothes are hardly used.

Resources

Further reading
Baby books are legion and approaches differ widely. The best thing you can do is browse and find the one that suits you (and your baby). Here are a few suggestions for starting places:

TWO BOOKS ABOUT YOU POSTPARTUM

The Year after Childbirth by Sheila Kitzinger (Prentice Hall & IBD, US, 1996) This one focuses on YOU (not babycare): anything from sex to childcare in the first year of your baby's life.

After the Baby's Birth: A Woman's Way to Wellness – A Complete Guide for Postpartum Women by Robin Lim (Celestial Arts, US, 2001) This is a good one for natural and wholesome types.

TWO GENERAL BOOKS WITH GOOD 'NEW BABY' INFORMATION

We keep recommending these two, but that's because they're good – in this case, particularly for immediate postpartum issues.

Pregnancy, Childbirth and The Newborn, revised and updated: The Complete Guide by Penny Simkin, Janet Whatlley, and Ann Keppler (Meadowbrook Press, US, 2001)

Birth and Beyond: Pregnancy, Birth, Your Baby and Family – The Definitive Guide by Dr Yehudi Gordon (Vermilion, UK, 2002)

THREE INTELLIGENT LOOKS AT MOTHERHOOD

They may make more sense once you're a mother.

Life After Birth by Kate Figes (Penguin, UK, 2000) A fairly solemn, thought-provoking look at the ups and downs of motherhood.

Life's Work: On Becoming a Mother by Rachel Cusk (Fourth Estate, UK, 2002) Novelist Cusk writes about becoming a first-time mother up to the time when her daughter takes her first steps, and she's not afraid of exploring the 'dark side' of motherhood.

Making Babies by Anne Enright (Jonathan Cape, UK, 2004) A lighter look at motherhood, and, as the publishers put it 'an antidote to the po-faced, polemical "How-to" baby books'.

ONE GOOD, POPULAR PARENTING GUIDE

Your Baby and Child: The Essential Guide for Every Parent by Penelope Leach (Penguin, UK, 1997) First published in the 80s this made Leach the 'new Dr Spock'. It's all about tolerant, loving parenting.

ONE BASIC BOOK ABOUT YOUR BABY'S HEALTH

Baby and Child Health Care by Dr Miriam Stoppard (Dorling Kindersley, UK, 1997) Basic, A–Z of common complaints, first aid and basic health care.

Online

Again, parenting and baby sites are legion. But here are some good starters:

Baby Centre www.babycentre.co.uk Tons of information on virtually any baby-related topic, plus chat rooms and shopping.

Mothers 35-Plus www.mothers35plus.co.uk Website aimed at older mothers, whether this is your first or tenth baby.

Working Families 020 7628 3565 www.workingfamilies.org.uk Gives practical help and information for parents about choices in childcare, employment rights, campaign for changes in the law, and to persuade employers to adopt practices which work for them and you alike.

Fathers Direct Herald House, Lambs Passage, Bunhill Row, London EC1Y 8TQ 0845 634 1328 www.fathersdirect.com Good on all issues, including meeting other dads.

Parentline Plus www.parentlineplus.org.uk 0808 800 2222 Good on anything from crying babies to how to keep your marriage on track.

For online health information try **Net Doctor**, an independent UK based health website with useful articles and good information about childhood illnesses and conditions. www.netdoctor.co.uk

www.webmd.com is comprehensive and **www.nhsdirect.nhs.uk** is usually worth a visit (includes a useful 'body key' tool for working out whether you need to call or not).

Finding help/friends

National Childbirth Trust (NCT) Alexandra House, Oldham Terrace, Acton London, W3 6NH 0870 444 8707 www.nctpregnancyandbabycare.com

TEN THINGS YOU MAY NOT KNOW ABOUT THE NCT

The NCT is a brilliant way to meet other mothers with similar age children in your area. You've probably heard about their childbirth classes, 'nearly new sales' and local groups, but here are some things you may not be aware of:

- **From the NCT you can hire equipment** such as hospital standard breast pumps and cushions especially designed to help you sit without pain after a vaginal birth.

- **The NCT is for Dads too:** there are local events specifically for Dads. It encourages dads to come to childbirth classes and all local groups welcome 'at home dads' (indeed, membership is for up to two people living at the same address so for the same fee you and your partner can join).

- **It has an active campaigning section** with policies, among other things, to increase the normal/straightforward birth rate in the UK.

- **It provides good quality, evidence based information** especially for parents. It has resources on tons of situations, concerns, options and issues to do with pregnancy, birth and parenthood.

- **It doesn't teach people how to be parents** but it helps parents explore parenthood and learn from each other.

- **Anyone can volunteer:** there are NCT opportunities that can help feed your brain when you're at home with kids (e.g. you can train, accompanied by your small infant, to be a breastfeeding counsellor or an antenatal teacher).

- **It's good for specific peer support:** it has an 'experience register' of women who have coped with unusual circumstances so that you can get in touch with other women who've been through the same thing as you – no matter how unusual it is.

- **You don't have to be an earth mother to benefit.** You'll hear people say that the NCT 'only' want you to have a natural birth and then breastfeed your baby, but the NCT should never censure your epidural, caesarean or bottle-feeding choices. According to Chief Executive Belinda Phipps, *'The NCT is there to support you, not judge you – no one should be questioning your decisions. We just want to help you inform yourself so you can make the right choices for you.'*

- **You don't have to be a 'group person'** or even a member to join in NCT activities (though joining, of course, helps the charity to fund its work).

- **No matter where you live** in the UK there will be an NCT branch that covers your area.

MAMA (meet-a-mum association) 26 Avenue Road, London SE25 4DX 0206 771 5595 www.mama.org.uk

Mumsnet THE place to chat with other mums, get information, support and have a laugh. www.mumsnet.co.uk They've also produced a book: *Mums on Babies* by Justine Roberts, Carrie Longton, Rachel Foster (Cassell, UK, 2003) a distillation of the comments, tips and 'wisdom' of mums who've mumsnetted.

Net Mums www.netmums.com Advice and information about 'being a mum with young children in your home town'.

FINALLY.......

Baby Blogs Baby Blogging ('or web-logging': keeping an on-line diary) is supposedly the baby book for the online generation. You keep a record of your baby's every burp, fart or poo for devoted family members to browse (and for posterity of course). Try: www.bloggingmommies.com for starters.

Notes

Introduction

1 Birth and Motherhood Survey, 2005, commissioned by motherandbabymagazine.com

Chapter One

1 The charity One Parent Families www.oneparentfamilies.org.uk
2 'The North Staffordshire Maternity Hospital prospective study of pregnancy-associated depression.' Johanson R., Chapman G., Murray D., Johnson I. and J. Cox *Psychosom Obstet Gynaecol.* 2000 Jun;21(2):93-7.
3 The *Top Santé* Women and Work survey in association with BUPA, June 2001
4 The organisation March of Dimes has a fact sheet *Stress and Pregnancy*, that lays out some of these. See www.marchofdimes.com
5 One study published in the *American Journal of Obstetrics and Gynecology*, January 2004, found that women with a history of eating disorders (in the past eight years) had a 70 per cent higher chance of having a pre-term baby, and an 80 per cent higher chance of a low birth-weight baby than women without a history of an eating disorder.
6 Multiply your height in metres by your height in metres. Then divide your weight in kg by this figure. Alternatively go to www.bbc.co.uk/health/yourweight/bmi.shtml and they'll do it for you.
7 SMA Parallel Lives survey, 2003
8 This list is taken from Tommy's the baby charity leaflet 'Healthy Eating: A guide for mums to be'.
9 British Pregnancy Advisory Service

Chapter Three

1 Green, J.M. and H.A. Baston (2003) 'Feeling in control in labor: concepts, correlates & consequences' *Birth* 30(4), 235-247
2 Terhi Saisto and Erja Halmesmäki ACTA REVIEW 'Fear of childbirth: a neglected dilemma', *Acta Obstetricia et Gynecologica Scandinavica* Volume 82 Issue 3 Page 201-8 March 2003

3 Clement, S. *Childbirth on television*. Br J Midwifery 1995; 5: 37-42.
4 Peterson, Gayle *An Easier Childbirth: a mother's guide for birthing normally* (Berkeley, CA; Shadow and Light Publications, 1993)
5 Shipman M.K., Boniface D.R., Tefft M.E., and F. McCloghry. 'Antenatal Perineal massage and subsequent perineal outcomes, a randomized controlled trial', *Br J Obstet Gynaecol.* 1997 Jul;104(7):787-91

Chapter Four

1 Abrams, Rebecca *Three Shoes, One Sock and No Hairbrush: Everything you need to know about having your second child.* (Cassel & Co, London, 2001)
2 *Listening to Mothers: Report of the first national US survey of women's childbearing experiences.* A Project of the Maternity Center Association in Collaboration with Harris Interactive. Declercq et al, October 2002. Online full Survey Report: maternitywise.org/listeningtomothers/
3 Hapidou E.G. and D. DeCatanzaro, 'Responsiveness to Laboratory Pain in Women as Function of Age and Childbirth Pain Experience', *Pain* 48 (2) February 1992: 177-181
4 Green, J.M. and H.A. Baston (2003) 'Feeling in control in labor: concepts, correlates & consequences' *Birth* 30(4), 235-247
5 NHS Maternity Statistics, England: 2002-03
6 NHS Maternity Statistics, England and Wales 1998-99 to 2000-01, 2.19.2 'Parity and age'
7 Kitzinger, Sheila *Episiotomy and the Second Stage of Labor* (Pennypress, Seattle, WA, 1990).
8 NHS Maternity Statistics, England 1998-99, 2000-01 and 2002-3
9 Ibid
10 Gordon, Yehudi *Birth and Beyond* (Vermilion, London, 2002) p.313
11 NHS Maternity Statistics, England 2002-03, p.6
12 The National Sentinel Caesarean Section Audit Report, 2001, p.17

13 NHS Maternity Statistics, England 1998-99, 2000-01. In 2000-01 about 16 per cent of deliveries were to women aged 35 or over, compared with 12 per cent in 1995-96 and 8 per cent in 1985.

14 Ibid: Singleton deliveries in 2000-01 were by elective caesarean for 5 per cent of women aged under 25; for 9 per cent aged 25-34 and for 15 per cent of those aged 35 or over.

15 Bell, et al. 'Do obstetric complications explain high caesarean section rates among women over 30? A retrospective analysis' *British Medical Journal* 2001; 322:894-895.

16 Gordon, Yehudi *Birth and Beyond*, p.505

17 NHS Maternity Statistics, England 2002-3, 2.15.2

Chapter Five

1 Green, J.M. and H.A. Baston (2003) 'Feeling in control in labour: concepts, correlates & consequences' *Birth* 30(4), 235-247

2 Gibbings J. and A.M. Thomson, 'Womens' expectations and experiences of childbirth' *Midwifery* 2001 Dec;17 (4): 302-13.

3 Newburn M. and D. Singh 'Creating a better birth environment: women's views about the design and facilities in maternity units: a national survey.' An audit toolkit (National Childbirth Trust: London, 2003)

4 NICE Caesarean Section guidelines April 2004 p.40.

5 Green J., Baston H., Easton S. and F. McCormick, 'Greater Expectations' Mother and Infant Research Unit, University of Leeds, 2003 p.13

6 Hofmeyr G.J. and M.E. Hannah, 'Planned caesarean section for term breech delivery' (Cochrane Review). In: *The Cochrane Library*, issue 2, 2004. Chichester, UK: John Wiley & Sons, Ltd

7 Simkin, Penny *Pregnancy, Birth and the Newborn*, p.178.

8 National Institute for Clinical Excellence (NICE) guidelines on Induction of Labour, June 2001. p4

9 NHS Maternity Statistics, England 1998-99 to 2000-01

10 National Institute for Clinical Excellence (NICE) guidelines on Induction of Labour, June 2001. p4

11 *Listening to Mothers*: Report of the first national US survey of women's childbearing experiences. Maternity Center Association in collaboration with Harris Interactive. Declercq et al, Oct 2002.

12 Olofsson C. et al. 'Lack of analgesic effect of systemically administered morphine or pethidine on labour pain' *British Journal of Obstetrics and Gynaecology* 1996 Oct; 103 (10); 968-72.

13 Howell, C.J. 'Epidural versus non-epidural analgesia for pain relief in labour' (Cochrane Review). In: *The Cochrane Library*, issue 2, 2004. Chichester UK: John Wiley & sons, Ltd.

14 Wilson M.J.et al. 'Randomised controlled trial comparing traditional with two 'mobile' epidural techniques: anesthetic and analgesic efficacy.' Comparative Obstetric Mobile Epidural Trial (COMET) Study Group UK. *Anesthesiology*. 2002 Dec;97(6):1567-75.

15 NICE guidelines on Caesarean Section, National Institute for Clinical Excellence (NICE) April 2004 p. 49.

16 Cluett E.R., Nikodem V.C., McCandlish R.E. and E.E. Burns. 'Immersion in water in pregnancy,labour and birth' (Cochrane Review). In: *The Cochrane Library*, Issue 2, 2004. Chichester, UK: John Wiley & Sons, Ltd

17 Gilbert R.E. and P.A.Tookey. 'Perinatal mortality and morbidity among babies delivered in water: national surveillance study.' *BMJ* 1999;319:483-7. Cited by the Royal College of Obstetricians and Gynaecologists *Birth in Water RCOG Statement No. 1* January 2001

18 Royal College of Midwives, Introduction to position paper No 1a, 'The Use of Water in Labour and Birth' Oct 2000

Chapter Six

1 Odent, Michel *The Caesarean* (Free Association Books, UK, 2004)

2 NHS Maternity Statistics, England 2002-03, 2.19.3

3 NICE guidelines on Caesarean Section, National Institute for Clinical Excellence (NICE) April 2004 p. 29

4 Ibid, p.30

5 Ibid, p 114

6 Chaffer & Royle 2000, Robinson 1999, Weaver et al 2001 cited in *Myles Textbook for Midwives* 14th edition. (Churchill Livingstone, Edinburgh, 2003) p 584-5.

7 NICE guidelines on Caesarean Section, National Institute for Clinical Excellence (NICE) April 2004 p.76

8 Ibid p. 95

Chapter Seven

1 *Listening to Mothers*: Report of the first
national US survey of women's childbearing
experiences. Maternity Center Association in
collaboration with Harris Interactive. Declercq
et al, Oct 2002.

2 Gibson, Fiona *Birth Plan: You're Joking?*
www.ivillage.co.uk

3 We have changed names and some
details for confidentiality.

Chapter Eight

1 *Junior Pregnancy and Baby Magazine*
Issue 8, Feb/Mar 2004, p.34

2 ibid

3 Quoted online by Fathers Direct 'What
good are dads?' report, 2001
www.fathersdirect.com

4 Survey by toy manufacturer Tomy,
reported in *Junior Pregnancy and Baby
Magazine*, issue 6, Oct/Nov 2003, p.14

5 Fathers Direct leaflet 'Father Facts', issue
1, vol 1

6 Brott A. and J. Ash *The Expectant Father:
facts, tips and advice for dads-to-be* (Abbeville,
1995) p.43.

7 Ibid. p.44.

8 Ibid. pp.25-6

9 Szeverényi P., Póka R., Hetey M. and Z.
Török 'Contents of childbirth-related fear
among couples wishing the partner's presence
at delivery' Department of Obstetrics and
Gynecology, University Medical School,
Debrecen, Hungary. Volume 19 Issue 1, March
1998

10 NCT Father's Survey 2000

11 www.homedad.org.uk

Chapter Nine

1 Hodnett E.D., Gates S., Hofmeyr G.J. and
C. Sakala 'Continuous support for women
during childbirth' (Cochrane Review). In: *The
Cochrane Library*, Issue 3, 2004.

2 Kennell J., Klaus M., McGrath S.,
Robertson S. and C. Hinkley 'Continuous
emotional support during labor in a US
hospital. A randomized controlled trial'.
Journal of the American Medical Association
1991 May 1;265(17):2197-201.

3 Quoted on the website of DUK
www.doula.org.uk.

4 Odent M. *The Caesarean* (Free
Association Books, UK, 2004) p. 19.

Chapter Ten

1 Moorhead, J 'What Lies Beneath', *Junior
Pregnancy and Baby Magazine*, Issue 7,
December/January 2004 p.33

2 Infant Feeding Survey 2000, Department
of Health. www.doh.gov.uk

3 WHO briefing *Mastitis: Causes and
management*. Available online at www.who.int

Index

role of, 267-9, 277-80
vaginal birth after
    caesarean, 208
see also birth partners
Down's syndrome, 47, 48,
    117-18
Down's Syndrome
    Association, 48
dream scenarios, birth plans,
    219-20
drugs:
    antidepressants, 10
    homebirth, 146
    in labour, 57-8, 96, 167
    over-the-counter drugs, 9,
        38
    recreational drugs, 9, 20,
        26
    street drugs, 9
dyes, hair, 20
dystocia, 37, 191-2, 209

e

ear infections, 311
eating see food
Eating Disorders Association,
    21
Eating for Pregnancy
    Helpline, 25
eclampsia, 190
eczema, 39, 311
effacement, cervix, 84
eggs, in diet, 27
electronic fetal monitoring
    (EFM), 160-1, 170, 205,
    208-9
emergencies:
    birth plans and, 222
    delivery, 80-2
    caesarean section, 103
emotions:
    after caesarean section,
        185, 188
    after miscarriage, 248
    effect on partner, 242
    overdue babies, 46
    partner's, 74
    in pregnancy, 10-11, 43, 44,
        45
    reasons for planned
        caesarean, 195-6
    see also worries
endorphins, 88, 89, 167
engorged breasts, 293, 298,
    312, 314-15

Entonox, 167-8
epidurals, 89, 166, 167,
    168-71
    caesarean section, 189
    description of, 168-9
    doulas and, 272
    induced labour, 158
    mobile epidurals, 169-70,
        209
    partner's reactions to, 252
    second births, 123
    vaginal birth after
        caesarean, 209
episiotomy:
    forceps delivery, 164, 165
    second births, 121, 122
    ways of avoiding, 103
    equipment, 284
    doula's, 278-80
    nappy bags, 259, 324
    shopping list, 323-4
    essential oils, 199, 279, 296
exercise:
    postpartum period, 301
    in pregnancy, 29-33
    for stress, 14
expressing milk, 315
external cephalic version
    (ECV), turning breech
    babies, 153

f

'failure to progress', 37, 162,
    185, 209
falls, 32, 33
family, support from, 14,
    288-9
fans, 279
fathers see partners
Fathers Direct, 263
fear, 88-96
    dealing with, 95-6
    of episiotomy or tearing,
        103-4
    loss of control, 54-5, 102-3
    media images of birth, 91-3
    'mind-body' ways of
        managing, 105-8
    other people's stories, 93-4
    and pain, 98
    partner's fears, 249
    problems with baby, 104-5,
        128
    second births, 114-16,
        125-6

sexual abuse and, 101-2
    understanding, 107-8
    writing birth plans, 221-2
feeds see bottle feeding;
    breastfeeding
feet:
    massage, 277
    swollen, 40
fentanyl, 169, 170
fetal alcohol syndrome, 16
fetal distress, 159-60, 161, 191
fetal scalp clips, 161
fetus:
    first trimester, 44
    movements, 51
    second trimester, 45
    third trimester, 46
    see also baby
fever, 302, 311
fibre, for constipation, 297
fibrogel, 297
finances:
    cost of a doula, 281
    worries, 243, 256-7
first trimester, 43-4
fish, 24, 27
fluid retention, 23
flying, 17
folic acid, 25, 26
fontanel, dehydrated babies,
    311
food:
    for breastfeeding, 301
    cravings, 38
    in labour, 175
    in 'latent labour', 64
    postpartum period, 287,
        301
    in pregnancy, 23-9
food poisoning, 24, 27
Food Standards Agency, 25
foot massage, 277
forceps delivery, 103, 121-2,
    164-5
Foundation for the Study of
    Infant Deaths (FSID), 235,
    309
freezing food, 287, 301
friends:
    as birth partners, 274
    postnatal help, 284, 288,
        289
    in pregnancy, 14
frozen food, 287, 301
frozen peas, soothing sore

l

La Leche League, 318
labour, 53–74
  active phase, 57, 67–74
  baby's position, 151–4, 190, 191
  'back labour', 162–3, 173
  birth plans, 102, 216–27
  doula's role, 277–8
  early phase, 57, 60–5
  'failure to progress', 37, 162, 185, 209
  fears, 11, 88–96
  first stage, 57
  induction, 61, 84, 122–3, 154–8
  losing control, 54–5, 102–3
  monitoring baby, 159–62, 170, 205, 208–9
  pain, 69, 96–100
  pain relief, 100, 166–74
  partners and, 248–53, 256
  positions, 158–9
  premature labour, 19
  pushing, 72–4, 103–4, 119–20
  rapid labour, 120–1
  second births, 58, 118–20, 129, 130–2
  second stage, 57, 192
  signs of progression, 68
  third stage, 57, 177, 227
  transition phase, 57
  travelling to hospital in labour, 232
  water birth, 175–6, 205
  when to call midwife, 60
  see also birth
labour bars, 174
lactulose, 297
latching on, breastfeeding, 293, 294, 313–14, 315, 317
'latent labour', 60–5
laughter, inducing labour, 155
lavender oil, 296
legs:
  blood clots, 302
  cramps, 39
  swollen ankles, 40
  varicose veins, 41
lemon, for nausea, 279
leukemia, 311
libido, 18–19, 245
life-coaching, 14

lifestyle changes, 243–4
lifting safely, 18
ligaments, loosening, 29
linseeds, 292, 293, 297
listeria, 24, 27
liver, eating, 27
liver problems, 39
lochia, 296
loo, sitting on in labour, 172
lotions, 20, 279
lubricants, 246, 295
lunges, during labour, 172
luring breech babies, 152–3
'lying-in period', 285, 290

m

macrosomia, 36–7, 84, 192
malposition, 84
malpresentation, 84
MAMA (meet-a-mum association), 10, 319
'mask of pregnancy', 298
massage:
  by doulas, 277
  inducing labour, 155
  in labour, 107
  perineal, 103
  postpartum period, 238
  in pregnancy, 13
mastitis, 287, 293, 302, 316–17
masturbation, 245, 246, 247
Maternity Alliance, 50
maternity bras, 49
maternity leave, 14, 50, 257
maternity nurses, 287–8
maternity pay, 50, 257
maternity units, 144, 253
mattresses, cot, 323
meat, 27
meconium, 84, 159, 309, 311
media images of birth, 91–3
medical intervention:
  birth plans, 228
  induction, 156–8
  instrumental birth, 164–5
  second births, 121–3
  see also caesarean section
meditation, 111, 155
Meet-a-Mum Association, 10, 319
membranes:
  artificial rupture, 156, 157
  waters breaking, 61–2, 69
meptid, 167

mercury, in fish, 24, 27
midwife units, 144
midwives, 267
  antenatal checks, 47
  birth plans, 218, 222
  communication with, 228–30
  discussing fears with, 89–90
  and doulas, 272
  homebirth, 145
  options, 147–50
  shortages, 148
  vaginal birth after caesarean, 207, 208, 210
  when to call, 60
Midwives Information and Resource Service: MIDIRS, 182
milk:
  breast, 246, 311, 314
  cow's, 27
  expressing, 315
MIND, 10
mind, postpartum period, 303–5
mints, 280
mirrors, 73, 279
miscarriage, 34–6
  and caesarean section, 187
  coping with, 35
  exercise and, 31–2
  partner's reactions to, 248
  past miscarriage, 11, 35
  signs of, 34–5, 42
mobile epidurals, 169–70, 209
money:
  cost of a doula, 281
  worries about, 243, 256–7
Mongolian marks, 76
monitors:
  baby monitors, 323
  in labour, 159–62, 170, 205, 208–9
  special care baby units, 234
mood swings, 10–11, 38, 43, 242, 304
morning sickness, 25, 39–40, 117
Moses baskets, 323
Mother@Work, 14
mothers:
  as birth partners, 274
  postnatal help, 288–9

rupture, 204, 206, 210
stitches, 190, 201, 202
'trial of labour', 205
scents, 279
second births, 58, 113–35
  age, 123–5
  caesarean section, 123, 125,
    192
  fears, 114–16, 125–6
  medical intervention, 121–3
  options, 140
  partner's role, 241
  planned caesarean, 211–12
  postpartum period, 318–20
  preparation for, 133–4
  speed of, 118–20
second trimester, 44–5
self-hypnosis, 108–11, 156
separation, 259
Serene, 307
sex:
  after birth, 261–2, 294, 295
  from partner's perspective,
    244–8
  inducing birth, 155
  in pregnancy, 18–20
sex of baby, 200
sexual abuse, 101–2, 191
shared care, 148
shellfish, 27
shopping:
  for baby, 323–4
  in postpartum period, 290,
    322
  in pregnancy, 18
shops, breastfeeding in, 316
shoulder dystocia, 37, 191–2,
  209
'show', signs of labour, 61
showers, 299–300
siblings *see* children
sickle cell disorders, 48
single mothers, 8–9
sitting position, in labour,
  172–3
sitzbaths, 296
skin:
  after birth, 298–9
  changes in pregnancy, 40,
    298
  eczema, 39
  itching, 39, 170
  jaundice, 310, 311
  newborn baby's, 76, 310
  skin-to-skin contact with

baby, 76–7, 198, 200, 203
stretchmarks, 40, 117,
  298–9
sleep:
  in labour, 71
  in 'latent labour', 63, 64
  newborn babies, 308
  partners, 260–1
  second pregnancy, 117
  sleep deprivation, 260–1,
    303
small babies, 233
smell, sense of, 8
smoking, 9, 20, 26, 34, 308
snacks, 28, 301–2
socks, rice, 278–9
soft drink cans, 279
soreness, soothing, 295–6
special care baby unit (SCBU),
  232–5
spicy foods, inducing labour,
  155
spina bifida, 26, 48
spinning, 32
sports, 30, 31, 33
spray bottles, 279
squatting, in labour, 174
squirty bottles, soothing sore
  bits, 295
stairs, 287
stations, progress of baby's
  head, 84–5
Stillbirth and Neonatal Death
  Society (SANDS), 235
stitches:
  caesarean section, 190,
    201, 202
  tears, 78, 177, 291
stomach, after birth, 116, 298
stress, 12–14, 254, 287
stress hormones, 88
stretch marks, 40, 117, 298–9
strollers, 323
superfoods, 28
supermarkets, breastfeeding
  in, 316
supplements, 25
support:
  birth defects, 104–5
  postpartum period, 287–8
surgeons, 190
surgical birth *see* caesarean
  section
sweating, after birth, 298,
  299

swimming, 30
swollen feet and ankles, 40
sympathetic pregnancy,
  241–2
symphysis pubis, 29
syntocinon, 157–8, 177,
  207–8
syntometrine, 177

t

TAMBA (Twins and Multiple
  Birth Association), 16
tampons, 295
team midwifery, 148
tears:
  how to avoid, 103–4
  stitches, 78, 177, 291
teeth, after birth, 300
television, images of birth,
  91–3
temperature:
  baby's, 258
  exercise and, 31
  fever, 302, 311
  hot baths, 18
TENS machines, 167, 296
terminations, 36
tests:
  antenatal, 47–8, 118
  consultation, 149
  pregnancy tests, 8, 239
tetanus, vaccination, 17
thalassaemia, 48
third trimester, 45–6
thrombosis, 187, 201
thrush, 41, 315
tiredness:
  after birth, 287, 294, 303
  after caesarean, 203
  sleep deprivation, 260–1,
    303
toilet, sitting on in labour,
  172
tokophobia, 90
toxic substances, 20–1
toxoplasmosis, 27–8
toys, 320
transition phase, 57
transverse lie, 190
travel:
  air travel, 17
  eating and, 28–9
  to hospital, 251
'trial of labour', 205–6, 210
trimesters, 43–6, 51

Acknowledgements

Lucy Atkins

Huge thanks to obstetrician Dr Lucy Chappell and head midwife Jenny Smith, both of Queen Charlotte's Hospital in London, two impressively busy women without whom this book would have been wholly inadequate; also to Dr Gary Stocks at Queen Charlotte's Hospital, Dr Eleri Adams, Dr Renée McCulloch and midwife Penny Green at the John Radcliffe Hospital in Oxford; midwives Sally Inch and Chloe Fisher of the breast-feeding clinic at the John Radcliffe Hospital; sex and relationships expert Dr Petra Boynton of University College, London, and to doula Julie Osborne – thank you all so much for your professional expertise and advice. Also thanks to George Capel and Denise Bates, for your enthusiasm, to Julia, of course – the blooming inspiration – and to the numerous mothers, fathers, doctors, midwives, doulas and patient friends who filled out questionnaires, answered random questions and agreed to be interviewed and quoted for this book. Finally, thank you John, Izzie, Sam and Ted for living with (and, in Ted's case, inside) me this past year: without you this book – quite literally – would not exist.

Julia Guderian

I wish to thank all of the women who have allowed me to be a witness to their growing families and those who supported the idea of this book with their honest stories and advice. Rhonda Griffin MSW, Annie Kennedy CD, Jenny Miller, Janelle Durham MSW, Carla Pedey-Braswell LMP, CBE, Kim Dolan CD, Mary Beth Rothnie CD, Michelle Kinner CCBE, Angie Dobbins CD, K.H. Railing CD, Michelle Smilowitz (ICAN Seattle), Jaye Barr, Barbara Elder CD, Amy DeLeva, Mara Williams, Ann Fulcher, DONA International, the wonderful women of ALACE, and all the others who helped that I've neglected to mention – I thank you all.

Special thanks to: Peggy Fitzgerald, M. Kelly Demetrio, Starbucks in Kenmore, Susan and Lorelei Gladstone, Meredith Bane, Georgina Capel, Denise Bates and of course Lucy.

Without the patience and professionalism of Dr. Kim Kelly ND, RN,LM, we would have never been able to trudge though the writing of this book. Thank you so much for everything, Kim.

Keaton and Larson, you are the source of my inspiration and I'm grateful for you both. Buckley, nobody but us will know how much of this book was possible because of you and I will never be able to thank you properly.

Finally, I dedicate my work on *Blooming Birth* to Gloria Fleischer. Girlie, we miss you dearly.

The authors

Lucy Atkins is an established journalist who regularly writes for the *Guardian*, *Red* magazine and *Junior Pregnancy* and *Baby* magazine. She has also written for a range of other publications including *The Times*, *The Sunday Times* and the *Telegraph*, and has been a book critic for the *Guardian*, the *Times Literary Supplement* and now *The Sunday Times*. Lucy has drawn on her own experiences as the inspiration for *Blooming Birth* – Julia Guderian was her doula with her second baby. She is a mother of three.

Julia Guderian is a childbirth educator and certified birth and post-labour doula. She founded and runs The New Hope Project, connecting volunteer doulas with women giving their babies up for adoption. She also founded a non-profit support group for women who have had caesareans (and are upset by them) and designed a network of mother's groups that has proved very popular across the us. She is a mother of two.